Myopathies

Editors

MAZEN M. DIMACHKIE
RICHARD J. BAROHN

NEUROLOGIC CLINICS

www.neurologic.theclinics.com

Consulting Editor
RANDOLPH W. EVANS

August 2014 • Volume 32 • Number 3

ELSEVIER

1600 John F. Kennedy Boulevard • Suite 1800 • Philadelphia, Pennsylvania, 19103-2899

http://www.theclinics.com

NEUROLOGIC CLINICS Volume 32, Number 3
August 2014 ISSN 0733-8619, ISBN-13: 978-0-323-32019-1

Editor: Joanne Husovski
Developmental editor: Donald Mumford

Neurologic Clinics (ISSN 0733-8619) is published quarterly by Elsevier Inc., 360 Park Avenue South, New York, NY 10010–1710. Months of issue are February, May, August, and November. Periodicals postage paid at New York, NY, and additional mailing offices. Subscription prices are $300.00 per year for US individuals, $517.00 per year for US institutions, $145.00 per year for US students, $375.00 per year for Canadian individuals, $627.00 per year for Canadian institutions, $415.00 per year for international individuals, $627.00 per year for international institutions, and $210.00 for Canadian and foreign students/residents. To receive student/resident rate, orders must be accompanied by name of affiliated institution, date of term, and the *signature* of program/residency coordinator on institution letterhead. Orders will be billed at individual rate until proof of status is received. Foreign air speed delivery is included in all *Clinics* subscription prices. All prices are subject to change without notice. **POSTMASTER:** Send address changes to *Neurologic Clinics*, Elsevier Health Sciences Division, Subscription Customer Service, 3251 Riverport Lane, Maryland Heights, MO 63043. **Customer Service: Telephone: 1-800-654-2452 (U.S. and Canada); 314-447-8871 (outside U.S. and Canada). Fax: 314-447-8029. E-mail: journalscustomerservice-usa@elsevier.com (for print support); journalsonlinesupport-usa@elsevier.com (for online support).**

Reprints. For copies of 100 or more of articles in this publication, please contact the Commercial Reprints Department, Elsevier Inc., 360 Park Avenue South, New York, New York, 10010-1710; Tel.: +1-212-633-3874; Fax: +1-212-633-3820, and E-mail: reprints@elsevier.com.

Neurologic Clinics is also published in Spanish by Nueva Editorial Interamericana S.A., Mexico City, Mexico.

Neurologic Clinics is covered in *Current Contents/Clinical Medicine, MEDLINE/PubMed (Index Medicus), EMBASE/Excerpta Medica, and PsycINFO, and ISI/BIOMED.*

Contributors

CONSULTING EDITOR

RANDOLPH W. EVANS, MD
Clinical Professor of Neurology, Baylor College of Medicine, Houston, Texas

EDITORS

MAZEN M. DIMACHKIE, MD
Director, Neuromuscular Section; Director, Neurophysiology Division; Professor, Department of Neurology, University of Kansas Medical Center, Kansas City, Kansas

RICHARD J. BAROHN, MD
Gertrude and Dewey Ziegler Professor and Chairman, Department of Neurology; University Distinguished Professor, Executive Vice Chancellor for Research, University of Kansas Medical Center, Kansas City, Kansas

AUTHORS

AHMAD ABUZINADAH, MD
Neuromuscular Medicine Fellow, Department of Neurology, University of Kansas Medical Center, Kansas City, Kansas

OSAMA ALMADHOUN, MD
Associate Professor, Department of Pediatrics, University of Kansas Medical Center, Kansas City, Kansas

ANTHONY A. AMATO, MD
Professor of Neurology, Vice-Chairman, Department of Neurology, Brigham and Women's Hospital, Harvard Medical School, Boston, Massachusetts

RICHARD J. BAROHN, MD
Gertrude and Dewey Ziegler Professor and Chairman, Department of Neurology; University Distinguished Professor, Executive Vice Chancellor for Research, University of Kansas Medical Center, Kansas City, Kansas

DIANA CASTRO, MD
Assistant Professor, University of Texas Southwestern Medical Center, Dallas, Texas

MAJED DASOUKI, MD
Professor, Department of Neurology, University of Kansas Medical Center, Kansas City, Kansas; Director, Newborn Screening & Biochemical Genetics Laboratory; Co-Director, Cytogenetics Laboratory, Department of Genetics, King Faisal Specialist Hospital & Research Center, Riyadh, Saudi Arabia

MAZEN M. DIMACHKIE, MD
Director, Neuromuscular Section; Director, Neurophysiology Division; Professor, Department of Neurology, University of Kansas Medical Center, Kansas City, Kansas

KEVIN M. FLANIGAN, MD
Professor of Pediatrics and Neurology, The Ohio State University; Investigator, Center for Gene Therapy Nationwide Children's Hospital, Columbus, Ohio

HEATHER R. GILBREATH, PA-C
Clinical Instructor, UT Southwestern Physician Assistant Program, Children's Medical Center of Dallas, Dallas, Texas

RONALD G. HALLER, MD
Department of Neurology and Neurotherapeutics, University of Texas Southwestern Medical Center; Neuromuscular Center, Institute for Exercise and Environmental Medicine, Texas Health Presbyterian Hospital; North Texas VA Medical Center, Dallas, Texas

LAURA HERBELIN, BS
Research Instructor, Department of Neurology, University of Kansas Medical Center, Kansas City, Kansas

SUSAN T. IANNACCONE, MD, FAAN
Jimmy Elizabeth Westcott Distinguished Chair in Pediatric Neurology; Professor of Pediatrics and Neurology and Neurotherapeutics, University of Texas Southwestern Medical Center, Dallas, Texas

CARLAYNE E. JACKSON, MD, FAAN
Professor of Neurology and Otolaryngology; Assistant Dean of Ambulatory Services; Chief Medical Officer, Division of Neurology, UT Medicine San Antonio, University of Texas Health Science Center, San Antonio, Texas

OMAR JAWDAT, MD
Neuromuscular Medicine Fellow, Department of Neurology, University of Kansas Medical Center, Kansas City, Kansas

JOHN T. KISSEL, MD, FAAN
Professor, Departments of Neurology and Pediatrics, The Ohio State University Wexner Medical Center, Columbus, Ohio

APRIL L. MCVEY, MD
Professor, Department of Neurology, University of Kansas Medical Center, Kansas City, Kansas

MAMATHA PASNOOR, MD
Associate Professor, Department of Neurology, University of Kansas Medical Center, Kansas City, Kansas

LAUREN PHILLIPS, MD
Assistant Professor, Department of Neurology and Neurotherapeutics, UT Southwestern Medical Center, Dallas, Texas

LYDIA J. SHARP, MD
Department of Neurology and Neurotherapeutics, University of Texas Southwestern Medical Center; Neuromuscular Center, Institute for Exercise and Environmental Medicine, Texas Health Presbyterian Hospital, Dallas, Texas

JEFFREY STATLAND, MD
Senior Instructor, Department of Neurology, University of Rochester Medical Center, Rochester, New York

RABI TAWIL, MD
Professor, Department of Neurology, University of Rochester Medical Center, Rochester, New York

CHARLES A. THORNTON, MD
Department of Neurology, Center for Neural Development and Disease, Center for RNA Biology, University of Rochester Medical Center, Rochester, New York

JAYA R. TRIVEDI, MD, FAAN
Associate Professor, Department of Neurology and Neurotherapeutics, UT Southwestern Medical Center, Dallas, Texas

MATTHEW P. WICKLUND, MD, FAAN
Professor, Departments of Neurology and Pediatrics, Penn State College of Medicine, Penn State University, Hershey, Pennsylvania

Contents

Myopathies are a heterogeneous group of disorders that can be challenging to diagnose. This review provides a diagnostic approach based predominantly on the clinical history and neurologic examination. Laboratory testing that can be used to confirm the suspected diagnosis based on this pattern recognition approach is also discussed. Careful consideration of the distribution of muscle weakness and attention to common patterns of involvement in the context of other aspects of the neurologic examination and laboratory evaluation should assist the clinician in making a timely and accurate diagnosis and can sometimes minimize the expense of further testing.

The idiopathic inflammatory myopathies (IIM) consist of rare heterogeneous autoimmune disorders that present with marked proximal and symmetric muscle weakness, except for distal and asymmetric weakness in inclusion body myositis. Despite many similarities, the IIM are fairly heterogeneous from the histopathologic and pathogenetic standpoints, and also show some clinical and treatment-response differences. The field has witnessed significant advances in our understanding of the pathophysiology and treatment of these rare disorders. This review focuses on dermatomyositis, polymyositis, and necrotizing myopathy, and examines current and promising therapies.

The idiopathic inflammatory myopathies (IIMs) are a heterogenous group of rare disorders that share many similarities. In addition to sporadic inclusion body myositis (IBM), these include dermatomyositis, polymyositis, and autoimmune necrotizing myopathy. IBM is the most common IIM after age 50 years. Muscle histopathology shows endomysial inflammatory exudates surrounding and invading nonnecrotic muscle fibers often accompanied by rimmed vacuoles and protein deposits. It is likely that IBM has a prominent degenerative component. This article reviews the evolution of knowledge in IBM, with emphasis on recent developments in the field, and discusses ongoing clinical trials.

Facioscapulohumeral Muscular Dystrophy

Jeffrey Statland and Rabi Tawil

Facioscapulohumeral muscular dystrophy (FSHD) is a common type of adult muscular dystrophy and is divided into types 1 and 2 based on genetic mutation. Clinically, both FSHD types often show asymmetric and progressive muscle weakness affecting initially the face, shoulder, and arms followed by the distal then proximal lower extremities. Approximately 95% of patients, termed FSHD1, have a deletion of a key number of repetitive elements on chromosome 4q35. The remaining 5%, termed FSHD2, have no deletion on chromosome 4q35. Nevertheless, both types share a common downstream mechanism, making it possible for future disease-directed therapies to be effective for both FSHD types.

The Limb-Girdle Muscular Dystrophies

Matthew P. Wicklund and John T. Kissel

A collection of more than 30 genetic muscle diseases that share certain key features, limb-girdle muscular dystrophies are characterized by progressive weakness and muscle atrophy of the hips, shoulders, and proximal extremity muscles with postnatal onset. This article discusses clinical, laboratory, and histologic features of the 6 most prevalent limb-girdle dystrophies. In this large group of disorders, certain distinctive features often can guide clinicians to a correct diagnosis.

Pompe Disease: Literature Review and Case Series

Majed Dasouki, Omar Jawdat, Osama Almadhoun, Mamatha Pasnoor, April L. McVey, Ahmad Abuzinadah, Laura Herbelin, Richard J. Barohn, and Mazen M. Dimachkie

Pompe disease is a rare multi-systemic metabolic myopathy caused by autosomal recessive mutations in the acidic alpha glucosidase (GAA) gene. Significant progress had been made in the diagnosis and management of patients with Pompe disease. Here, we describe our experience with 12 patients with various forms of Pompe disease including 4 potentially pathogenic, novel GAA variants. We also review the recent advances in the pathogenesis, diagnosis, and treatment of individuals with Pompe disease.

Metabolic and Mitochondrial Myopathies

Lydia J. Sharp and Ronald G. Haller

Metabolic and mitochondrial myopathies encompass a heterogeneous group of disorders that result in impaired energy production in skeletal muscle. Symptoms of premature muscle fatigue, sometimes leading to myalgia, rhabdomyolysis, and myoglobinuria, typically occur with exercise that would normally depend on the defective metabolic pathway. But in another group of these disorders, the dominant muscle symptom is weakness. This article reviews the clinical features, diagnosis, and management of these diseases with emphasis on the recent literature.

> Skeletal muscle channelopathies are rare heterogeneous diseases with marked genotypic and phenotypic variability. Despite advances in understanding of the molecular pathology of these disorders, the diverse phenotypic manifestations remain a challenge in diagnosis and therapeutics. These disorders can cause lifetime disability and affect quality of life. There is no treatment of these disorders approved by the US Food and Drug Administration at this time. Recognition and treatment of symptoms might reduce morbidity and improve quality of life. This article summarizes the clinical manifestations, diagnostic studies, pathophysiology, and treatment options in nondystrophic myotonia, congenital myasthenic syndrome, and periodic paralyses.

> In this article, distal myopathy syndromes are discussed. A discussion of the more traditional distal myopathies is followed by discussion of the myofibrillar myopathies. Other clinically and genetically distinctive distal myopathy syndromes usually based on single or smaller family cohorts are reviewed. Other neuromuscular disorders that are important to recognize are also considered, because they show prominent distal limb weakness.

NEUROLOGIC CLINICS

RELATED INTEREST

In Physical Medicine and Rehabilitation Clinics of North America,
February 2013 (Vol. 24, No. 1)
Electrodiagnostic Evaluation of Myopathies
Sabrina Paganoni, and Anthony Amato, *Editors*

NOW AVAILABLE FOR YOUR iPhone and iPad

Preface

Myopathies

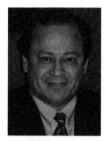 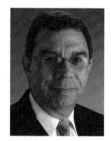

Mazen M. Dimachkie, MD   Richard J. Barohn, MD
Editors

Busy clinicians can often be challenged by patients with skeletal muscle disorders. In this issue of *Neurologic Clinics,* we provide an approach and information that we believe will help clinicians take care of patients with myopathies. We begin with a practical pattern recognition approach that we have developed and which allows the clinician to narrow down the diagnostic possibilities by placing the symptoms and signs in one of the ten patterns. We then have a series of articles that discuss a variety of acquired and inherited muscle disorders. We provide updates on the latest genetic developments for the hereditary myopathies. Drug therapies are discussed as well, and this applies primarily to acquired muscle diseases; however, interventional treatments for many muscular dystrophies are currently in research trials, and we believe some of these novel therapeutic approaches will be in the clinics very soon.

The contributors are in the neuromuscular services at major academic centers (such as the University of Kansas Medical Center, the University of Rochester Medical Center School of Medicine and Dentistry, the University of Texas-Southwestern, the Milton S. Hershey Medical Center–Pennsylvania, the Ohio State University, and Nationwide Children's Hospital–Center for Gene Therapy). The authors are all colleagues who have worked together for many years. As in our recent issue on neuropathies, our goal has been to push the envelope toward phenotype identification to perform selective diagnostic tests that lead us to optimal management of patients with neuromuscular disorders. We hope this issue complements the neuropathy issue and assists physicians in their approach and management of these diseases. In the current issue, we did not discuss the various neuromuscular junction disorders, which we hope to address in a future *Neurologic Clinics* issue. We would like

Neurol Clin 32 (2014) xiii–xiv
http://dx.doi.org/10.1016/j.ncl.2014.06.001
0733-8619/14/$ – see front matter © 2014 Elsevier Inc. All rights reserved.

to express our appreciation to all of the authors who have worked so hard to make this issue a success.

Mazen M. Dimachkie, MD
Neurophysiology Division
Neuromuscular Section
Department of Neurology
University of Kansas Medical Center
3901 Rainbow Boulevard, Mail Stop 2012
Kansas City, KS 66160, USA

Richard J. Barohn, MD
Department of Neurology
University of Kansas Medical Center
3901 Rainbow Boulevard, Mail Stop 2012
Kansas City, KS 66160, USA

E-mail addresses:
mdimachkie@kumc.edu (M.M. Dimachkie)
rbarohn@kumc.edu (R.J. Barohn)

A Pattern Recognition Approach to Patients with a Suspected Myopathy

Richard J. Barohn, MD[a],*, Mazen M. Dimachkie, MD[b],
Carlayne E. Jackson, MD[c]

KEYWORDS

- Myopathy • Limb-girdle • Distal myopathy • Inflammatory myopathy
- Metabolic myopathy • Myotonia

KEY POINTS

- The initial key to the diagnosis of myopathies is recognition of a clinical pattern.
- There are 6 key questions the clinician should consider in arriving at the pattern that fits the patient.
- After arriving at the pattern that fits best, then the clinician can better determine the most appropriate diagnostic tests and management.

INTRODUCTION

Myopathies are disorders affecting the channel, structure, or metabolism of skeletal muscle. Myopathies can be distinguished from other disorders of the motor unit, including the neuromuscular junction, peripheral nerve, or motor neuron, by characteristic clinical and laboratory features. Therefore, the first goal in approaching patients with a suspected muscle disease is to determine the correct *site* of the lesion. Once the lesion is localized to the muscle, the next step is to identify whether the myopathy is caused by a defect in the muscle channel, muscle structure, or a dysfunction in muscle metabolism. The second goal is to determine the *cause* of the myopathy. In general, myopathies can be classified into acquired or hereditary disorders (**Box 1**).

This publication (or project) was supported by an Institutional Clinical and Translational Science Award, National Institutes of Health/National Center for Advancing Translational Sciences grant number UL1TR000001. Its contents are solely the responsibility of the authors and do not necessarily represent the official views of the National Institutes of Health.

[a] Department of Neurology, University of Kansas Medical Center, 3901 Rainbow Boulevard, Mail Stop 2012, Kansas City, KS 66160, USA; [b] Neuromuscular Section, Neurophysiology Division, Department of Neurology, University of Kansas Medical Center, 3901 Rainbow Boulevard, Mail Stop 2012, Kansas City, KS 66160, USA; [c] Division of Neurology, UT Medicine San Antonio, University of Texas Health Science Center, 8300 Floyd Curl Drive, Mail Code 7883, San Antonio, TX 78229-3900, USA
* Corresponding author.
E-mail address: rbarohn@kumc.edu

Box 1
Classification of myopathies

Acquired

  Drug-induced myopathies

  Endocrine myopathies

  Inflammatory/immune myopathies

  Myopathies associated with other systemic illness

  Toxic myopathies

Hereditary

  Channelopathies

  Congenital myopathies

  Metabolic myopathies

  Mitochondrial myopathies

  Muscular dystrophies

  Myotonias

Finally, the third goal in the authors' approach is to determine if there is a specific treatment and, if not, to optimally manage the patients' symptoms in order to maximize their functional abilities and enhance their quality of life.

CLINICAL EVALUATION

The most important component of evaluating patients with a suspected myopathy is obtaining a comprehensive medical history. The history should allow the clinician to make a reasonable preliminary diagnosis that places patients into one of the categories in **Box 1**. The findings on the physical examination, in particular the distribution of muscle weakness, should provide additional information in determining the correct diagnosis. The results of laboratory studies (blood tests, electrodiagnostic studies, muscle biopsy, molecular genetic studies) then play a confirmatory diagnostic role.[1–4]

The first step in this clinical approach is to ask 6 key questions regarding the patients' symptoms.

1. Which Negative and/or Positive Symptoms Do Patients Demonstrate?
2. What is the Temporal Evolution?
3. Is There a Family History of a Myopathic Disorder?
4. Are There Precipitating Factors That Trigger Episodic Weakness or Stiffness?
5. Are There Associated Systemic Symptoms or Signs?
6. What is the Distribution of Weakness?

Which Negative and/or Positive Symptoms Do Patients Demonstrate?

Symptoms of muscle disease (**Box 2**) can be divided into negative complaints, such as exercise intolerance, fatigue, muscle atrophy and weakness, and positive complaints, such as contractures, cramps, myalgias, muscle stiffness, and myoglobinuria.

Weakness is by far the most common negative symptom reported by patients with muscle disease. When the upper extremities are involved, patients notice trouble brushing their teeth, combing their hair, or lifting objects overhead. If the weakness involves the lower extremities, patients will complain of difficulty arising from a low chair

---

Box 2
Symptoms associated with myopathies

Negative

  Exercise intolerance

  Fatigue

  Muscle atrophy

  Weakness

Positive

  Cramps

  Contractures

  Muscle hypertrophy

  Myalgias

  Myoglobinuria

  Stiffness

---

or toilet, getting up from a squatted position, or climbing stairs. These symptoms in the arms and legs indicate proximal muscle weakness, which is probably the most common distribution of weakness in a myopathic disorder (see later discussion). Less commonly, patients with myopathies can complain of distal weakness manifested as difficulty turning a key in the ignition, opening jars, or gait instability caused by foot drop. Some myopathies may also result in cranial muscle weakness resulting in complaints of slurred speech, difficulty swallowing, or double vision.

Fatigue is a much less useful negative symptom because it may be a result of patients' overall health, cardiopulmonary status, level of conditioning, sleeping habits, or emotional state. Many patients who complain of generalized weakness or fatigue do not have a myopathy, particularly if the neurologic examination is normal. However, it is important to define the intensity and duration of exercise that provokes the fatigue because metabolic and mitochondrial myopathies can cause abnormal fatigability after exercise.

Positive symptoms associated with myopathies may include cramps, contractures, myalgias, muscle stiffness, or myoglobinuria. Myalgia, like fatigue, is another nonspecific symptom of some myopathies (**Box 3**). Myalgias may be episodic such as in metabolic myopathies or nearly constant such as in inflammatory muscle diseases. However, muscle pain is usually not common in most muscle diseases; pain is more likely to be caused by orthopedic or rheumatologic disorders. It is extremely uncommon for a myopathy to be responsible for vague aches and muscle discomfort in the presence of a normal neuromuscular examination and laboratory studies.

Muscle cramps are a specific type of muscle pain. They are typically benign, occurring frequently in normal individuals, and are seldom a feature of a primary myopathy. Cramps commonly occur because of dehydration, hyponatremia, azotemia, myxedema, and disorders of the nerve or motor neuron (especially amyotrophic lateral sclerosis) or most often are benign and not related to an underlying disease process. Cramps may last from seconds to minutes and are usually localized to a particular muscle region, typically the calves. Cramps are characterized by rapidly firing motor unit discharges on needle electromyography.

Muscle contractures are uncommon but can superficially resemble a cramp. They are typically provoked by exercise in patients with glycolytic enzyme defects. Contractures

---

Box 3
Muscle diseases associated with myalgias

Toxic/drug-induced myopathies (statins and others)

Eosinophilia-myalgia syndrome

Hypothyroid myopathy

Inflammatory myopathies (dermatomyositis, polymyositis)

Myotonic disorders

Mitochondrial myopathies

Tubular aggregate myopathy

Muscular dystrophies, examples

   X-linked myalgia and cramps/Becker dystrophy variant

Infectious myositis (especially viral)

Myoadenylate deaminase deficiency (controversial)

---

differ from cramps in that they usually last longer and are electrically silent with needle electromyography. Muscle contractures should not be confused with fixed tendon contractures. Muscle disorders that are associated with contractures are listed in **Box 4**.

Myotonia is caused by repetitive depolarization of the muscle membrane and results in impaired relaxation of muscle after forceful voluntary contraction. Myotonia most commonly involves the eyelids and hands. As a result, patients may complain of muscle stiffness or tightness resulting in difficulty releasing their handgrip after a handshake, unscrewing a bottle top, or opening their eyelids if they forcefully shut their eyes. Myotonia classically improves with repeated exercise. In contrast, patients with paramyotonia congenita demonstrate paradoxic myotonia in that symptoms are typically worsened by exercise or repeated muscle contractions. Exposure to cold results in worsening of both myotonia and paramyotonia. The muscle disorders associated with muscle stiffness are listed in **Box 5**. Sometimes patients with myotonia also complain of myalgias and fatigue.

Myoglobinuria is caused by the excessive release of myoglobin from muscle during periods of rapid muscle destruction (rhabdomyolysis) and is a relatively uncommon

---

Box 4
Myopathies associated with muscle contractures

Brody disease

Glycolytic/glycogenolytic enzyme defects

   Myophosphorylase deficiency (McArdle disease)

   Phosphofructokinase deficiency

   Phosphoglycerate kinase deficiency

   Phosphoglycerate mutase deficiency

   Lactate dehydrogenase deficiency

   Debrancher enzyme deficiency

Hypothyroid myopathy

Rippling muscle disease

Box 5
Myopathies associated with muscle stiffness

Hypothyroid myopathy

Myotonia congenita

Paramyotonia congenita

Myotonic dystrophy type 1

Proximal myotonic myopathy (myotonic dystrophy type 2)

Hyperkalemic periodic paralysis

---

manifestation of muscle disease. Severe myoglobinuria can result in renal failure caused by acute tubular necrosis. If patients complain of exercise-induced weakness and myalgias, they should be asked if their urine has ever turned cola colored or red during or after these episodes. Isolated episodes or myoglobinuria, particularly occurring after unaccustomed strenuous exercise, are frequently idiopathic, whereas recurrent episodes are usually caused by an underlying metabolic myopathy (**Box 6**).

What is the Temporal Evolution?

It is obviously important to determine the onset, duration, and evolution of patients' symptoms and signs of muscle disease. Did the weakness (or other symptoms) first manifest at birth, or was the onset in the first, second, third, or later decade (**Box 7**)? Identifying the age that symptoms began can provide crucial information leading to the correct diagnosis. For example, the symptoms of Duchenne muscular dystrophy are usually identified by 3 years of age, whereas most facioscapulohumeral and limb-girdle muscular dystrophies (LGMD) begin in adolescence or later. For further discussion of these diseases, the reader is referred to the corresponding

---

Box 6
Causes of myoglobinuria

Prolonged, intensive exercise

Drugs and toxin

Metabolic myopathies

   Glycogenoses (myophosphorylase deficiency)

   Lipid disorders (carnitine palmitoyltransferase deficiency)

   Malignant hyperthermia (central core myopathy, Duchenne muscular dystrophy)

Heat stroke

Some muscular dystrophies (eg, limb-girdle muscular dystrophy 2C-F [sarcoglycanopathies], 2I [FKRP], dystrophinopathies)

Neuroleptic malignant syndrome

Severe metabolic disturbances, including prolonged fever

Trauma (crush injuries)

Viral and bacterial infections (rare)

Inflammatory myopathies (rare)

Abbreviation: FKRP, fukutin-related protein.

Box 7
Diagnosis of myopathy based on age of onset

Myopathies Presenting at Birth

   Central core disease

   Centronuclear (myotubular) myopathy

   Congenital fiber-type disproportion

   Congenital muscular dystrophy

   Congenital myotonic dystrophy

   Glycogen storage diseases (acid maltase and phosphorylase deficiencies)

   Lipid storage diseases (carnitine deficiency)

   Nemaline (rod) myopathy

Myopathies Presenting in Childhood

   Congenital myopathies: nemaline myopathy, centronuclear myopathy, central core

   Endocrine-metabolic disorders: hypokalemia, hypocalcemia, hypercalcemia

   Glycogen storage disease (acid maltase deficiency)

   Inflammatory myopathies: dermatomyositis, polymyositis (rarely)

   Lipid storage disease (carnitine deficiency)

   Mitochondrial myopathies

   Muscular dystrophies: congenital, Duchenne, Becker, Emery-Dreifuss, facioscapulohumeral, limb-girdle

Myopathies Presenting in Adulthood

   Centronuclear myopathy

   Distal myopathies

   Endocrine myopathies: thyroid, parathyroid, adrenal, pituitary disorders

   Inflammatory myopathies: polymyositis, dermatomyositis, inclusion body myositis, viral (human immunodeficiency virus)

   Metabolic myopathies: acid maltase deficiency, lipid storage diseases, debrancher deficiency, phosphorylase b kinase deficiency

   Mitochondrial myopathies

   Muscular dystrophies: limb-girdle, facioscapulohumeral, Becker, Emery-Dreifuss

   Myotonic dystrophy

   Nemaline myopathy

   Toxic myopathies: alcohol, corticosteroids, local injections of narcotics, colchicine, chloroquine

---

articles by Wicklund and Kissel in this issue. Of the inflammatory myopathies, dermatomyositis occurs in children and adults; polymyositis rarely occurs in children as a benign childhood myositis but is primarily at any decade in the adult years; and inclusion body myositis occurs most commonly in the elderly.

It is also imperative to determine the evolution and duration of the disease. Myopathies can present with either *constant* weakness (inflammatory myopathies, muscular dystrophies) or *episodic* periods of weakness with normal strength interictally (metabolic myopathies caused by certain glycolytic pathway disorders, periodic paralysis).

The episodic disorders are characterized by acute loss of strength that can return to normal within hours or days. The tempo of the disorders with constant weakness can vary from (1) acute or subacute progression in some inflammatory myopathies (dermatomyositis and polymyositis), (2) chronic slow progression over years (most muscular dystrophies), or (3) nonprogressive weakness with little change over decades (congenital myopathies). Finally, both constant and episodic myopathic disorders can have symptoms that may be monophasic or relapsing. For example, polymyositis can occasionally have an acute monophasic course with complete resolution of strength within weeks or months. Patients with periodic paralysis or metabolic myopathies can have recurrent attacks of weakness over many years, whereas patients with acute rhabdomyolysis caused by cocaine may have a single episode.

Is There a Family History of a Myopathic Disorder?

Because many myopathies are inherited, obtaining a thorough family history is of tremendous importance in making a correct diagnosis. A detailed family tree should be completed to evaluate for evidence of autosomal dominant, autosomal recessive, and X-linked patterns of transmission. Questions regarding family members' use of canes or wheelchairs, skeletal deformities, or functional limitations are usually more informative than vague questions, such as asking whether any family members have a muscle disease. Identifying a particular hereditary pattern can not only help in correctly diagnosing the specific myopathy (**Box 8**) but is also of critical importance in providing appropriate genetic counseling.

Are There Precipitating Factors That Trigger Episodic Weakness or Stiffness?

A history of precipitating factors that might trigger or exacerbate symptoms of weakness or myotonia should be explored. It is important to ask patients if there is any history of using either illegal drugs or prescription medications that might produce a myopathy. Drugs that can cause toxic myopathies are listed in **Box 9**, and further discussion of this topic by Pasnoor, Barohn, and Dimachkie is found elsewhere in this issue. A history of weakness, pain, and/or myoglobinuria that is provoked by exercise might suggest the possibility of a glycolytic pathway defect. Episodes of weakness that occur in association with a fever would be supportive of a diagnosis of carnitine palmityl transferase deficiency. Periodic paralysis is characteristically provoked by exercise and ingestion of a carbohydrate meal followed by a period of rest. Patients with

---

Box 8
Diagnosis of myopathy based on pattern of inheritance

X-linked

  Becker muscular dystrophy, Duchenne muscular dystrophy, Emery-Dreifuss muscular dystrophy

Autosomal dominant

  Central core myopathy, FSH, limb-girdle muscular dystrophy type 1, oculopharyngeal MD, myotonic dystrophy, paramyotonia congenita, periodic paralysis, thomsen disease

Autosomal recessive

  Becker myotonia, limb-girdle muscular dystrophy type 2, metabolic myopathies

Maternal transmission

  Mitochondrial myopathies

Box 9
Drugs that can cause toxic myopathies

Inflammatory

　Cimetidine

　D-penicillamine

　Procainamide

　L-tryptophan

　L-dopa

Noninflammatory necrotizing or vacuolar

　Alcohol

　Cholesterol-lowering agents

　Chloroquine

　Colchicine

　Cyclosporine and tacrolimus

　Emetine

　ε-aminocaproic acid

　Isoretinoic acid (vitamin A analogue)

　Labetalol

　Vincristine

Rhabdomyolysis and myoglobinuria

　Alcohol

　Amphetamine

　Cholesterol-lowering drugs

　Cocaine

　Heroin

　Toluene

　ε-aminocaproic acid

Myosin loss

　Nondepolarizing neuromuscular blocking agents

　Steroids

---

paramyotonia congenita frequently report that cold exposure may precipitate their symptoms of muscle stiffness.

Are There Associated Systemic Symptoms or Signs?

Involvement of organs or tissues other than muscle may also provide helpful clues in making the appropriate diagnosis. Cardiac disease (**Box 10**) may be associated with Andersen-Tawil syndrome, Duchenne or Becker muscular dystrophies, Emery-Dreifuss muscular dystrophy, LGMD 1B (laminopathy), LGMD 2I (Fukutin related protein), LGMD 2C-F (sarcoglycanopathies), LGMD 2G (telethoninopathies), and myotonic dystrophy (types 1 and 2).

Box 10
Myopathies associated with cardiac disease
Arrhythmias
Andersen-Tawil syndrome
Kearns-Sayre syndrome
Polymyositis
Muscular dystrophies: myotonic, limb-girdle 1B, 2C-F, 2G, Emery-Dreifuss
Congestive heart failure
Acid maltase deficiency
Carnitine deficiency
Muscular dystrophies: Duchenne, Becker, Emery-Dreifuss, myotonic, limb-girdle 1B, 2C-F, 2G
Nemaline myopathy
Polymyositis

Respiratory failure may be the presenting symptom of acid maltase deficiency, centronuclear myopathy, myotonic dystrophy, or nemaline myopathy (**Box 11**). Eventually, many myopathies will affect respiratory muscle strength, highlighting the need for consistent monitoring of pulmonary function studies throughout the disease course. Once symptoms of hypoventilation are evident, supportive care should be initiated with noninvasive positive pressure ventilation and assistive devices for clearance of upper airway secretions.

Box 11
Myopathies associated with respiratory insufficiency
Muscular dystrophies
Becker
Duchenne
Congenital
Emery-Dreifuss
Limb-girdle 2A, 2I
Myotonic
Facioscapulohumeral muscular dystrophy
Metabolic myopathies
Acid maltase deficiency
Debrancher deficiency
Mitochondrial myopathies
Congenital myopathies
Centronuclear
Nemaline
Inflammatory myopathies
Polymyositis

Hepatomegaly may be seen in myopathies associated with deficiencies in acid maltase, carnitine, and debranching enzyme. The presence of cataracts, frontal balding, and mental retardation strongly suggests the diagnosis of myotonic dystrophy. Dysmorphic features may be associated with the congenital myopathies. The presence of a rash is extremely helpful in confirming the diagnosis of dermatomyositis. Musculoskeletal contractures can occur in many myopathies of a longstanding duration. However, contractures developing early in the course of the disease, especially at the elbows, can be a clue to Bethlem myopathy, Emery-Dreifuss dystrophy, and LGMD 1B (laminopathy). Evidence of diffuse systemic disease can indicate amyloidosis, sarcoidosis, an endocrinopathy, collagen-vascular disease, infectious disease, or a mitochondrial disorder.

What is the Distribution of Weakness?

In order to determine the distribution of muscle weakness, it is important to know which muscles to test and how to grade their power. Muscle strength can be tested by manual testing and from observation of functional activity (**Box 12**). Functional testing is particularly informative in young children who cannot usually cooperate with formal manual muscle testing and in adults with give-way weakness who present with complaints of muscle pain.

Assessment of muscle strength is usually based on the expanded Medical Research Council of Great Britain (MRC) grading scale of 0 to 5 (**Box 13**). In performing manual muscle testing of the upper extremities, it is necessary to assess shoulder abduction, external and internal rotation; elbow flexion and extension; wrist flexion and extension; and finger and thumb extension, flexion, and abduction.[5] Muscle groups that should be tested in the lower extremities include hip flexion, extension, and abduction; knee flexion and extension; ankle dorsiflexion, plantar flexion, inversion, and eversion; and toe extension and flexion. All muscle groups should be tested bilaterally and preferably against gravity. Neck flexors should be assessed in the supine position and neck extensors in the prone position. Knee extension and hip flexion should be tested in the seated position; knee flexion should be tested prone; and hip abduction should be tested in the lateral decubitus position. If testing against gravity is not done, the presence of significant muscle weakness can escape recognition.

The MRC grading system has being criticized because of the unequal width of response options. For instance, a one-point change from MRC 2 to 1 does not have

---

Box 12
Functional assessment of muscle weakness

Location	Signs or Symptoms of Weakness
Facial	Inability to bury eyelashes, horizontal smile, inability to whistle
Ocular	Double vision, ptosis, disconjugate eye movements
Bulbar	Nasal speech, weak cry, nasal regurgitation of liquids, poor suck, difficulty swallowing, recurrent aspiration pneumonia, cough during meals
Neck	Poor head control
Trunk	Scoliosis, lumbar lordosis, protuberant abdomen, difficulty sitting up
Shoulder girdle	Difficulty lifting objects overhead, scapular winging
Forearm/hand	Inability to make a tight fist, finger or wrist drop, inability to prevent escape from hand grip
Pelvic girdle	Difficulty climbing stairs, waddling gait, Gower sign
Leg/foot	Foot drop, inability to walk on heels or toes
Respiratory	Use of accessory muscles

Box 13
Expanded MRC scale for manual muscle testing

Modified MRC Grade	Degree of Strength
5	Normal power
5−	Equivocal, barely detectable weakness
4+	Definite but slight weakness
4	Able to move the joint against combination of gravity and some resistance
4−	Capable of minimal resistance
3+	Capable of transient resistance but collapses abruptly
3	Active movement against gravity
3−	Able to move against gravity but not through full range
2	Able to move with gravity eliminated
1	Trace contraction
0	No contraction

the same significance as far as the amount of motor unit or muscle loss as a change from 5 to 4. Using Rasch analysis[6] in more than 1000 patients with a variety of neuro-muscular disorders, disordered thresholds were demonstrated in 74% to 79% of the muscles examined, indicating the physicians' inability to discriminate between most MRC categories regardless of the physicians' experience or illness type. Thresholds were restored after rescoring the MRC grades from 6 to 4 options (0, paralysis; 1, severe weakness; 2, slight weakness; 3, normal strength). The modified MRC sum score acceptably fulfilled Rasch model expectations.

Finally, cranial nerve muscles such as the orbicularis oculi and oris, extraocular muscles, tongue, and palate should be examined. These muscles may be best tested by observation of functional activities such as asking patients to whistle, suck from a straw, and smile.

In addition to manual muscle testing and functional testing, muscles should be inspected for evidence of atrophy or hypertrophy. Atrophy of proximal limb muscles is common in most chronic myopathies. However, certain myopathies may demonstrate atrophy in specific groups that correspond to severe weakness in those muscles and provide additional diagnostic clues. For example, atrophy of the peri-scapular muscles associated with scapular winging is characteristic of faciosca-pulohumeral dystrophy. Scapular winging is also seen in patients with LGMD 1B (laminopathy), LGMD 2A (calpainopathy), Pompe disease, and LGMD 2C-F (sarcogly-canopathies). Selective atrophy of the quadriceps muscles and forearm flexor muscles is highly suggestive of inclusion body myositis. Distal myopathies may have profound atrophy of the anterior or posterior lower extremity compartments. However, muscles can show evidence of hypertrophy in some myotonic conditions, such as myotonia congenita. Muscle hypertrophy is also characterized by disorders including amyloidosis, sarcoidosis, and hypothyroid myopathy. In Duchenne and Becker dystrophy, the calf muscles demonstrate pseudohypertrophy caused by replacement with connective tissue and fat. Calf muscle hypertrophy is also characteristically seen in LGMD 2C-F (sarcoglycanopathies) early on in the course of Miyoshi myopathy and anoctamin-5 defect and in LGMD 2I (fukutin-related protein). In LGMD 2G (telethoninopathy), 50% of the patients will show calf hypertrophy and 50% will demonstrate calf atrophy. Focal muscle enlargement can also be caused by a neoplastic or inflammatory process, ectopic ossification, tendon rupture, or partial denervation.

PATTERN RECOGNITION APPROACH TO MYOPATHIC DISORDERS

After answering the 6 key questions outlined earlier from the history and neurologic examination, one can attempt to classify a myopathic disorder into one of 10 distinctive patterns of muscle weakness, each with a specific differential diagnosis. The final diagnosis can then be confirmed based on information from a *selective* number of laboratory evaluations.

Pattern 1: Proximal Limb-Girdle Weakness

The most common pattern of muscle weakness in myopathies is symmetric weakness affecting predominantly the proximal muscles of the legs and arms or the so-called limb-girdle distribution. The distal muscles are usually involved but to a much lesser extent. Neck extensor and flexor muscles are also frequently affected. This pattern of weakness is seen in most hereditary and acquired myopathies and, therefore, is the least specific in arriving at a particular diagnosis.

Pattern 2: Distal Weakness

This pattern of weakness predominantly involves the distal muscles of the upper or lower extremities (anterior or posterior compartment muscle groups) (**Box 14**) (see the article by Dimachkie and Barohn elsewhere in this issue). Depending on the diagnosis and severity of disease, proximal muscles may also be affected. The involvement is usually, although not invariably, symmetric. Selective weakness and atrophy in distal extremity muscles is more commonly a feature of neuropathies; therefore, a careful sensory and reflex examination must always be performed in patients presenting with this phenotype.

Pattern 3: Proximal Arm/Distal Leg Weakness (Scapuloperoneal)

This pattern of weakness affects the peri-scapular muscles of the proximal arm and the anterior compartment muscles of the distal lower extremity or the so-called scapuloperoneal distribution (**Box 15**). The scapular muscle weakness is usually characterized by scapular winging. Weakness can be very *asymmetric*. When this pattern is associated with facial weakness, it is highly suggestive of a diagnosis of

---

Box 14
Myopathies with distal weakness

Distal myopathies

    Late adult onset distal myopathy type 1 (Welander)

    Late adult onset distal myopathy type 2 (Udd-Markesbery)

    Early adult onset distal myopathy type 1 (Nonaka)

    Early adult onset distal myopathy type 2 (Miyoshi)

    Early adult onset distal myopathy type 3 (Laing)

Centronuclear myopathy

Debrancher deficiency

Hereditary inclusion body myopathy

Inclusion body myositis

Myofibrillar myopathy

Myotonic dystrophy

Box 15
Pattern 3: scapuloperoneal pattern of weakness

Acid maltase deficiency

Central core myopathy

Emery-Dreifuss humeroperoneal dystrophy

Facioscapulohumeral dystrophy

Limb-girdle dystrophy 2A (calpain), 2C-F (sarcoglycans), 2I (FKRP)

Nemaline myopathy

Scapuloperoneal dystrophy

---

facioscapulohumeral muscular dystrophy (see Statland and Tawil in this issue). More detailed discussion of this entity can be found in the section of this issue by Statland and Tawil. Other hereditary myopathies that are associated with a scapuloperoneal distribution of weakness include acid maltase deficiency, congenital myopathies, Emery-Dreifuss dystrophy, LGMD 1B (laminopathies), LGMD 2A (calpain), LGMD 2C-F (sarcoglycans), and scapuloperoneal dystrophy.

Pattern 4: Distal Arm/Proximal Leg Weakness

This pattern is associated with distal arm weakness involving the distal forearm muscles (wrist and finger flexors) and proximal leg weakness involving the knee extensors (quadriceps). The facial muscles are typically spared, and involvement of other muscles is extremely variable. In addition, the weakness is often *asymmetric* between the two sides, which is uncommon in most myopathies. This pattern is essentially pathognomonic for *inclusion body myositis*. For further discussion of this disease, the reader is referred to the article by Barohn and Dimachkie in this issue. This pattern may also represent an uncommon presentation of myotonic dystrophy; however, unlike inclusion body myositis, muscle weakness is symmetric.[7]

68-year old with slowly progressive muscle weakness

A 68-year-old man without significant past medical history is referred for evaluation of slowly progressive muscle weakness for the past 5 years. His symptoms initially began with difficulty walking down stairs caused by his right knee giving out. He currently has difficulty arising from a chair and grasping objects with his right hand. He was evaluated by a neurologist 2 years ago whose work-up included a creatine phosphokinase (CPK) of 500 IU/L and a left quadriceps muscle biopsy that was consistent with polymyositis. The patient has been treated with a variety of immunosuppressive medications, including prednisone, methotrexate, and azathioprine, with continued progression of his weakness. The current examination reveals intact cranial nerves, sensation, and muscle stretch reflexes. Motor examination in the right upper extremity shows MRC grade 5 shoulder abduction, 5 elbow flexion/extension, 4 wrist flexion, 5 wrist extension, and 3− finger flexion. The strength in the left upper extremity is normal except for grade 4+ finger flexion. In the left lower extremity, the patient exhibits grade 4+ hip flexion, 3+ knee extension, and 4+ ankle dorsiflexion with thigh muscle atrophy. In the right lower extremity, the strength is normal except for grade 4+ knee extension.

Comment

The chronic onset, asymmetric distribution of weakness, and selective involvement of wrist/finger flexion and knee extension is most consistent with a diagnosis of inclusion body myositis (IBM). In many cases, the initial muscle biopsy fails to identify vacuoles; patients are inappropriately treated with immunosuppressant medications for presumptive polymyositis. In patients with a phenotype consistent with IBM, particularly if they are refractory to immunosuppressive treatment, a repeat biopsy may be necessary to clarify the diagnosis.

Pattern 5: Ptosis with or Without Ophthalmoparesis

Myopathies presenting with predominant involvement of ocular and/or pharyngeal muscles represent a relatively limited group of disorders (**Box 16**). The ocular involvement principally results in ptosis and ophthalmoparesis, which usually, although not always, occurs *without* symptoms of diplopia. Facial weakness is not uncommon; extremity weakness is extremely variable, depending on the diagnosis.

The combination of ptosis, ophthalmoparesis without diplopia, and dysphagia should suggest the diagnosis of oculopharyngeal dystrophy, especially if there is a positive family history and the onset is in middle age or later. Ptosis and ophthalmoparesis without prominent pharyngeal involvement is a hallmark of many of the mitochondrial myopathies. Ptosis and facial weakness without ophthalmoparesis is a common feature of myotonic dystrophy and facioscapulohumeral dystrophy. Ptosis has diurnal variation in ocular myasthenia gravis and is often associated with diplopia.

70-year old with progressive dysphagia and weakness
A 70-year-old white woman with a family history of myasthenia gravis presents for the evaluation of a 10-year history of progressive dysphagia and weakness. She specifically denies any symptoms of diplopia and states that her symptoms do not fluctuate during the day or when she becomes fatigued. She has noted no improvement with a course of prednisone 60 mg/d and pyridostigmine 60 mg 4 times a day. Cranial nerve examination is remarkable for bilateral ptosis, incomplete abduction/adduction of both eyes, mild orbicularis oris weakness, and mild tongue weakness. The motor examination reveals MRC grade 4 neck flexion, 4 shoulder abduction, 4+ elbow flexion, 5 finger extension, 4 hip flexion, 5 knee extension, and 5 ankle dorsiflexion and plantar

---

Box 16
Pattern 5: myopathies with ptosis or ophthalmoparesis

Ptosis without ophthalmoparesis

  Congenital myopathies

    Nemaline myopathy

    Central core myopathy

  Desmin (myofibrillar) myopathy

  Myotonic dystrophy

Ptosis with ophthalmoparesis

  Centronuclear myopathy

  Mitochondrial myopathy

  Multicore disease

  Oculopharyngeal muscular dystrophy

  Oculopharyngodistal myopathy

  Neuromuscular junction disease (myasthenia gravis, Lambert-Eaton, botulism)

flexion. Sensory, cerebellar, and reflex examinations are normal. The work-up by a referring physician was remarkable for a creatine kinase (CK) of 350 IU/L and a negative acetylcholine receptor antibody.

Comment

The patient's distribution of weakness (ptosis, ophthalmoparesis, dysphagia, and proximal weakness), age of onset, and positive family history would be most suggestive of a diagnosis of oculopharyngeal muscular dystrophy (OPMD). The absence of symptoms of diplopia and muscle fatigue and the patient's slowly progressive course strongly argues against a diagnosis of a neuromuscular junction disorder, such as myasthenia gravis.

Pattern 6: Prominent Neck Extensor Weakness

This pattern is characterized by severe weakness of the neck extensor muscles. The term *dropped head syndrome* has been used in this situation (**Box 17**). Involvement of the neck flexors is variable. Extremity weakness depends on the diagnosis and may follow one of the previously outlined phenotypic patterns. For example, patients with a limb-girdle pattern of weakness may also have significant neck extensor involvement. Isolated neck extension weakness represents a distinct muscle disorder called isolated neck extensor myopathy (INEM).[8] Prominent neck extensor weakness is also common in 2 other neuromuscular diseases: amyotrophic lateral sclerosis and myasthenia gravis.

Pattern 7: Bulbar Weakness

Bulbar weakness (ie, tongue and pharyngeal weakness) is manifested by symptoms of dysarthria and dysphagia. Although several myopathies can have some bulbar involvement, the muscular dystrophy that has bulbar involvement as a primary manifestation is OPMD. Limb-girdle muscular dystrophy type 1A (myotilinopathy) can present with isolated bulbar weakness, and the inflammatory myopathies may rarely present in this manner. Neuromuscular junction disorders, such as myasthenia gravis and Lambert-Eaton myasthenic syndrome, also frequently have bulbar symptoms and signs. This pattern is considered an overlap pattern with amyotrophic lateral sclerosis and other motor neuron disorders that can have significant bulbar involvement.

Box 17
Pattern 6: myopathies with prominent neck extensor weakness

Isolated neck extensor myopathy

Dermatomyositis

Polymyositis

Inclusion body myositis

Carnitine deficiency

Facioscapulohumeral dystrophy

Myotonic dystrophy

Congenital myopathy

Hyperparathyroidism

Pattern 8: Episodic Pain, Weakness, and Myoglobinuria

This pattern is characterized by a history of episodic pain, weakness, and myoglobinuria and may be related to a variety of conditions, many of which are not caused by an underlying muscle disorder (**Box 18**). When these symptoms are triggered by exercise, a metabolic myopathy is most likely. However, several patients may develop myoglobinuria because they are inactive individuals who are suddenly required to do an overwhelming amount of exercise (ie, the couch potato syndrome).

Pattern 9: Episodic Weakness Delayed or Unrelated to Exercise

This pattern applies to the disorders of periodic paralysis, both the genetic autosomal dominant channelopathies (**Box 19**) and the secondary periodic paralyses, such as those caused by thyrotoxicosis. Also, for completeness sake, it is reasonable to include the neuromuscular junction disorders in this pattern. In all of these conditions, the weakness can occur during or after exercise, or often the weakness is unrelated to physical exertion.

Pattern 10: Stiffness and Decreased Ability to Relax

This pattern includes all of the disorders that produce myotonia and paramyotonia and includes the hereditary disorders involving skeletal muscle sodium and chloride channels (**Box 20, Table 1**) as well as myotonic dystrophy types 1 and 2 (see the articles by Trivedi and Thornton elsewhere in this issue). Both myotonic dystrophies usually also have fixed muscle weakness, with predominantly distal weakness in myotonic dystrophy type 1 and proximal weakness in myotonic dystrophy type 2. The autosomal recessive form of chloride channelopathies, Becker disease, also has fixed proximal weakness. In addition, other less common disorders that fit this pattern include Brody disease, neuromyotonia, and the central nervous system disorder, stiff-person syndrome (see **Table 1**).

Table 2 summarizes these 10 patterns of presentation of muscle disease. Once the key questions reviewed earlier have been answered and patients have been placed

---

Box 18
Pattern 8: myopathies with episodic pain, weakness, and myoglobinuria/rhabdomyolysis

Related to exercise

    Couch potato syndrome

    Glycogenoses (McArdle and so forth)

    Lipid disorders (CPT deficiency)

Not related to exercise

    Central non-neuromuscular causes

        Neuroleptic malignant syndrome

        Status epilepticus

    Drugs/toxins

    Malignant hyperthermia

    Polymyositis/dermatomyositis (rarely)

    Viral/bacterial infections

Abbreviation: CPT, carnitine palmitoyltransferase.

Box 19
Pattern 9: episodic weakness: delayed or unrelated to exercise

Periodic paralysis

  Ca^{++} channelopathies (hypokalemic)

  Na^{++} channelopathies (hyperkalemic)

  Andersen-Tawil syndrome

  Secondary PP (thyrotoxicosis)

Other: neuromuscular junction diseases

Abbreviation: PP, periodic paralysis.

---

into one of these 10 patterns of weakness, laboratory studies can then be used to confirm the diagnosis.

LABORATORY APPROACH IN THE EVALUATION OF A SUSPECTED MYOPATHY
CK

CK is an extremely useful laboratory study for the evaluation of patients with a suspected myopathy (**Box 21**). The CK is elevated in most patients with muscle disease but may be normal in slowly progressive myopathies. The degree of CK elevation can also be helpful in distinguishing different forms of muscular dystrophy. For example, in Duchenne dystrophy, the CK is invariably at least 10 times (and often up to 100 times) normal, whereas there are less significant elevations in most other myopathies. The other exceptions are LGMD 1C (caveolinopathy), 2A (calpainopathy), and 2B (dysferlinopathy) whereby CK may also be markedly elevated. The CK level may not be

---

Box 20
Pattern 10: stiffness/decreased ability to relax

Improves with exercise

  Myotonia: Na^{++} or Cl^- channelopathy

Worsens with exercise/cold sensitivity

  Paramyotonia: Na^{++} channelopathy

  Brody disease

With fixed weakness

  Myotonic dystrophy (DM 1)

  Proximal myotonic myopathy (DM 2)

  Becker disease (AR Cl^- channelopathy)

Other

  Malignant hyperthermia

  Neuromyotonia

  Rippling muscle

  Stiff-person syndrome

Abbreviation: AR, autosomal recessive.

Table 1
Channelopathies and related disorders

Disorder	Clinical Features	Pattern of Inheritance	Chromosome	Gene
Chloride channelopathies	Myotonia	Autosomal dominant	7q35	CLC-1
Myotonia congenita				
Thomsen disease	Myotonia	Autosomal dominant	7q35	CLC-1
Becker type	Myotonia + weakness	Autosomal recessive		
Sodium channelopathies				
Paramyotonia congenita	Paramyotonia	Autosomal dominant	17q13.1–13.3	SCNA4A
Hyperkalemic periodic paralysis	Periodic paralysis and myotonia and paramyotonia	Autosomal dominant	17q13.1–13.3	SCNA4A
Potassium-aggravated myotonias				
Myotonia fluctuans	Myotonia	Autosomal dominant	17q13.1–13.3	SCNA4A
Myotonia permanens	Myotonia	Autosomal dominant	17q13.1–13.3	SCNA4A
Acetazolamide responsive	Myotonia	Autosomal dominant	17q13.1–13.3	SCNA4A
Calcium channelopathies				
Hypokalemic periodic paralysis	Periodic paralysis	Autosomal dominant	1a31–32	Dihydropyridine receptor
Schwartz-Jampel syndrome (chondrodystrophic myotonia)	Myotonia, dysmorphic	Autosomal recessive	1p34.1–36.1	Perlecan
Rippling muscle disease	Muscle mounding/stiffness	Autosomal dominant	1q41 3p25	Unknown Caveolin-3
Anderson-Tawil syndrome	Periodic paralysis, cardiac arrhythmia, dysmorphic	Autosomal dominant	17q23	KCMJ2-Kir 2.1
Brody disease	Delayed relaxation, no myotonia	Autosomal recessive	16p12	Calcium-ATPase
Malignant hyperthermia	Anesthetic-induced delayed relaxation	Autosomal dominant	19q13.1	Ryanodine receptor

Table 2
Clinical patterns of muscle disorders

	Weakness				Episodic	Trigger	Diagnosis
	Proximal	Distal	Asymmetric	Symmetric			
Pattern 1 Limb-girdle	+	—	—	+	—	—	Most myopathies, hereditary and acquired
Pattern 2a Distal	—	+	—	+	—	—	Distal myopathies (also neuropathies)
Pattern 3 Proximal arm/distal leg scapuloperoneal	+ Arm	+ Leg	+ (FSH)	+ (Others)	—	—	FSH, Emery-Dreifuss, acid maltase, congenital scapuloperoneal
Pattern 4 Distal arm/proximal leg	+ Leg	+ Arm	+	—	—	—	IBM Myotonic dystrophy
Pattern 5 Ptosis/ophthalmoplegia	+	—	+ (MG)	+ (Others)	—	—	OPMD, MG, myotonic dystrophy, mitochondria
Pattern 6a Neck, extensor	+	—	—	+	—	—	INEM, MG (also ALS)
Pattern 7a Bulbar (tongue, pharyngeal)	+	—	—	+	—	—	MG, LEMS, OPMD (also ALS)
Pattern 8 Episodic weakness/pain/ rhabdomyolysis + trigger	+	—	—	+	+	+	McArdle, CPT, drugs, toxins
Pattern 9 Episodic weakness Delayed or unrelated to exercise	+	—	—	+	+	+/−	Primary periodic paralysis Channelopathies Na++ Ca++ Secondary periodic paralysis
Pattern 10 Stiffness/inability to relax	—	—	—	—	+	+/−	Myotonic dystrophy, channelopathies, PROMM, rippling (also stiff-person, neuromyotonia)

Abbreviations: ALS, amyotrophic lateral sclerosis; CPT, carnitine palmityl transferase; FSH, facioscapulohumeral muscular dystrophy; LEMS, lambert-eaton myasthenic syndrome; MG, myasthenia gravis; OPMD, oculopharyngeal muscular dystrophy; PROMM, proximal myotonic myopathy.
a Overlap pattern with neuropathy/motor neuron disease.

| **Box 21** |
| **Differential diagnosis of CK elevation** |
| Myopathies |
| Carrier state (dystrophinopathies) |
| Channelopathies |
| Congenital myopathies |
| Drug/toxin induced |
| Inflammatory myopathies |
| Metabolic myopathies |
| Muscular dystrophies |
| Motor neuron diseases |
| Amyotrophic lateral sclerosis |
| Postpolio syndrome |
| Spinal muscular atrophy |
| Neuropathies |
| Charcot-Marie-Tooth disease |
| Guillain-Barré syndrome |
| Others |
| Idiopathic hyperCKemia |
| Increased muscle mass |
| Hypothyroidism/hypoparathyroidism |
| Medications |
| Race |
| Sex |
| Strenuous exercise |
| Surgery |
| Trauma (electromyography studies, intramuscular, or subcutaneous injections) |

elevated in some myopathies or may even by lowered by several factors, including profound muscle wasting, corticosteroid administration, collagen diseases, alcoholism, or hyperthyroidism.

It is also important to remember than an elevation of serum CK does not necessarily imply a primary myopathic disorder. Many times the CK will increase modestly (usually to <10 times normal) in motor neuron disease; uncommonly, CK elevations may be seen in Charcot-Marie-Tooth disease and Guillain-Barré syndrome. Endocrine disorders, such as hypothyroidism and hypoparathyroidism, can also be associated with high CK levels. The causes of CK elevation other than neuromuscular disease include muscle trauma (falls, intramuscular or subcutaneous injections, electromyography [EMG] studies), viral illnesses, seizures, or strenuous exercise. In these cases, CK elevations are usually transient and less than 5 times normal.

Race and sex can also affect serum CK (**Box 22**). CK levels are frequently more than the normal range in some black individuals and in patients with enlarged muscles. Occasionally, benign elevations of CK appear on a hereditary basis. It is extremely

Box 22		
Effect of race and sex on CK measurements		
Group	**Constituents**	**ULN (IU/L)**
High	Black men	1201
Intermediate	Nonblack men	504
	Black women	621
Low	Nonblack women	325

Abbreviation: ULN, upper limit of normal.

Adapted from Silvestri NJ, Wolfe GI. Asymptomatic/pauci-symptomatic creatine kinase elevations (hyperckemia). Muscle Nerve 2013;47(6):813; with permission.

unusual for a slightly elevated CPK (3-fold or less) to be associated with an underlying myopathy in the absence of objective muscle weakness or pain. Recent data suggest that even higher cutoff values than those listed in **Box 22** may be found in otherwise normal individuals based on sex and ethnicity.[9] For black men, an upper normal limit of 1201 IU/L was suggested, 621 for black women, and 504 nonblack men; the lowest cutoff is for nonblack women at 325 IU/L. In the absence of muscle weakness on examination, these patients can be observed as long as the history does not suggest a metabolic myopathy.[10]

Serum tests for other muscle enzymes are significantly less helpful than the determination of the CK. Enzymes such as aldolase, aspartate aminotransferase (AST, serum glutamic-oxaloacetic transaminase), alanine aminotransferase (ALT, serum glutamic-pyruvic transaminase), and lactate dehydrogenase (LDH) may be slightly elevated in myopathies. Because AST, ALT, and LDH are often measured in screening chemistry panels, their elevation should prompt CK measurement to determine if the source is muscle or liver. If patients with an inflammatory myopathy are treated with an immunosuppressive agent that may cause hepatotoxicity, the liver-specific enzyme, gamma glutamic transferase, should be followed.

In general, CK isoenzymes are not helpful in evaluating myopathies. CK-MM elevations are typical of muscle disease, but CK-MB is also elevated in myopathies and does not indicate that cardiac disease is present.

Electrophysiologic Studies

Electrophysiologic studies, consisting of both nerve conduction studies (NCS) and EMG, should be part of the routine evaluation of patients with a suspected myopathy.[11,12]

These studies are helpful in confirming that the muscle is indeed the correct site of the lesion and that weakness is not the result of an underlying motor neuron disease, neuropathy, or neuromuscular junction disorder. NCS are typically normal in patients with myopathy except in distal myopathies. Needle EMG examination showing evidence of brief-duration, small-amplitude motor units with increased recruitment can be extremely helpful in confirming the presence of a myopathy. Needle EMG can also provide a clue as to which muscles have had recent or ongoing muscle injury and can be a guide as to which muscle to biopsy. It is important to realize, however, that the EMG can be normal in patients with myopathy; the results of electrodiagnostic studies need to be evaluated in the context of the patients' history, neurologic examination, and other laboratory studies.

The Muscle Biopsy

If the clinical features and/or electrodiagnostic features suggest the possibility of a myopathy, a muscle biopsy may be an appropriate test to confirm the diagnosis.[13]

However, many forms of hereditary muscle disorders can now be diagnosed with molecular genetic testing, eliminating the need for performing a muscle biopsy in every patient. A muscle specimen can be obtained through either an open or closed (needle or punch) biopsy procedure. The advantage of a needle or punch biopsy is that it is minimally invasive, is cosmetically more appealing, and multiple specimens can be obtained. The disadvantage of the closed biopsy procedure is that not all laboratories have the expertise to adequately process the muscle tissue acquired with this approach for all the necessary studies.

Selection of the appropriate muscle to biopsy is critical. Muscles that are severely weak (MRC grade 3 or less) should not be biopsied because the results are likely to only show evidence of end-stage muscle. In addition, muscles that have recently been studied by needle EMG should be avoided because of the possibility of artifacts created by needle insertion. Biopsies should generally be taken from muscles that demonstrate MRC grade 4 strength. For practical purposes, in the upper extremities, the muscles of choice are either the biceps or deltoid; in the lower extremities, the best choice is the vastus lateralis. The gastrocnemius should be avoided because its tendon insertion extends throughout the muscle and inadvertent sampling of a myotendinous junction may cause difficulty with interpretation. Occasionally, an imaging procedure, such as muscle ultrasound, computed tomography, or magnetic resonance imaging, can be used to guide the selection of the appropriate muscle to biopsy.

Biopsy specimens can be analyzed by light microscopy, electron microscopy, biochemical studies and immune staining (**Box 23**). In most instances, light microscopic observations of frozen muscle tissue specimens are sufficient to make a pathologic diagnosis. Typical myopathic abnormalities include central nuclei, both small and large hypertrophic round fibers, split fibers, and degenerating and regenerating fibers. Inflammatory myopathies are characterized by the presence of mononuclear inflammatory cells in the endomysial and perimysial connective tissue between fibers and occasionally around blood vessels. In addition, in dermatomyositis, atrophy of fibers located on the periphery of a muscle fascicle, perifascicular atrophy, is a common finding. Chronic myopathies frequently show evidence of increased connective tissue and fat.

For general histology, the hematoxylin and eosin and modified Gomori trichrome are the most useful. The latter is particularly helpful in identifying ragged-red fibers that

---

Box 23
Utility of muscle biopsy stains and histochemical reactions

Histochemical Reactions and Stains	Clinical Utility
ATPase	Distribution of fiber types
Gomori trichrome	General histology and mitochondrial disease
Hematoxylin and eosin	General histology
NADH, succinate dehydrogenase, cytochrome oxidase	Myofibrillar and mitochondrial abnormalities
Oil red O	Lipid storage diseases
Periodic acid-Schiff	Glycogen storage diseases
Congo red, crystal violet	Detection of amyloid deposition
Myophosphorylase	McArdle disease
Phosphofructokinase	Phosphofructokinase deficiency
Myoadenylate deaminase	Myoadenylate deaminase deficiency
Dystrophin immunostain	Duchenne and Becker muscular dystrophy
Dysferlin immunostain	Limb-girdle MD 2B
Membrane attack complex immunostain	Dermatomyositis

might suggest a mitochondrial disorder. In addition to these standard stains, other histochemical reactions can be used to gain additional information (see **Box 23**). The myosin ATPase stains (alkaline at pH 9.4 and acidic at pH 4.3 and 4.6) allow a thorough evaluation of histochemistry fiber types. Type 1 fibers (slow-twitch, fatigue-resistant, oxidative metabolism) stain lightly at alkaline and darkly at acidic pH. Type 2 fibers (fast-twitch, fatigue-prone, glycolytic metabolism) stain darkly at alkaline and lightly at acidic pH. Normally, there is a random distribution of the 2 fiber types; there are generally twice as many type 2 as type 1 fibers. In several myopathies, there is a nonspecific type 1 fiber predominance. Oxidative enzyme stains (NADH dehydrogenase, succinate dehydrogenase, cytochrome-c oxidase) are useful for identifying myofibrillar and mitochondrial abnormalities. Periodic acid–Schiff stains can be helpful in identifying glycogen storage diseases, and oil red O stains may assist with the diagnosis of a lipid storage disease. Acid and alkaline phosphatase reactions can highlight necrotic and regenerating fibers, respectively. Qualitative biochemical enzyme stains can be performed for myophosphorylase (McArdle disease), phosphofructokinase deficiency, and myoadenylate deaminase deficiency. Amyloid deposition can be assayed with Congo red or crystal violet staining. Finally, immunohistochemical techniques can stain for muscle proteins that are deficient in some muscular dystrophies (eg, dystrophin in Duchenne and Becker dystrophy) or for products that are increased in certain inflammatory myopathies, such as the membrane attack complex in dermatomyositis or p62 in inclusion body myositis.[14]

Electron microscopy (EM) evaluates the ultrastructural components of muscle fibers and is not required in most myopathies to make a pathologic diagnosis. EM is important, however, in the diagnosis of some congenital myopathies and mitochondrial disorders. Findings detected only by EM are seldom of clinical importance.

The muscle tissue can also be processed for biochemical analysis to determine a specific enzyme defect in the evaluation of a possible metabolic or mitochondrial myopathy. In addition, Western blot determinations from muscle tissue can be performed for certain muscle proteins. This type of analysis is usually limited to the dystrophin assays when the immune stains and the molecular genetic studies are inconclusive in establishing a diagnosis of either Duchenne or Becker dystrophy. This method has recently been expanded to calpainopathies and the dysferlin defect, though gene sequencing is more definitive.

Molecular Genetic Studies

The specific molecular genetic defect is now known for a large number of hereditary myopathies, and mutations can be identified by peripheral blood DNA analysis. Examples of molecular genetic studies that are commercially available are included in **Box 24**. This list is continually updated on www.genetests.org. Molecular genetic testing frequently eliminates the need for muscle biopsy. This technology is also extremely helpful for determining the carrier status and for performing prenatal testing. For Pompe disease, dry blood spot assay is a good screening test that must be followed by confirmation of acid alpha-glucosidase enzymatic activity in blood lymphocytes or other tissues (muscle or skin fibroblasts) or through gene sequencing (please refer to the article by Majed Dasouki and colleagues in this issue).

Other Tests

In addition to CK determinations, additional blood tests that can be extremely helpful in the evaluation of patients with a suspected myopathy include serum electrolytes, thyroid function tests, parathyroid hormone levels, vitamin D levels, and human immunodeficiency virus. In patients with an inflammatory myopathy, serologic

---

Box 24
Commercially available molecular genetic studies performed with peripheral blood samples

Chronic progressive external ophthalmoplegia (POLG, TWINKLE, ANT1, OPA1)

Collagen VI disorders (COL61, COL62, COL63)

Congenital muscular dystrophy (FKRP, FCMD, LAMA2, POMGNT, POMT1, POMT2)

Duchenne and Becker muscular dystrophy (DMD sequencing)

Emery-Dreifuss muscular dystrophy (EMD, FHL1)

Facioscapulohumeral muscular dystrophy (FSHD)

Hypokalemic and hyperkalemic periodic paralysis (CACNA1S, SCN4A)

Limb-girdle muscular dystrophy (CAPN3, CAV3, DYSF, FKRP, LMNA, SGCA, B, D, G, CAPN3, SGCA)

Mitochondrial myopathy, encephalopathy, lactic acidosis, and stroke (MELAS)

Myoclonic epilepsy and ragged red fibers (MERRF)

Myotonic dystrophy (DM1, DM2)

Myofibrillar myopathy (CRYAB, DES, FLNC, LDB3, MYOT, BAG3)

Myotubular myopathy (MTM1 mutations)

Nemaline myopathy (ACTA1 mutations)

OPMD

---

determinations for systemic lupus erythematosus, rheumatoid arthritis, and other immunologic markers (eg, Jo-1 antibodies) can occasionally be useful. A urine analysis can also be performed to detect the presence of myoglobinuria. This condition should be suspected if the urine tests positive for blood but no red blood cells are identified.[10]

Forearm exercise testing can often be an important part of the evaluation of patients with a suspected metabolic myopathy. The exercise test should be carried out without the blood pressure cuff because ischemic exercise may be hazardous in patients with defects in the glycolytic enzyme pathway. The test is performed by asking patients to perform isometric contractions using a handgrip dynamometer for 1.5 seconds separated by rest periods of 0.5 seconds for 1 minute. A resting blood sample for venous lactate and ammonia is obtained at baseline and subsequently at 1, 2, 4, 6, and 10 minutes following the completion of exercise. A 3-fold increase in the lactate level represents a normal response. The characteristic elevation of serum lactate after exercise is absent (phosphofructokinase deficiency, myophosphorylase deficiency) or reduced (phosphoglycerate mutase deficiency). Forearm testing is normal in all disorders of fat metabolism and is also in some glycolytic disorders with fixed muscle weakness, such as acid maltase deficiency.

SUMMARY

Although this pattern recognition approach to myopathy may have limitations, it can be extremely helpful in narrowing the differential diagnosis and, therefore, minimizing the number of laboratory studies that must be ordered to confirm the diagnosis. There will always be patients with muscle disease who will not fit neatly into any of these 10 categories. In addition, patients with involvement of other areas of the neuraxis, such as the motor neuron, peripheral nerve, or neuromuscular junction, may also frequently present with one of these patterns. For example, although proximal greater than distal weakness is most often seen in a myopathy, patients with acquired demyelinating neuropathies (Guillain-Barré syndrome and chronic inflammatory demyelinating polyneuropathy) often have proximal as well as distal muscle involvement. Careful consideration of the distribution of muscle weakness and attention to these common patterns of involvement in the context of other aspects of the neurologic examination and laboratory evaluation will usually, however, lead the clinician to a timely and accurate diagnosis.

WEB SITES

NIH/Gene Reviews: genetic testing and reviews: http://www.ncbi.nlm.nih.gov/sites/GeneTests/review

Muscular Dystrophy Association: http://mdausa.org/

Washington University Neuromuscular Disease Center: http://neuromuscular.wustl.edu/

REFERENCES

1. Amato AA, Russell JA. Neuromuscular disorders. New York: McGraw Hill; 2008.
2. Barohn RJ. General approach to muscle diseases. Cecil textbook of medicine. 23rd edition. Philadelphia: Goldman & Bennett ; 2008. p. 2816–34.
3. Brooke MH. A clinician's view of neuromuscular disease. 2nd edition. Baltimore (MD): Williams & Wilkins; 1986.
4. Griggs RC, Mendell JR, Miller RG. Evaluation and treatment of myopathies. Philadelphia: FA Davis; 1995.
5. Medical Research Council. Aids to the examination of the peripheral nervous system. London: Balliere Tindall; 1986.
6. Vanhoutte EK, Faber CG, van Nes SI, et al, PeriNomS Study Group. Modifying the Medical Research Council grading system through Rasch analyses. Brain 2012; 135(Pt 5):1639–49.
7. Barohn RJ. Myotonic dystrophy with quadriceps and finger flexor weakness: the inclusion body myositis phenotype. J Child Neurol 2002;17:15.
8. Katz JS, Wolfe GI, Burns DK, et al. Isolated neck extensor myopathy: a common cause of dropped head syndrome. Neurology 1996;46:917–21.
9. Silvestri NJ, Wolfe GI. Asymptomatic/pauci-symptomatic creatine kinase elevations (hyperckemia). Muscle Nerve 2013;47(6):805–15.
10. Martin A, Haller RG, Barohn RJ. Metabolic myopathies. Curr Opin Rheumatol 1994;6:552–8.
11. Amato AA, James A, Russell JA. Testing in neuromuscular disease – electrodiagnosis and other modalities. In: Anthony AA, Russell JA, editors. Neuromuscular disorders. New York: McGraw-Hill Professional; 2008. p.17–70.
12. Preston DC, Shapiro BE. Myopathy. In: Preston DC, Shapiro BE, editors. Electromyography and neuromuscular disorders: clinical-electrophysiological correlations. London: Butterworth-Heinemann; 1998. p. 525–39.
13. Dubowitz V, Sewery CA. Muscle biopsy: a practical approach. 3rd edition. London: Saunders; 2007.
14. Dubourg O, Wanschitz J, Maisonobe T, et al. Diagnostic value of markers of muscle degeneration in sporadic inclusion body myositis. Acta Myol 2011;30(2): 103–8.

Idiopathic Inflammatory Myopathies

Mazen M. Dimachkie, MD[a],*, Richard J. Barohn, MD[b], Anthony A. Amato, MD[c]

KEYWORDS

- Polymyositis • Dermatomyositis • Necrotizing myopathy • Inclusion body myositis
- Clinical presentation • Diagnosis • Pathology • Treatment

KEY POINTS

- The idiopathic inflammatory myopathies (IIM) consist of rare heterogeneous autoimmune disorders that present with marked proximal and symmetric muscle weakness, except for distal and asymmetric weakness in inclusion body myositis (IBM).
- Besides frequent creatine kinase (CK) elevation, the electromyogram confirms the presence of an irritative myopathy.
- Extramuscular involvement affects a significant number of cases with interstitial lung disease (ILD), cutaneously in dermatomyositis (DM), systemic or joint manifestations, and increased risk of malignancy, especially in DM.
- Myositis-specific autoantibodies influence the phenotype of the IIM. Jo-1 antibodies are frequently associated with ILD and the newly described HMG-CoA reductase antibodies are characteristic of autoimmune necrotizing myopathy (NM).
- Muscle abnormality ranges from inflammatory exudates of variable distribution to intact muscle fiber invasion, necrosis, phagocytosis, and, in the case of IBM, rimmed vacuoles and protein deposits.
- Despite many similarities, the IIM are fairly heterogeneous from the histopathologic and pathogenetic standpoints, and show some clinical and treatment-response differences.

EPIDEMIOLOGY

The idiopathic inflammatory myopathies are rare sporadic disorders with an overall annual incidence of approximately 1 in 100,000 (**Table 1**). Except for juvenile dermatomyositis (JDM), the IIM are diseases of the adult, and besides IBM these affect more

This publication was supported by an Institutional Clinical and Translational Science Award, National Institutes of Health/National Center for Advancing Translational Sciences Grant Number UL1TR000001. Its contents are solely the responsibility of the authors and do not necessarily represent the official views of the NIH.

[a] Neurophysiology Division, Neuromuscular Section, Department of Neurology, University of Kansas Medical Center, 3901 Rainbow Boulevard, Mail Stop 2012, Kansas City, KS 66160, USA; [b] Department of Neurology, University of Kansas Medical Center, 3901 Rainbow Boulevard, Mail Stop 2012, Kansas City, KS 66160, USA; [c] Department of Neurology, Brigham and Women's Hospital, Harvard Medical School, 75 Francis Street, Boston, MA 02115, USA
* Corresponding author.
E-mail address: mdimachkie@kumc.edu

Neurol Clin 32 (2014) 595–628
http://dx.doi.org/10.1016/j.ncl.2014.04.007
0733-8619/14/$ – see front matter © 2014 Elsevier Inc. All rights reserved.

neurologic.theclinics.com

Acronym	
APCs	Antigen-Presenting Cells
AZA	Azathioprine
BAFF	B Cell-Activating Factor
CK	Creatine Kinase
CMAP	Compound Muscle Action Potential
CS	Corticosteroids
DC	Dendritic Cells
DM	Dermatomyositis
EMG	Electromyography
IBM	Inclusion Body Myositis
IFIH1	Interferon-Induced Helicase
ILD	Interstitial Lung Disease
IVIG	Intravenous Immunoglobulin
JDM	Juvenile Dermatomyositis
MSAs	Myositis-Specific Antibodies
MTX	Methotrexate
MUAPs	Motor Unit Action Potentials
NM	Necrotizing Myopathy
PCP	Pneumocystis Carinii Pneumonia
PDC	Plasmacytoid Dendritic Cells
PM	Polymyositis
RA	Rheumatoid Arthritis
SANAM	Statin-Associated Autoimmune
SRP	Signal Recognition Particle
TGF	Transforming Growth Factor

women than men. In a Dutch study that excluded IBM, necrotizing myopathy (NM) represented 19%, whereas dermatomyositis (DM) and nonspecific myositis accounted for 36% and 39% of all IIM, respectively.[1] Unlike findings from other studies, polymyositis (PM) was reported to be uncommon, accounting for only 2% of IIM cases.[1] However, a PM clinical phenotype was the most common cause of PM disorder in the Mayo Clinic case series.[2] Indeed, 27 of 43 cases with pathologic PM had clinical features of PM, whereas 37% had phenotypic IBM with tissue inflammation but no rimmed vacuoles. Studies of the combined incidence of PM and DM from Israel, South Australia, and the United States (Allegheny County, Pennsylvania and Olmstead County, Minnesota) have yielded rates ranging from 2.2 to 7.0 per million population using a variety of methods.[3] The incidence of DM in South Australia is to 1.0 to 1.4 per million, whereas in Olmstead County it is 9.6 per million inhabitants. The incidence of PM in South Australia derived from muscle biopsy findings and review of medical records is 4 times higher than that of DM, respectively 4.1 to 6.6 per million versus 1.0 to 1.4 per million. A recent study indicates the prevalence rates in South Australia to be 1.97 and 7.2 per 100,000 for DM and PM, respectively. In a nationwide Taiwanese population survey between 2003 and 2007, the overall annual incidences of DM and PM were 7.1 (95% confidence interval [CI] 6.6–7.6) and 4.4 (95% CI 4.0–4.8) cases per million population. The incidence of DM and PM increased with advancing age and reached a peak at age 50 to 59 years.[4]

Table 1
Idiopathic inflammatory myopathies: clinical and laboratory findings

	Typical Age of Onset	Rash	Pattern of Weakness	Creatine Kinase	Muscle Biopsy	Cellular Infiltrate	Response to Immunosuppressive Therapy	Common Associated Conditions
Dermatomyositis	Childhood and adult	Yes	Proximal > distal	Normal or elevated up to 50× normal	Perimysial and perivascular inflammation; perifascicular atrophy; MAC	CD4+ T cells; B cells; plasmacytoid dendritic cells	Yes	Malignancy, ILD, CTD, myocarditis, vasculitis, calcinosis (juvenile)
Polymyositis	Adult (>18 y)	No	Proximal > distal	Elevated up to 50× normal	Endomysial inflammation surrounding and invading nonnecrotic myofibers	CD8+ T cells; macrophages; myeloid dendritic cells	Yes	Cancer, ILD, CTD, myocarditis
Inclusion body myositis	Elderly (>50 y)	No	Finger flexors, knee extensors, asymmetry, dysphagia	Normal or mildly elevated up to 15–20× normal	Rimmed vacuoles; endomysial inflammation surrounding and invading nonnecrotic myofibers	CD8+ T cells; macrophages; myeloid dendritic cells	No	Autoimmune disorders: Sjögren, SLE, thrombocytopenia, sarcoidosis
Autoimmune necrotizing myopathy	Adult and elderly	No	Proximal > distal	Elevated (>10× normal)	Necrotic muscle fibers; absent inflammatory infiltrate	Abundant macrophages, lymphocytes none to mild	Yes	Malignancy, CTD, drug-induced

Abbreviations: CTD, connective tissue disease; ILD, interstitial lung disease; MAC, membrane attack complex; SLE, systemic lupus erythematosus.
Adapted from Amato AA, Barohn RJ. Idiopathic inflammatory myopathies. Neurol Clin 1997;15:616; with permission.

CLINICAL PRESENTATION
Dermatomyosis

The presentation of DM is cutaneous, muscular, or both, with acute to insidious progressive proximal muscle weakness. As in PM and NM, patients with DM describe difficulty using their arms while elevated above the head, and being unable to get up from a deep chair, rise off the floor, or climb stairs. Formal grip-force measures are reduced in chronic DM and PM in comparison with controls.[5] Weakness is painless except in patients with acute disease and/or subcutaneous calcifications. DM may result in bulbar muscle weakness manifesting as dysphagia, chewing difficulty, jaw-opening weakness, and sometimes dysarthria. In addition, multisystem involvement is common in JDM, which frequently presents as an insidious muscle weakness and pain after a febrile episode and rash.

The characteristic rash antedates or occurs concurrently with the onset of muscle weakness, thereby providing early clues to the diagnosis of classic DM. Adermatopathic DM is more difficult to recognize, as it is histopathologically proven DM without the rash. Amyopathic DM presents with only the rash and no weakness, although muscle histology may show some inflammation. Although classic DM rash can be subtle, a heliotrope rash is typical and consists of purplish discoloration of the eyelids often associated with periorbital edema (**Fig. 1**). However, generalized or limb edema is an uncommon manifestation of DM. Gottron papules (see **Fig. 1**), a violaceous lichenoid papular pathognomonic scaly rash, appear on the extensor surface of the hands, fingers, elbows, and, at times, toes. When occasionally located on the volar aspects, the papules are referred to as inverse Gottron papules.[6] A macular erythematous rash may affect the face, neck, and anterior chest (V-sign), upper back (shawl sign), and the extensor surface of the elbows, knuckles (see **Fig. 1**), knees, or toes (Gottron sign). At times, the nail beds have dilated capillary loops with importantly periungual hyperemia (see **Fig. 1**). Nailfold capillary density is a reduced in JDM and is inversely associated over time with muscle and skin disease activity.[7] Subcutaneous calcinosis of the elbows and knees, sometimes with ulceration, often occurs in JDM but is uncommon in adult DM. "Mechanic's hands," manifesting as thickened and cracked skin on the

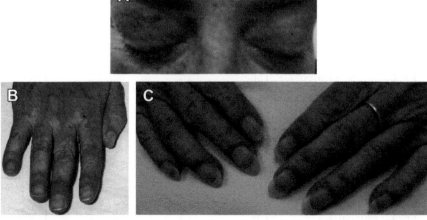

Fig. 1. (*A*) Heliotrope rash and periorbital edema and erythema in dermatomyositis (DM). (*B*) Violaceous erythematous scaly papular rash in DM (Gottron papules), with cutaneous ulceration and periungual hyperemia. (*C*) Periungual hyperemia in DM.

dorsal and ventral surfaces of the hands, is encountered in patients with the antisynthetase syndrome (arthritis, Raynaud phenomenon, ILD). Cutaneous symptoms, including prominent pruritus, have a significant impact on quality of life.[8,9]

In 1975 Bohan and Peter[10,11] described 5 criteria that when present support definite DM, including:

1. Proximal weakness
2. Elevated creatine kinase (CK)
3. Myopathic electromyogram (EMG)
4. Inflammation
5. Typical rash, which sets it apart from PM

A modification of the Bohan and Peter criteria has since been reported by Targoff and colleagues,[12] who introduced a sixth criterion of myositis-specific autoantibodies as performed by a validated assay, thus allowing patients who fulfilled 4 of 6 criteria to be diagnosed with definite DM or PM. A group of international experts met in Naarden, the Netherlands and published proposed classification criteria of the IIM to improve diagnosis specificity.[13] This system is based on clinical criteria, CK elevation, other laboratory criteria, and better defined muscle biopsy criteria, as detailed in **Box 1**. DM is classified as definite, probable, amyopathic, and possible DM sine dermatitis (**Box 2**). Definite DM requires pathologic evidence of perifascicular atrophy, whereas probable DM is based on either perivascular perimysial inflammatory cell infiltrate, membrane attack complex (MAC) depositions on small blood vessels, reduced capillary density, tubuloreticular inclusions in endothelial cells on electron microscopy (EM), or major histocompatibility complex class 1 (MHC-1) expression on perifascicular fibers. These pathologic features in the absence of typical rash are sufficient for the diagnosis of possible DM sine dermatitis. Muscle biopsy in amyopathic DM does not reveal features compatible with definite or probable DM.

Polymyositis

Since the Bohan and Peter criteria publication nearly 4 decades ago,[11] PM has been defined as an exclusionary diagnosis in patients who do not have a rash or alternative muscle or nerve disease. Although the existence of PM was recently brought into question,[1,14] recent studies have confirmed it as a distinct clinical entity accounting for most (63%) patients with histologically demonstrable findings of PM.[2] Revised classification criteria (see **Boxes 1** and **2**) were recently advanced to factor in advances in the understanding of PM immunopathogenesis.[13]

PM affects adults older than 20 years, and is more common in women than in men.[11,15,16] Because there is no pathognomonic rash, diagnosis is often more delayed in PM in comparison with DM. Patients develop progressive neck flexor and symmetric proximal limb muscle weakness subacutely or insidiously over weeks to months. Distal muscles are relatively spared. Although myalgias and muscle tenderness are common, these are not presenting complaints; rather, weakness or dysphagia occurs in one-third of patients. In patients with acute quadriparetic presentation, weakness of jaw-opening was noted in 71% of PM/DM cases, whereas this was rarely present (4%) in those with Guillain-Barré syndrome.[17] Although mild facial weakness is occasionally present, extraocular muscles and sensation are spared. Tendon reflexes are normal except in severely weak muscles, where they may be reduced.

Necrotizing Myopathy

Whereas NM may be due to toxic exposure, autoimmune NM is a unique progressive myopathy with distinct pathologic features, namely little or no inflammatory infiltrate

---

Box 1
Components of classification criteria for the idiopathic inflammatory myopathies (except IBM), proposed by Anthony A. Amato, and approved by the Muscle Study Group (MSG) and the European Neuromuscular Centre (ENMC) workshop

1. Clinical criteria

    Inclusion criteria

    a. Onset usually beyond 18 years (postpuberty); onset may be in childhood in DM and nonspecific myositis

    b. Subacute or insidious onset

    c. Pattern of weakness: symmetric proximal > distal, neck flexor > neck extensor

    d. Rash typical of DM: heliotrope (purple) periorbital edema; violaceous papules (Gottron papules) or macules (Gottron sign), scaly if chronic, at metacarpopharyngeal and interpharyngeal joints and other bony prominences; erythema of chest and neck (V-sign) and upper back (shawl sign)

    Exclusion criteria

    a. Clinical features of IBM[148]: asymmetric weakness, wrist/finger flexors same or worse than deltoids; knee extensors and/or ankle dorsiflexors same or worse than hip flexors

    b. Ocular weakness, isolated dysarthria, neck extensor worse than neck flexor weakness

    c. Toxic myopathy (eg, recent exposure to myotoxic drugs), active endocrinopathy (hyper- or hypothyroid, hyperparathyroid), amyloidosis, family history of muscular dystrophy or proximal motor neuropathies (eg, SMA)

2. Elevated serum creatine kinase level

3. Other laboratory criteria

    a. Electromyography:

        Inclusion criteria

        I. Increased insertional and spontaneous activity in the form of fibrillation potentials, positive sharp waves, or complex repetitive discharges

        II. Morphometric analysis reveals the presence of short duration, small amplitude, polyphasic MUAPs

        Exclusion criteria

        I. Myotonic discharges that would suggest proximal myotonic dystrophy or other channelopathy

        II. Morphometric analysis reveals predominantly long duration, large amplitude MUAPs

        III. Decreased recruitment pattern of MUAPs

    b. MRI: diffuse or patchy increased signal (edema) within muscle tissue on STIR images

    c. Myositis-specific antibodies detected in serum

4. Muscle biopsy inclusion and exclusion criteria

    a. Endomysial inflammatory cell infiltrate (T cells) surrounding and invading nonnecrotic muscle fibers

    b. Endomysial CD8+ T cells surrounding, but not definitely invading nonnecrotic muscle fibers, or ubiquitous MHC-1 expression

    c. Perifascicular atrophy

    d. MAC depositions on small blood vessels, or reduced capillary density, or tubuloreticular inclusions in endothelial cells on EM, or MHC-1 expression of perifascicular fibers

e. Perivascular, perimysial inflammatory cell infiltrate

f. Scattered endomysial CD8⁺ T-cell infiltrate that does not clearly surround or invade muscle fibers

g. Many necrotic muscle fibers as the predominant abnormal histologic feature. Inflammatory cells are sparse or only slight perivascular; perimysial infiltrate is not evident. MAC deposition on small blood vessels or pipe-stem capillaries on EM may be seen, but tubuloreticular inclusions in endothelial cells are uncommon or not evident.

h. Rimmed vacuoles, ragged red fibers, cytochrome oxidase–negative fibers that would suggest IBM

i. MAC deposition on the sarcolemma of nonnecrotic fibers and other indications of muscular dystrophies with immunopathology

Abbreviations: DM, dermatomyositis; EM, electron microscopy; IBM, inclusion body myositis; MAC, membrane attack complex; MHC, major histocompatibility complex; MRI, magnetic resonance imaging; MUAPs, motor unit action potentials; STIR, short-tau inversion recovery.

Adapted from Hoogendijk JE, Amato AA, Lecky BR, et al. 119th ENMC international workshop: trial design in adult idiopathic inflammatory myopathies, with the exception of inclusion body myositis, 10–12 October 2003, Naarden, The Netherlands. Neuromuscul Disord 2004;14(5):337–45; with permission.

besides intense myophagocytosis (see **Boxes 1** and **2**).[13] As in PM, NM presents as a subacute to insidious progressive proximal muscle weakness without a rash, but is more severe in tempo and in 30% of patients more marked in severity.[1] There may be associated myalgia and, in some cases, dysphagia. In the Dutch case series,[1] NM occurred in 19% of 165 IIM cases, and affected adults older than 30, with a female-to-male ratio of 2:1. In an Australian case series, the mean age of diagnosis was 57 years for NM and 61 years for the IIM, with a wide range.[18] Strangely there were more males than females in this series but, as expected, median CK with NM (1941 U/L) was significantly higher than in the other IIM.

Besides rheumatologic disorders, autoimmune NM may be associated with neoplasms, thick pipe stems on muscle abnormality, the signal recognition particle (SRP) autoantibody, statin therapy, or may be, by exclusion, idiopathic. Paraneoplastic NM is a rare, rapidly progressive, severe variant of NM that affects adults older than 40 years. NM with pipe-stem capillaries affects a similar age group and is associated with subacute weakness, brain infarction caused by vasculitis, or connective tissue disease. SRP autoantibodies affect younger NM patients, women more so than men, with typical onset of severe fulminant weakness in the fall season. Although the original report suggested an increased risk for congestive heart failure, this has not been supported by other studies. Treatment-refractory SRP-associated NM cases have been reported in childhood as young as age 5 years, with initial misdiagnosis including facioscapulohumeral muscular dystrophy (asymmetric shoulder girdle muscle involvement) and limb girdle muscular dystrophy.[19]

The authors have coined the term statin-associated autoimmune NM (SANAM)[20] to refer to patients in whom statins induce an autoimmune NM that progresses beyond 3 to 6 months after drug discontinuation.[21] Although statins are ubiquitously used, 82% of NM patients had history of statin use, compared with 18% in DM, 24% in PM, and 38% for IBM.[21] SANAM affects individuals between 46 and 89 years of age (mean 65.5 years), with onset of SANAM being at times delayed by up to 10 years following statin initiation. Although it commonly begins during statin use, onset in one-third of cases may be 0.5 to 20 months after statin cessation for an elevated CK. Most patients required immunosuppressive therapy, suggesting an autoimmune mechanism.

Box 2
Classification criteria for the idiopathic inflammatory myopathies, proposed by Anthony A. Amato, and approved by the MSG and the ENMC workshop

Inclusion body myositis as per Griggs and colleagues[148]

Polymyositis

Definite polymyositis

1. All clinical criteria with the exception of rash

2. Elevated serum creatine kinase (CK)

3. Muscle biopsy criteria include a; and exclude c; d; h; i

Probable polymyositis

1. All clinical criteria with the exception of rash

2. Elevated serum CK

3. Other laboratory criteria (1 of 3)

4. Muscle biopsy criteria include b; and exclude c; d; g; h; i

Dermatomyositis

Definite dermatomyositis

1. All clinical criteria

2. Muscle biopsy criteria include c

Probable dermatomyositis

1. All clinical criteria

2. Muscle biopsy criteria include d or e, or elevated serum CK, or other laboratory criteria (1 of 3)

Amyopathic dermatomyositis

1. Rash typical of DM: heliotrope, periorbital edema, Gottron papules/sign, V-sign, shawl sign, holster sign

2. Skin biopsy demonstrates a reduced capillary density, deposition of MAC on small blood vessels along the dermal-epidermal junction, and variable keratinocyte decoration for MAC

3. No objective weakness

4. Normal serum CK

5. Normal electromyogram

6. Muscle biopsy, if done, does not reveal features compatible with definite or probable DM

Possible dermatomyositis sine dermatitis

1. All clinical criteria with the exception of rash

2. Elevated serum CK

3. Other laboratory criteria (1 of 3)

4. Muscle biopsy criteria include c or d

Nonspecific myositis

1. All clinical criteria with the exception of rash

2. Elevated serum CK

3. Other laboratory criteria (1 of 3)

4. Muscle biopsy criteria include e or f; and exclude all others

Immune-mediated necrotizing myopathy

1. All clinical criteria with the exception of rash

2. Elevated serum CK

3. Other laboratory criteria (1 of 3)

4. Muscle biopsy criteria include g; and exclude all others

Adapted from Hoogendijk JE, Amato AA, Lecky BR, et al. 119th ENMC international workshop: trial design in adult idiopathic inflammatory myopathies, with the exception of inclusion body myositis, 10–12 October 2003, Naarden, The Netherlands. Neuromuscul Disord 2004;14(5): 337–45; with permission.

Otherwise, NM may be idiopathic in the remainder of cases. Anti–HMG coenzyme A reductase (HMG-CoAR) antibodies have recently been described in SANAM and idiopathic NM (see later discussion).

CONDITIONS ASSOCIATED WITH DERMATOMYOSITIS, POLYMYOSITIS, AND NECROTIZING MYOPATHY

There is an increased incidence of interstitial lung disease (ILD), autoimmune disorders, cancer, and, possibly, cardiac involvement in the IIM. In JDM, necrotizing vasculitis may complicate the gastrointestinal system with bowel ischemia, necrosis, and perforation with associated petechial rash or even muscle infarcts. In the IIM, inflammation of gastrointestinal tract smooth muscles results in dysphagia, aspiration pneumonia, and delayed gastric emptying. In JDM cases there is a strong family history of other autoimmune disease, particularly type 1 diabetes and systemic lupus erythematosus.[22]

Polyarthritis

Polyarthritis has been reported in nearly half of patients with PM at the time of diagnosis.[23] Scleroderma and mixed connective tissue disease are frequently associated with NM.

Interstitial Lung Disease

Ten percent to 25% of adult IIM patients have ILD, which manifests as dyspnea and cough.[24] In most instances the diagnosis of ILD is made concurrently with that of the muscle disease, but in one-third of ILD cases it may antecede or follow the diagnosis of PM or DM. Including the 5% asymptomatic myositis subjects despite evidence of ILD on pulmonary function testing and chest imaging, ILD may affect up to 30% of DM and PM cases.[24] A chronic progressive course is most common, whereas 5% may have an acute presentation. ILD may occur in JDM and has been reported in upward of 10% of PM cases, with most having histidyl tRNA synthetase (Jo-1) antibodies,[12,25] which are associated more with DM than PM.[1]

Malignancy

Although rates of malignancy have been reported to be as high as 45%,[26] most studies suggest that 15%[27] to 25%[28] of adult DM cases, especially in those who are older than 40 years, have preexisting, concurrent, or future malignancies. In women the most common DM-associated malignancy is ovarian cancer[29] and in men it is small cell lung cancer, whereas nasopharyngeal carcinoma in common in Southeast Asia, Southern China, and Northern Africa. Treatment of the malignancy, which may present 2 years after the onset of DM, improves muscular involvement. Rarely, malignancies including hematologic disorders have been reported in JDM.[30] In comparison with the general population, the risk of malignancy is modestly increased in patients with PM and NM.[31] In Taiwan, 13.8% of DM patients and 6.2% of PM patients had cancers. Overall standardized incidence ratios for cancer were 5.36 for DM cases and 1.80 among PM patients, but were even higher in the first year, at 24.55 and 9.17, respectively.[4] Gastrointestinal tract adenocarcinoma and small cell and non–small cell carcinoma of the lung are common malignancies in paraneoplastic autoimmune NM.

Autoimmune Necrotizing Myopathy

Statins can trigger SANAM, an autoimmune NM, which is rare and distinct from the more common toxic NM with statin use.[22,32] Other drugs associated with toxic NM include fibrates, ezetimibe, cyclosporine, labetolol, propofol, and alcohol. In the Dutch case series,[1] 10% of NM cases were associated with collagen vascular disease and in an Australian case series, systemic lupus erythematosus occurred in 21%.[18] In addition there are patients with NM who have no known associated conditions or precipitating factors, and these are considered to have an idiopathic immune-mediated myopathy.[33]

Cardiac Defects

Whereas cardiac conduction defects and arrhythmias may occur in the IIMs, pericarditis and congestive heart failure have been less commonly described. Up to one-third of PM patients may have myocarditis, which manifests primarily as conduction abnormalities and much less commonly as congestive heart failure. SRP autoantibodies predict a fulminant form of refractory PM or NM that rapidly progresses over 1 month to severe weakness and, although this point has become controversial, may be associated with myocarditis.[34] There is an overall increase in the risk for cardiovascular disease with the IIM.[35,36]

LABORATORY STUDIES IN DERMATOMYOSITIS, POLYMYOSITIS, AND NECROTIZING MYOPATHY

Serum CK level is increased up to 50 times the upper limit of risk in most DM patients. However, 10% of DM patients have a normal CK level regardless of severity, especially adults with insidious disease and in JDM patients. By contrast, CK is always elevated in active PM in the range of 5 to 50 times the upper normal limit, and is increased at least 10-fold in NM. Although the degree of CK abnormality does not correlate well with the severity of weakness, a decrease or increase in CK level generally correlates with good treatment response or relapse, respectively, and is a useful measure of disease activity in conjunction with manual muscle testing. It is rare for serum aldolase to be elevated without a CK abnormality. The erythrocyte sedimentation rate may be elevated, but does not correlate with disease activity. Isolated antinuclear antibody positivity, as occurs in some IIM patients, is of unclear significance.

Cancer Screening

Screening for malignancy is important in DM but also in NM and PM, especially in the first few years following diagnosis. In a study of 618 Caucasian patients with DM, Hill and colleagues[37] found that DM was strongly associated with various types of malignancies (odds ratio [OR] 3), including especially ovarian (OR 10.5) and lung (OR 5.9), but also pancreatic, stomach, and colorectal cancers. In 914 Caucasian patients with PM, these investigators also reported that PM was associated with lung (OR 2.8) and bladder cancers (OR 2.4). More recently, an increased risk of hematologic malignancies, mostly B-cell lymphoma, has been reported in older DM patients.[38] Data on cost-effectiveness of cancer screening in DM are limited to retrospective case series. Some have suggested that further testing, beyond a thorough evaluation by an internist, a chest radiograph, and in women a pelvic examination and mammogram, should be guided by abnormal symptoms or results. Others, however, have found that routine computed tomography (CT) scans of the chest and abdomen and, in women, pelvic CT optimize cancer detection.[39] The authors approach includes a careful skin examination for melanoma, CT scan of the chest, abdomen, and pelvis, and, in women, a mammogram and pelvic examination; in men, testicular and prostate examinations are indicated. In women a pelvic sonogram is advocated for better evaluation for the most common associated malignancy, ovarian cancer. In those older than 50 years, a colonoscopy rather than a stool occult blood test is recommended. More recently, the European Federation of Neurological Societies Task Force recommended that in DM, patients should have CT of the chest/abdomen, pelvic ultrasonography and mammography in women, ultrasonography of testes in men younger than 50 years, and colonoscopy in men and women older than 50. If primary screening is negative, repeat screening is recommended after 3 to 6 months, after which screening is every 6 months up until 4 years.[40] The authors consider that repeat screening decisions are best guided by the clinical context.

Pulmonary Function Testing

Symptoms of ILD should prompt pulmonary consultation, including chest imaging and pulmonary function testing. A chest radiograph is less sensitive than a CT scan but reveals diffuse reticulonodular infiltrates and, in more severe ILD cases, a ground-glass appearance. High-resolution chest CT has higher sensitivity in detecting milder ILD changes. Pulmonary function testing reveals abnormal forced vital capacity and lung diffusion. The course of ILD is variable and may be static and asymptomatic (30%), slowly progressive (50%), or fulminant (20%).[41] Jo-1 antibody occurs in 50% of myositides afflicted with ILD,[12,25] and progressive ILD cases incur high mortality. Of the antisynthetase antibodies, anti–PL-7 and anti–PL-12 antisynthetase antibodies are strongly associated with ILD in 90% to 100% of cases and with gastrointestinal complications.[42,43] Presence of anti–PL-12 antibody is associated with less frequent though severe/steroid-refractory myositis, and ILD that is both frequent and severe.[44] In clinically amyopathic DM, anti–CADM-140 (MDA5/IFIH1) antibodies were thought originally to be markers of acute rapidly progressive ILD with very poor prognosis.[45] In another case series, however, MDA-5 autoantibodies were found in DM patients presenting with the antisynthetase syndrome, but in the absence of antisynthetase autoantibodies.[46] Most anti–MDA-5 positive patients had ILD, which was occasionally severe yet typically resolved with immunosuppressive therapy.

Biomarker Monitoring

The G allele of interferon-induced helicase (IFIH1) was found to be protective against ILD, whereas the AA genotype was identified as a risk factor for lung injury in PM.[47] The combination of anti–Jo-1 and anti–SSA/Ro antibodies is a marker of severe ILD.[42] Besides serial imaging and pulmonary function testing, serum KL-6,[48] SP-D, interleukin (IL)-18, and ferritin levels may be useful biomarkers for monitoring the activity and severity of ILD.[49] The lower consolidation/ground-glass attenuation pattern and the presence of anti–CADM-140 were significantly associated with 90-day mortality.[50] There is a positive correlation of B-cell–activating factor (BAFF) and ΔBAFF expression with PM/DM disease activity measures assessed by the International Myositis Assessment and Clinical Studies core set tool.[51] Upregulation of resistin in muscle tissue and elevated serum resistin levels in the IIM reflected global disease activity, including extramuscular organ involvement. However, there are currently no sufficient data to distinguish the features of resistin that cause injury of muscle tissue from those that promote muscle regeneration and repair.[52]

Antibody Identification

Although there are no published prospective studies, current experience suggests that most of the so-called myositis-specific antibodies (MSAs) predict poor treatment response because of the association with ILD. However, these antibodies, which are only present in a minority of DM patients, have an unknown and controversial pathogenetic role in the IIM. The MSAs include 2 classes of cytoplasmic antibodies: those directed against Mi-2 and Mas antigens and others targeting translational proteins, such as various tRNA synthetases, the SRP, transcriptional intermediary factor 1 (TIF1; anti-155/140 antibody), and the melanoma differentiation-associated gene 5 (MDA5; anti–CADM-140 antibody).[53] Although most patients have no detectable MSAs and a rare case may have 2 detectable MSAs,[54,55] those who do have it carry mostly 1 MSA type in association with specific human leukocyte antigen (HLA) haplotypes.[1,56]

The Jo-1 antibody is associated with ILD, arthritis, Raynaud phenomenon, and mechanic's hand,[12] and is seen in up to 20% of IIM.[12,25] The frequent association of Jo-1 antibodies with ILD may be the basis for moderate treatment response and poor long-term prognosis.[57] The other antisynthetases (PL-7, PL-12, EJ, KS, OJ) are less common, occurring in fewer than 2% to 3% of IIM cases. Anti-OJ ILD positive patients with PM/DM lack the manifestations of Raynaud phenomenon and sclerodactyly, and show good prognoses and responses to glucocorticoid therapy.[58] Antibodies to nuclear matrix protein NXP2, previously known as MJ antibodies, are among the most common MSAs in JDM but occur in fewer than 2% of adult DM cases, with up to 50% having an associated adult malignancy.[53]

Nonsynthetase antibodies to Mi-2 are found in 15% to 30% of DM patients and are associated with acute onset, an erythematous rash, nail-bed capillary dilation, good response to therapy, and favorable prognosis.[12,57] However, it is unknown whether DM cases with Mi-2 antibody respond differently from those without this antibody.

Whereas anti–Mi-2 is associated with classic DM without ILD or malignancy, anti-155/140 is associated with malignancy in adults, and patients with anti–CADM-140 frequently had clinically amyopathic DM and rapidly progressive interstitial lung disease. Upward of 70% of Japanese adult DM cases harboring anti-TIF1 have a malignancy.[59] However, a subgroup with anti-p155/140 autoantibody in juvenile myositis included Gottron papules, malar rash, shawl-sign rash, photosensitivity, cuticular overgrowth, low CK levels, and a predominantly chronic course of illness without malignancy.[60] In a DM case series, 20 of 55 patients had ILD, but rapidly progressive ILD was present in 3 cases, all of whom had anti–CADM-140 antibodies, whereas those with anti-tRNA synthetase antibodies had slow progression of ILD.[61] Nearly half of DM ILD cases have serologic evidence of these autoantibodies.[62] Although most patients with clinically amyopathic DM do not harbor anti–CADM-140, the prevalence of muscle involvement in patients with anti–CADM-140 may be up to 83%.[61] In a JDM series, CADM-140 antibody was positive in 5 of 6 patients with ILD but was absent in all 7 patients without ILD.[63]

SRP antibodies have been reported in up to 5% to 8% of PM cases, and are mostly associated with the phenotype of NM.[64] Patients present in the fall with rapidly progressive proximal severe weakness that often responds poorly to steroid therapy.[65] There is associated ILD and possible cardiac involvement. Rarely, PM patients may be positive for both the SRP antibody and a non–Jo-1 antisynthetase antibody,[1] and an MSA may be present in up to one-third of NM cases. In a case series, one NM patient harbored antibodies to both Mi-2 and a non–Jo-1 antisynthetase.[1] SRP antibodies may be nonspecifically positive in patients with alternative muscle diagnosis or no evidence of muscle involvement.[66]

The authors routinely obtain Jo-1 antibodies on all IIM cases. Because 50% of Jo-1–positive cases either already have or will develop ILD, use of methotrexate is avoided in such patients. Antibodies to SRP are especially indicated in severe fulminant PM or NM because they predict a rapid course leading to muscle fibrosis and marked cardiac involvement, dictate the need for aggressive and swift pharmacotherapy, and may portend a poor prognosis.

Anti-200/100 autoantibodies characterized a unique subset of patients with myopathies, representing 62% of patients with idiopathic necrotizing myopathies.[67] Of the 16 antibody-positive cases, 10 were previously exposed to statins. The target antigen has been identified as HMG-CoAR.

ELECTROPHYSIOLOGY OF DERMATOMYOSITIS, POLYMYOSITIS, AND NECROTIZING MYOPATHY

Nerve conduction studies are normal, except for compound muscle action potential (CMAP) amplitude reduction in fulminant cases associated with severe diffuse muscle weakness. This finding should prompt the electromyographer to evaluate for the Lambert-Eaton myasthenic syndrome. Needle EMG at rest shows increased insertional, small-amplitude, low-frequency fibrillation potentials, and occasionally scattered pseudomyotonic or complex repetitive discharges indicating chronicity. Besides proximal myotonic myopathy, diffuse electrical myotonia is a prominent finding in SANAM. On activation, the proficient electromyographer readily identifies polyphasic motor unit action potentials (MUAPs) of low amplitude and, more importantly, of reduced duration, especially in the proximal musculature. The crisp sound of these MUAPs is distinctive, in addition to direct visualization and measurement of MUAP duration. Activation of MUAPs shows an early recruitment pattern resulting from central compensation, except in severe cases where recruitment might be reduced. With chronicity, reinnervation of split fibers produces MUAPs of increased duration.

In addition to its diagnostic utility and ability to target muscle biopsy, EMG is helpful in assessing relapsing weakness during treatment with corticosteroids. In previously responsive myositis, worsening strength in the absence of fibrillation potentials on needle electromyography examination (NEE) suggests steroid-induced myopathy/type 2 muscle fiber atrophy, which is a rare entity. Fibrillation potentials would confirm active myositis and the need for more immunosuppression.

MUSCLE IMAGING

In the absence of typical NEE findings, newer diagnostic criteria may allow the use of muscle magnetic resonance imaging (MRI) signal abnormality or the presence of MSAs to support probable PM or DM (see **Box 1**).[13] Fat-suppressed and short-tau inversion recovery skeletal muscle MRI may show fibrosis, and diffuse or patchy signal symmetric increase in the proximal muscles and intermuscular fascia indicates muscle edema caused by inflammation. There is a relative sparing of the adductor, obturator, and pectineus muscles.[68] Fat deposition on T1-weighted images usually appears after 3 to 5 months of disease duration and preferentially involves the hamstrings. Whereas others may use muscle MRI, it is the authors' experience that a proficiently performed EMG and clinical evaluation are sufficient for the selection of the optimal muscle for biopsy.

MUSCLE HISTOPATHOLOGY AND PATHOGENESIS OF DM, PM, AND NM
Dermatomyositis

Except for amyopathic cases, muscle biopsy is critical for the diagnosis of DM. The earliest detectable histologic abnormality on light microscopy in DM is deposition of the C5b-9 or MAC of complement around small blood vessels.[69,70] This humorally mediated microangiopathy leads to decreased capillary density, especially at the periphery of the fascicle. It is fairly characteristic of DM, and may explain the occasional infarction of muscle fibers in JDM. MAC deposition is highly sensitive and specific in differentiating DM from other IIM. Capillary damage and myofiber atrophy are concentrated in regions distant from the affected intermediate-sized perimysial vessels, leading to the suggestion that watershed ischemia is the cause of myofiber atrophy and capillary damage in regions of muscle near the avascular perimysium.[71] The interferon (IFN)-α/β–inducible protein, myxovirus resistance (MxA), was recently found to be expressed in 90% of capillaries.[72,73]

Nearly half of muscle biopsies demonstrate perifascicular atrophy (**Fig. 2**), often without an inflammatory infiltrate. When present, the inflammatory infiltrate consists of predominantly perimysial and perivascular macrophages and B cells presenting a putative antigen to naïve CD4$^+$ cells, some of which are T lymphocytes but most of which are plasmacytoid dendritic cells (pDC) (see **Fig. 2**). Invasion of nonnecrotic fibers is not common. The incidence of rare infiltrative lesions in those with malignant tumors (45%) was significantly higher than in those without such tumors (14%). The end result of this humoral microangiopathy is myofibril necrosis in groups, and regeneration. The presentation is HLA class II restricted, and leads to the maturation of CD4$^+$ T cells and pDC, depending on the cytokine environment, into T-helper type 1 (Th1), Th2, Th17, or regulatory T cells (Treg). Th1 and Th17 activation produce proinflammatory cytokines present in myositis tissues, and are associated with the migration, differentiation, and maturation of inflammatory cells, including dendritic cells (DC). Natural Tregs are CD4$^+$CD25$^+$ FoxP3$^+$, whereas adaptive Tregs are induced in the peripheral immune system after encountering foreign antigens and have 2 distinct cytokine profiles. Type 1 Tregs secrete high levels of IL-10, whereas Th3 cells secrete high levels of the profibrotic agent transforming growth factor (TGF)-β.[74] Antiga and colleagues[75] found that the number of Treg cells in the peripheral blood of patients with DM was significantly reduced when compared with healthy controls, with a reduction in TGF-β and IL-10 serum levels suggesting that Treg depletion may be an important factor in the pathogenesis of the disease. FOXP3$^+$ Tregs are found in close proximity to effector cells, and serve to counterbalance muscle destruction by cytotoxic T cells in myositis.[76] Fascin-positive DC predominance in inflammatory infiltrates in both PM and DM muscles confirms the prevalence of mature forms and indicates that there is stimulation of DC maturation.[77]

On EM, the earliest recognized changes are tubuloreticular inclusions in the intramuscular arterioles and capillaries.[78] MxA colocalizes to the small intramuscular blood vessel inclusions, and is thought to form tubuloreticular inclusions around RNA viruses.[72] Therefore, the endothelial cell tubuloreticular inclusions present in affected

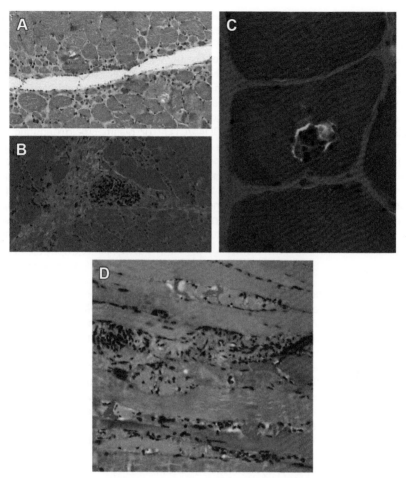

Fig. 2. (A) DM: perifascicular atrophy (hematoxylin and eosin [H&E], original magnification 20×). (B) DM: perimysial inflammation (H&E, original magnification 20×). (C) Polymyositis: central invasion of nonnecrotic fibers by inflammatory infiltrates (H&E, original magnification 40×). (D) Necrotizing myopathy: multiple necrotic fibers undergoing phagocytosis (H&E, original magnification 40×).

DM muscle are thought to be biomarkers of type 1 IFN (IFN1) exposure (see later discussion).

Recent evidence from DM muscle–derived microarray studies has uncovered an increase in MHC-1 and immunoglobulin gene transcripts[79] and a robust increase in the expression of IFN1-inducible genes up to 570-fold, in addition to an abundant immunoglobulin gene transcript.[72] The expression of MxA is localized to 50% perifascicular muscle fibers in addition to diffuse perifascicular MHC-1 positivity. MxA, as the name indicates, is inducible by IFN1s. IFN1s are known to upregulate MHC expression, activate natural killer cell cytotoxicity, promote activated T-cell survival, and support DC maturation. Analysis of peripheral blood mononuclear cells demonstrates a high IFN-α/β signature, which parallels disease activity in DM.[80] IL-6, a proinflammatory cytokine, plays central roles in the regulation of both innate and adaptive inflammatory and immune responses, in addition to both humoral and cell-mediated autoimmune reactions. Prominent IFN1 signatures, manifesting as both transcript upregulation and elevated levels of serum proteins, and elevated IL-6 levels in the patients' serum correlated strongly with DM disease activity.[81,82] Comparing IFNα, IFNβ, and IFNω in DM, PM, and IBM blood samples with those of healthy volunteers, the IFNβ signature was uniquely associated with DM. It was detectable in 64% of samples from patients with untreated or minimally treated DM and in 35% of all DM samples, compared with 6% of other inflammatory myopathy samples and 6% of healthy volunteer samples.[83,84]

In addition, evidence has emerged suggesting that not all CD4$^+$ cells are T cells, and that 30% to 90% of these cells are CD4$^+$/CD3$^-$ or plasmacytoid dendritic cells (pDC).[72] The pDC are part of the innate immune system response to viral antigens, and respond by producing a large amount of IFN1 once their toll-like receptors (TLR-7 and TLR-9) bind to viral nucleic acids. TLR activation leads to the generation of cytokines and chemokines and to the maturation of antigen-presenting cells (APCs) by upregulating costimulatory molecules that promote efficient interactions between APCs and T cells. This IFN signature was also noted in the active phase of other autoimmune disorders. IFN signature is seen in DM skin, similar to that found in the blood and muscle of DM patients.[83]

Polymyositis

Muscle biopsy is critical for the confirmation of PM and exclusion of mimics such as IBM, but also muscular dystrophy, acid maltase deficiency, and NM (**Table 2**). The histologic features of PM are distinct from those seen in DM because PM is the result of an HLA-restricted cell-mediated cytotoxic immune response directed at muscle fibers. Prominent microscopic features are variability in fiber size, scattered necrotic and regenerating fibers, and endomysial inflammation, which consists primarily of activated CD8$^+$ cytotoxic T cells and macrophages that in 63% of cases invade non-necrotic muscle fibers[2] expressing MHC-1 antigens (see **Fig. 2**). This histologic pattern is not distinctive, as it also occurred in IBM patients.[2] MHC-1 antigens, which are not constitutively expressed, decorate the surface of noninvaded intact myocytes. Surface expression of MHC-1 is not specific to the IIM and can be seen in faciosca-pulohumeral muscular dystrophy, Duchenne and Becker muscular dystrophy, statin-associated myopathy, dysferlinopathy, and, rarely, other limb-girdle muscular dystrophies and merosin deficiency. A sarcoplasmic reticular pattern of internal MHC-1 reactivity was recently reported to be 70% sensitive and 100% specific to

Table 2	
Polymyositis mimics	
Age ≤40	**Age >40**
Fibromyalgia	Inclusion body myositis
Dermatomyositis, necrotizing myopathy	Overlap syndrome: RA, SLE
Dystrophin, dysferlin, calpain-3, FSHD, Pompe disease, etc	Myotonic dystrophy 2
Myotonic dystrophy 2	Polymyalgia rheumatica
Overlap syndrome: RA, SLE, juvenile RA	Dermatomyositis, necrotizing myopathy
Inclusion body myositis	Fibromyalgia
Influenza A or B	Pompe disease

Abbreviations: FSHD, facioscapulohumeral muscular dystrophy; RA, rheumatoid arthritis; SLE, systemic lupus erythematosus.

Adapted from Dimachkie MM. Idiopathic inflammatory myopathies. J Neuroimmunol 2011;231(1–2):32–42; with permission.

the IIM when using a cutoff value of 50%.[76] It is thought that MHC-1 antigens express an unknown endogenous peptide, which acts as the autoantigen. The endomysial CD8[+] cytotoxic T cells are antigen specific and destroy myocytes through the perforin pathway. These cells are accompanied by abundant myeloid DCs that surround non-necrotic fibers and act as antigen-presenting cells.[85] The authors demonstrated increased immunoglobulin gene expression on muscle microarray experiments in PM.[79,86] The immunoglobulins are secreted by endomysial plasma cells but, unlike DM, are not deposited in the muscle blood vessels.[86] IFN1 signature is significantly overexpressed in the blood of both DM and PM patients,[87] and significantly correlates with disease activity as measured by the modified Myositis Intention to Treat scale.

Necrotizing Myopathy

Muscle histopathology is central to the diagnosis of NM. The hallmark of all autoimmune NM is the presence of scattered necrotic myofibers with myophagocytosis, and either absence or paucity of T-lymphocytic inflammatory exudates (see **Fig. 2**). In addition, microvascular deposition of complement MAC suggests a humorally mediated microangiopathy. Unlike DM, perivascular inflammation is scant, and there are no endothelial tubuloreticular inclusions on EM.

In addition to these common pathologic features, a variety of distinctive findings occur in specific subtypes of NM. Demonstration of thick-walled and enlarged pipe-stem capillaries of normal number is diagnostic of NM with pipe-stem capillaries.[88] Muscle connective tissue positively staining for alkaline phosphatase has been described in malignancy-associated NM. The SRP-associated NM demonstrates early in the course a bimodal distribution of fiber sizes in addition to increased endomysial connective tissue and reduced number, together with enlargement and thickening of endomysial capillaries. Marked fibrosis is noted 6 months after its onset. The deposition of MAC on endomysial capillaries has been shown in biopsy specimens obtained from SRP-positive patients. Upregulation of MHC-1 antigens was present in a 9% of idiopathic NM cases[18] while in another case series, 75% of NM cases demonstrated this upregulation in 10% or more of the nonnecrotic fibers.[89]

Muscle fibers of SANAM express on their surfaces MHC-1 antigens in all 8 biopsy specimens, supporting the notion of an immune-mediated NM induced by endoplasmic reticulum stress.[32] It is thought that the latter leads to exposure of neoantigens, thereby activating the immune system despite statin cessation. Although the pathophysiology of SANAM is uncertain, it is likely NM mediated humorally via cytokine expression and complement activation.[22] The pathophysiology of NM has witnessed marked advances with the discovery of the anti-200/100 autoantibodies, which target HMG-CoAR.[67] These autoantibodies were identified 17 IIM cases; 16 had pathologic features of NM and 1 had extensive inflammatory infiltrates. Of a total 38 NM cases, 12 had SRP antibodies, and 16 of the 26 remaining NM cases had the newly described 200/100 autoantibodies. Of these 16 NM cases, 10 were exposed to statins and 6 were not. Although close examination revealed endomysial and/or perivascular collections of inflammatory cells in 5 of the 16 muscle biopsy specimens, the degree of inflammation was mild compared with that seen in typical muscle biopsy specimens obtained from patients with PM or DM. Examination of frozen muscle tissue samples available in 8 of 16 patients revealed abnormally enlarged endomysial capillaries with thickened walls in 5 specimens with preservation of capillary density. Although endomysial capillaries were not recognized by the MAC, small perimysial vessels stained positive in 6 of 8 muscle biopsy specimens. Unlike the findings of Needham and colleagues,[32] only 4 of 8 specimens demonstrated sarcolemmal MHC-1 positivity. Mamen and colleagues[90] subsequently identified the 100-kDa antigen to be the 3-hydroxy-3-methylglutarylcoenzyme A reductase (HMGCR) protein. In muscle biopsy tissues from antibody-positive patients, HMGCR expression was upregulated in cells expressing neural cell adhesion molecule, a marker of muscle regeneration. After statin cessation, high levels of HMGCR expression in regenerating muscle tissue might continue to drive the autoimmune response. Although others have reported genetic variants and mutations in the SLCO1B1, CYP, and COQ2 genes as determinants to individual statin myopathy susceptibility, the prevalence of the rs4149056 C allele was not increased in patients with anti-HMGCR. In summary, the HMGCR autoantibody is present in 63% of NM cases with high specificity approaching 100%. However, a puzzling finding is that 33% of antibody-positive NM cases are statin-naïve.

THERAPY FOR DERMATOMYOSITIS, POLYMYOSITIS, AND NECROTIZING MYOPATHY

Immunosuppressive therapy is the mainstay of treatment in patients with active disease related to DM, PM, and NM (**Table 3**).[91] Autoimmune NM is often more resistant than DM and PM to immunosuppressive therapy, particularly if there is an underlying malignancy or a statin trigger. The overwhelming majority (23/25) of SANAM cases required more than one immunosuppressive agent, with relapse in 12 cases following tapering of immunosuppressive therapy.[22] However, as in DM and PM, immunosuppressants such as prednisone in combination with methotrexate (MTX) or azathioprine (AZA) are the first-line therapies in autoimmune NM. For resistant or severe cases, adding intravenous immunoglobulin (IVIG) may be helpful. Third-line drugs include mycophenolate mofetil, cyclosporine, tacrolimus, rituximab, etanercept, and cyclophosphamide.

The few published randomized controlled trials of immunosuppression in DM or PM compared placebo with AZA,[92] plasma exchange,[93] or IVIG.[94] In addition, randomized controlled trials compared MTX with AZA,[95] cyclosporine with MTX,[96] and intravenous MTX with oral MTX plus AZA.[97] The only positive controlled trials are a small crossover study of IVIG in DM[94] and a randomized, double-blind, placebo-controlled trial of etanercept (50 mg subcutaneously weekly) for 52 weeks in 16 DM subjects.[98]

Corticosteroids

Although no controlled trial using corticosteroids (CS) has been conducted, there is general agreement that these are effective in DM, PM, and NM. CS can be used in a wide range of regimens and routes of administration. The authors administer prednisone 1 mg/kg/d (60–100 mg) for 4 weeks followed by an abrupt or tapered conversion to an every-other-day (QOD) schedule. This taper is slower in patients with severe disease. A daily CS schedule is necessary in well-controlled hypertensive or nonbrittle diabetic patients. Although most patients feel immediately better after taking CS, strength improvement is delayed by 2 to 3 months after the onset of treatment. An immediate response may suggest an alternative diagnosis such as polymyalgia rheumatica (see **Table 2**). For the first 3 months, the typical adult patient remains on prednisone 60 to 100 mg QOD or its equivalent. If no improvement is noted after 3 to 6 months, or if weakness reoccurs during the taper, a second-line immunosuppressive agent such as AZA, MTX, or IVIG is started. The authors do initiate CS therapy early on in high-risk patients such as those with uncontrolled hypertension, diabetes, osteoporosis, obesity, and baseline severe weakness. For good responders, a taper by 20 mg per month until 40 mg QOD then by 10 mg per month will reduce the prednisone dose to 20 mg QOD after 6 to 8 months from the initiation of therapy. Thereafter, the taper is by 5 mg and the interval is every 3 months to reach the minimal effective dose. In severe cases, the authors prefer starting with 5-day intravenous pulse methylprednisolone therapy followed by high-dose oral prednisone in combination with a second-line drug. Recently, a randomized, multicenter, double-blind clinical trial compared oral dexamethasone pulse therapy with daily prednisolone in 62 patients with subacute-onset myositis.[99] The pulsed regimen consisted of 6 cycles of dexamethasone given monthly as 40 mg/d for 4 consecutive days. The main issue is that there was a large number of early discontinuations in both groups for a variety of reasons. Although pulsed high-dose oral dexamethasone was not found to be superior to daily prednisolone as first-line treatment of IIM, it also caused substantially fewer side effects. Ten patients (33%) treated with prednisolone and 1 patient (4%) treated with pulsed dexamethasone developed diabetes mellitus. Mood changes occurred in 20 (67%) and 8 (29%) patients, respectively. Treatment adjustments for comorbid conditions (hypertension, diabetes mellitus) were needed in 1 patient in the dexamethasone group, compared with 15 patients in the prednisolone group.

Because the risks of long-term CS therapy are numerous, discussing risk with the patient and establishing a monitoring plan in collaboration with the primary care physician are integral to the management plan. Before CS initiation, the authors place a PPD skin test or obtain a QuantiFERON-TB Gold test to identify the need for isoniazid in previously exposed cases. As CS is being initiated, a baseline bone dual-energy x-ray absorptiometry scan is obtained and the patient is requested to seek an ophthalmologic examination, with yearly follow-up for both. The authors maintain patients on oral calcium, 500 to 600 mg 2 to 3 times daily with vitamin D 400 IU daily. In JDM, the incidence of vertebral fracture 12 months following steroid initiation was 6%, and these were mostly asymptomatic.[100] The risk of fracture increased with higher steroid dose, and in the first 6 months, with greater increases in body mass index or greater declines in spine Z scores. The authors ask patients and their families to be alert about personality changes and psychiatric side effects. Patients are instructed to reduce salt and carbohydrates in their diet and visit regularly with the primary care physician for blood pressure, serum glucose, and potassium measurements. Pneumococcal vaccine and yearly influenza shots are advocated. Given the immunosuppressed state, evidence has suggested that seroprotection of the influenza A/H1N1 vaccine is significantly reduced in DM patients compared with controls.[101] However, another study showed adequate immunogenicity despite IIM therapy, and no harmful effects over the short term.[102] In a retrospective study of 279 PM/DM cases over 15 years, 37% were admitted for a severe pyogenic infection (n = 71) mostly because of aspiration pneumonia or an opportunistic infection (n = 33).[103] There are currently no consensus criteria to identify patients who are at high risk for *Pneumocystis carinii* pneumonia (PCP) infection and who would therefore benefit from prophylaxis. Patients with total lymphocyte counts less than 800/μL and/or CD4 lymphocyte counts less than 200 to 400/μL are likely to benefit from PCP prophylaxis before initiation of and in the course of immunosuppressive therapy.[104]

Methotrexate

MTX, an antifolate that inhibits lymphocyte proliferation, is an effective, more rapidly acting second-line steroid-sparing immunosuppressant. The authors start oral MTX at 7.5 mg/wk, and in 2 weeks increase it to 15 mg/wk in 2 divided doses. The dose is then increased by 2.5 mg per week every 3 months to reach the maximum weekly dose of 25 mg. Folic acid, 0.8 to 1 mg/d orally is also coadministered to prevent stomatitis.

Table 3
Immunosuppressive therapy for inflammatory myopathies

Therapy	Route	Dose	Side Effects	Monitor
Azathioprine	PO	2–3 mg/kg/d; single AM dose	Influenza-like illness, hepatotoxicity, pancreatitis, leukopenia, macrocytosis, neoplasia, infection, teratogenicity	Monthly blood count, liver enzymes
Chlorambucil	PO	4–6 mg/d, single AM dose	Bone marrow suppression, hepatotoxicity, neoplasia, infertility, teratogenicity, infection	Monthly blood count, liver enzymes
Cyclophosphamide	PO	1.5–2 mg/kg/d; single AM dose	Bone marrow suppression, infertility, hemorrhagic cystitis, alopecia, infections, neoplasia, teratogenicity	Monthly blood count, urinalysis
	IV	1 g/m^2	Same as PO (although more severe), and nausea/vomiting, alopecia	Daily to weekly blood count, urinalysis
Cyclosporine	PO	4–6 mg/kg/d, split into 2 daily doses	Nephrotoxicity, hypertension, infection, hepatotoxicity, hirsutism, tremor, gum hyperplasia, teratogenicity	Blood pressure, monthly cyclosporine level, creatinine/BUN, liver enzymes
Intravenous immunoglobulin	IV	2 g/kg over 2–5 d; then 1 g/kg every 2–4 wk or 2 g/kg monthly as needed	Hypotension, arrhythmia, diaphoresis, flushing, nephrotoxicity, headache, nausea, aseptic meningitis, anaphylaxis, stroke	Heart rate, blood pressure, creatinine/BUN
Methotrexate	PO	7.5–25 mg weekly, single or divided doses; 1 d a week dosing	Hepatotoxicity, pulmonary fibrosis, infection, neoplasia, infertility, leukopenia, alopecia, gastric irritation, stomatitis, teratogenicity	Monthly liver enzymes, blood count; consider liver biopsy at 2 g accumulative dose
	IV/IM	20–50 mg weekly; 1 d a week dosing	Same as PO	Same as PO

Drug	Route	Dosage	Adverse effects	Monitoring
Methylprednisone	IV	1 g in 100 mL/normal saline over 1–2 h, daily or every other day for 2–6 doses	Arrhythmia, flushing, dysgeusia, anxiety, insomnia, fluid and weight gain, hyperglycemia, hypokalemia, infection	Heart rate, blood pressure, serum glucose/potassium
Mycophenolate mofetil	PO	1–1.5 g twice a day	Myelosuppression, GI (diarrhea, nausea, abdominal pain), peripheral edema, fever, infection, opportunistic infection, malignancy, teratogenicity	Monthly blood count
Prednisone	PO	60–100 mg/d for 2–4 wk, then 100 mg every other day; single AM dose	Hypertension, fluid and weight gain, hyperglycemia, hypokalemia, cataract, glaucoma, gastric irritation, osteoporosis, infection, aseptic femoral necrosis, psychiatric	Weight, blood pressure, serum glucose/potassium, cataract formation
Rituximab	IV	2 doses of 750 mg/m^2 administered 2 wk apart	Mild infusion-related adverse events (headache, nausea, chills, hypotension), anaphylaxis, infection	CD19 counts (<5%), IgG level (keep above 30% of the lower normal limit)
Tacrolimus	PO	0.1–0.15 mg/kg/d, split into 2 daily doses	Nephrotoxicity, GI (diarrhea, abdominal pain), hypertension, electrolyte imbalance, tremor, infection, hepatotoxicity, teratogenicity	Blood pressure, creatinine/BUN, electrolytes, monthly trough level (aim 5–15 ng/mL)

Abbreviations: BUN, blood urea nitrogen; GI, gastrointestinal; IgG, immunoglobulin G; IM, intramuscularly; IV, intravenously; PO, by mouth.
Adapted from Dimachkie MM. Idiopathic inflammatory myopathies. J Neuroimmunol 2011;231(1–2):32–42; with permission.

Besides stomatitis, potential adverse events include alopecia, pneumonitis, teratogenicity, induction of malignancy, susceptibility to infections, and renal insufficiency. For bone marrow suppression and liver toxicity, the authors monitor complete blood count, differential count, and liver function tests every week in the first 4 weeks, then monthly for 6 months and every 3 months thereafter while on a stable dose. MTX-induced pneumonitis can be difficult to distinguish from myositis-associated ILD. MTX is not used in patients with known ILD or in those with the Jo-1 antibodies.

Therapeutic effects of oral MTX are often noticeable after 4 to 8 weeks. If no improvement is observed by that time, the dose is escalated. In nonresponders and in more severe cases, the authors recommend intravenous or intramuscular MTX treatment at a dose of 0.4 to 0.8 mg/kg in weekly infusions, increasing it by 5 mg every week to reach up to 60 mg weekly. Leucovorin rescue on the day after parenteral MTX administration is needed for doses as high as 50 mg.

Azathioprine

AZA, an antimetabolite that blocks T-lymphocyte proliferation, is a very effective second-line steroid-sparing immunosuppressant with delayed onset of response. AZA is administered in divided doses of 2 to 3 mg/kg/d, ranging from 100 to 250 mg/d. The authors start with 50 mg/d for a week before gradually increasing the dose over 1 to 2 weeks to 100 to 150 mg/d. In 3 to 6 months it may be increased to the maximum range of 200 to 250 mg/d. Onset of response is delayed to at least 4 to 8 months and peaks at 1 to 2 years. It is therefore not surprising that the 3-month placebo-controlled trial of AZA did not show any efficacy.[92] However, hand-grip strength improvement after 1 year was no different when comparing AZA and MTX recipients.[95] Before AZA initiation, it has been suggested to test for thiopurine methyltransferase activity because its deficiency predicts an increased risk of leukopenia. AZA is contraindicated in homozygous cases, whereas in heterozygous patients lower doses may be carefully tried.[105] A meta-analysis of 54 observational studies and 1 randomized controlled trial did not demonstrated sufficient evidence to address the effectiveness of pretesting thiopurine methyltransferase activity. In clinical practice, the authors monitor patients' blood cell counts weekly at the initiation of AZA, then monthly.[106]

An influenza-like reversible acute hypersensitivity reaction affects 12% of users in the first 2 weeks of therapy. It is associated with a rash, elevation in liver enzymes, and pancreatitis. Some may tolerate a rechallenge after recovery. Delayed adverse events include myelosuppression, hepatotoxicity, susceptibility to infection, malignancy, teratogenicity, rash, alopecia, fever, and arthralgia.

The authors monitor complete blood count and liver enzymes every week for 4 weeks, then monthly for 6 months, then every 3 months as long as the patient remains on stable AZA doses. When liver enzymes are markedly elevated (>2 times the normal limit), AZA should be stopped for several months until enzymes normalize before the patient may be rechallenged, at times successfully. It is important to obtain levels of liver-specific γ-glutamyltransferase because transaminases may be released from necrotic muscle fibers.

The dose is adjusted according to treatment response, and to maintain the white blood cell (WBC) count above 3500 and the absolute lymphocyte count below 1000. AZA administration must be interrupted if the WBC count falls below 2500 or the absolute neutrophil count is less than 1000. Patients taking allopurinol, an inhibitor of the main detoxification pathway, require AZA dose reduction to 25% to 33% of the aforementioned. Angiotensin-converting enzyme inhibitors must be avoided because of the serious risk of severe leukopenia.

Intravenous Immunoglobulin

IVIG, a pooled γ-globulin product from several thousand blood donors, has a complex immunomodulatory mechanism of action. It is thought to involve modulation of pathogenic autoantibody production and binding inhibition, proinflammatory cytokine suppression, Fc-receptor blockade, increase in macrophage colony stimulating factor and monocyte chemoattractant protein 1, alteration in T-cell function, decrease in circulating CD54 lymphocytes, and inhibition of cell transmigration into the muscle. A randomized controlled trial with optional crossover showed that IVIG, 2 g/kg administered monthly for 3 months, was very effective in 9 of 12 treatment-resistant cases of DM.[94] Although prospective controlled trials are lacking, IVIG is also thought to be effective in PM[107,108] and NM. The American Academy of Neurology 2012 guidelines recommend IVIG as possibly effective and to be considered for treating nonresponsive DM cases.[109] There was insufficient evidence to support or refute the use of IVIG in PM or IBM. In a recent retrospective inception cohort, 78 JDM patients were treated with steroids, of whom 30 were treated additionally with IVIG.[110] The IVIG group maintained similar or lower disease activity than controls. The authors institute IVIG in addition to intravenous solumedrol as initial therapy in severely affected patients to achieve a more rapid improvement. Occasionally IVIG is administered as maintenance therapy in otherwise refractory patients, or more commonly to reduce long-term CS dose. Dosing is 2 g/kg total initially, given divided over 2 to 5 days, after which infusions are repeated every 2 to 4 weeks, with a total monthly dosage of 0.4 to 2 g/kg.

The authors closely monitor patients with the first infusion, starting at a very slow rate of 25 to 50 mL/h for 30 minutes and increasing it progressively by 50 mL/h every 15 to 20 minutes up to 150 to 200 mL/h. Mild reactions (headache, nausea, chills, myalgia, chest discomfort, back pain) occur in 10% and are improved with slowing the infusion rate, and are preventable with premedication with acetaminophen, benadryl, and, if necessary, intravenous methylprednisolone. Moderate rare reactions include chemical meningitis and delayed red, macular skin reaction of the palms, soles, and trunk, with desquamation. Acute renal failure is uncommon and is related to patient dehydration and the sucrose or maltose diluent. Other severe and rare reactions are anaphylaxis, stroke, myocardial infarction, or pulmonary emboli resulting from hyperviscosity syndrome. The latter is more likely to occur in elderly patients and in those with immobility, diabetes, thrombocytopenia, hypercholesterolemia, hypergammaglobulinemia, and cryoglobulinemia. The authors avoid using IVIG in patients with several of these risk factors, and place IVIG recipients on low-dose aspirin prophylactically. The extremely rare patients with total immunoglobulin A deficiency should not receive IVIG. In an uncontrolled preliminary report, 7 Caucasian women (4 DM and 3 PM) with median disease duration of 72 months were treated with subcutaneous immunoglobulin.[111] Over a median follow-up period of 14 months all patients showed a favorable clinical response, leading to reduction of the daily maintenance prednisone dose by a mean of 23 mg, and 3 patients were able to discontinue prednisone altogether.[111] These encouraging findings have not been not been validated in a controlled study.

Treatment of Refractory Patients

In refractory patients who have not responded to second-line agents or mycophenolate mofetil,[112] the authors initiate rituximab[113,114] or cyclophosphamide as third-line drugs. If patients fail to respond to these agents or cannot tolerate them, etanercept,[98] cyclosporine, tacrolimus,[115] and chlorambucil are considered (see **Table 3**).[116] A large multicenter clinical trial to clarify the role of CD20 depletion using rituximab in adults and children with refractory PM and DM was conducted.[117] Two hundred patients with DM, JDM, or PM were randomized to receive rituximab early (Group A) or late (8 weeks later, Group B) in the course of this 44-week trial. This study was negative, but problems with design limit its conclusions. It is likely that the study's delayed treatment design hampered the detection of a significant benefit of rituximab, as 83% of refractory cases met the definition of improvement following rituximab treatment. In a small uncontrolled study, rituximab improved 6 of 8 refractory SRP-positive patients on manual muscle strength and/or resulted in CK decline as early as 2 months after treatment.[118] Quantitative levels of serum anti-SRP antibodies also decreased after rituximab treatment. Furthermore, anti-SRP-positive myositis appears to be one of the few autoimmune diseases in which specific autoantibody levels are correlated with surrogate disease activity markers.[119]

In a controlled trial of etanercept, 5 of 11 subjects in the etanercept arm were successfully weaned off prednisone, whereas none of the 5 placebo-recipient could be weaned off.[98] The median of the average prednisone dosage after week 24 was lower in the etanercept group (1.2 mg/d) than in the placebo group (29.2 mg/d). Five etanercept-treated subjects and 1 placebo-treated patient developed worsening DM rash. In an uncontrolled study of refractory JDM, etanercept did not demonstrate appreciable improvement, and some patients noted worsening of disease. Therefore, caution should be taken when recommending tumor necrosis factor (TNF)-receptor inhibitors to patients with active symptoms of JDM.[120]

Although a case of refractory DM ILD was successfully treated with adalimumab,[121] another patient with rheumatoid arthritis developed DM 4.5 years after treatment with this anti–TNF-α drug.[122] TNF antagonists are widely used for the treatment of rheumatoid arthritis in addition to inflammatory bowel disease, psoriasis, psoriatic arthritis, and ankylosing spondylitis. Lupus-like symptoms have been reported in less than 0.2% of patients within 4 to 9 months of treatment of these diseases, but development of PM/DM is limited to patients with underlying rheumatoid arthritis. It is likely in the latter case that DM is a manifestation of overlap syndrome rather than it being induced by adalimumab. Until an association of PM/DM with TNF antagonists is demonstrated in patients who do not have rheumatoid arthritis, it is premature to ascertain a causal relationship.

IIM Associated with ILD

CS are the first-line drug for IIM associated with ILD, but most patients require adjuvant immunomodulating drugs.[45] In cases of ILD refractory to steroids, mycophenolate mofetil,[123] cyclosporine,[124,125] and tacrolimus have been shown to be effective second-line agents.[115] Early intervention with prednisolone and cyclosporine combination therapy, and tight control of daily cyclosporine dose by monitoring the blood level 2 hours after dosing, has improved pulmonary function tests and chest imaging findings in DM cases with acute to subacute ILD.[124] Cyclosporine is effective and substantially safe in patients with anti-Jo1 antisynthetase syndrome and corticosteroid-refractory ILD.[125] Side effects were hypertension (5 of 18 patients) and creatinine increase (6 of 18 patients). Cyclosporine withdrawal may be associated with ILD relapse, and low-dose chronic maintenance was effective in ILD control. Rituximab and cyclophosphamide are third-line options to arrest progression in cases of refractory ILD. One-third of treated cases experienced resolution of pulmonary involvement, whereas 16% deteriorated.[24] Factors predictive of poor ILD prognosis include older age, symptomatic ILD, lower values of vital capacity and diffusing capacity for carbon monoxide, a pattern of interstitial pneumonia on high-resolution CT scan and lung biopsy, and steroid-refractory ILD. There is an increased mortality rate in patients with deteriorating ILD in comparison with those without ILD deterioration (47.1% vs 3.3%).

Promising Therapies

Tocilizumab, a humanized anti–IL-6 receptor antibody, is approved by the Food and Drug Administration (FDA) for the treatment of moderate to severe rheumatoid arthritis.[126] Ogata and Tanaka[126] recently reported the first 2 patients with refractory PM who responded to tocilizumab with reduction in CK; in one case there was resolution of myalgia and stabilization of disease activity, and in the other disappearance of the high-intensity zones in the thigh muscles on MRI. Abatacept, a fusion protein between immunoglobulin and the extracellular domain of cytotoxic T-lymphocyte antigen 4, exerts its anti-inflammatory effect by downregulating T-cell activation and is approved by the FDA for moderate to severe rheumatoid arthritis. A patient with refractory JDM responded to intravenous abatacept and vasodilation with topical sodium thiosulfate, with significant reductions in muscle and skin inflammation, decreased corticosteroid dependence, and an arrest of calcinosis progression.[127] A bedridden PM patient had a very good clinical response to abatacept.[128] Abatacept may therefore hold promise as a steroid-sparing agent for the treatment of refractory DM.

There are anecdotal reports of immune ablation similar to that achieved following myeloablative autologous hematopoietic stem cell transplantation through the intensive administration of alemtuzumab, an anti-CD52 antibody. A patient with refractory PM responded rapidly to a single course of treatment with alemtuzumab.[129] Another case of refractory JPM treated with alemtuzumab had stable clinical improvement for more than 6 years.[130] However, a refractory adult patient with PM developed Epstein-Barr virus–driven lymphoproliferative disorder 9 weeks after alemtuzumab therapy.[131] In a preliminary report, 10 patients with refractory or severe DM/PM underwent allogeneic mesenchymal stem cell transplantation, all of whom showed initial improvement in their serum CK, patient global assessment by visual analog scale, and muscle strength by manual muscle test.[132] However, 3 had recurrence of disease activity 6 to 8 months after the transplant, of whom 2 underwent a second transplant with good clinical response in 1 case. The efficacy of allogeneic mesenchymal stem cell transplantation in DM or PM has yet to be confirmed in controlled trials.

Physical Therapy

In addition to pharmacotherapy, it is generally agreed that physical therapy, orthotic devices, occupational therapy, and exercise are beneficial in DM, PM, and NM as early as 2 to 3 weeks from the acute phase.[133] A long-term follow-up study demonstrated that patients who have had JDM have persistently impaired fitness on maximal exercise using a cycle ergometer, which is related to duration of active disease.[134] Although other studies have reported the safety and benefits of resistive exercise in active patients 1 to 3 months into their treatment,[135] most of the studies have been in chronic PM or DM.[136] All studies demonstrated the efficacy and safety of exercise as measured by the Functional Index, 36-item Short Form, muscle histology, muscle MRI scanning, or creatine phosphokinase levels. Besides improved muscle strength and increased maximal oxygen uptake, resistance exercise training of 8 myositis patients resulted in marked reductions in gene expression, reflecting reductions in proinflammatory and profibrotic gene networks, together with a reduction in tissue fibrosis.[137] In severe cases, the authors start with passive range of motion exercises, and will usually wait for the first month to 3 months for strength and CK to start responding to pharmacotherapy before subjecting severely weakened muscles to a rigorous strengthening exercise program. In patients with mild to moderate weakness, a strengthening program is started after steroid initiation. Because pain from arthralgia and, possibly, arthritis is relieved by joint flexion, early mobilization is important to prevent flexion contractures of the large and small joints, especially in JDM. There may also be a role for creatine monohydrate supplementation, as it improves functional performance without significant adverse effects.[138]

PROGNOSIS

In general the prognosis of DM, PM, and NM is favorable, with some exceptions. An associated malignancy portends a poor prognosis for recovery and increases mortality. SANAM is resistant to treatment. Concomitant ILD or autoantibodies to Jo-1 or SRP predict a poorer prognosis. Overall, drug-free remissions are rare except in JDM. Recent series underline that only 20% to 40% of treated PM/DM patients will achieve remission, whereas 60% to 80% will experience a polycyclic or chronic continuous course of the disease.[139,140] On medium-term and long-term follow-up, up to 80% of treated PM/DM patients are still disabled based on Health Assessment Questionnaire scores.[141] The overall mortality ratio in PM/DM patients also remains 2- to 3-fold higher compared with the general population, with cancer, lung, and cardiac complications and infections being the most common causes of deaths.[142,143] Poor prognostic factors in PM/DM patients include older age,[144] male gender, non-Caucasian ethnicity, longer symptom duration before diagnosis, ILD,[145] cardiac involvement, dysphagia,[146] cancer,[143] and serum MSAs (including coexistence of anti-Ro52 and anti-Jo1 antibodies, SRP, anti-155/140, or anti–CADM-140 antibodies). Complete remission of PM/DM was less frequent (13.6% vs 41.1%) and the mortality rate (47.8% vs 7.3%) was higher in elderly patients than in their younger counterparts.[144] In a recent series the coexistence of Ro52 and Jo1 antibodies was associated with more severe myositis/joint impairment, symptomatic ILD, increased risk of cancer, and higher mortality.[147] Anti-SRP antibody is associated with acute onset of refractory necrotizing myositis, and antibody titers correlate with CK levels and disease activity.[119] Anti-155/140 antibody is associated in adults with malignancy, whereas the presence of anti–CADM-140 antibody is associated with amyopathic DM and rapidly progressive ILD.

REFERENCES

1. van der Meulen MF, Bronner IM, Hoogendijk JE, et al. Polymyositis: an overdiagnosed entity. Neurol 2003;61:316–21.
2. Chahin N, Engel AG. Correlation of muscle biopsy, clinical course, and outcome in PM and sporadic IBM. Neurol 2008;70(6):418–24.
3. Tan JA, Roberts-Thomson PJ, Blumbergs P, et al. Incidence and prevalence of idiopathic inflammatory myopathies in South Australia: a 30-year epidemiologic study of histology-proven cases. Int J Rheum Dis 2013;16(3):331–8.
4. Kuo CF, See LC, Yu KH, et al. Incidence, cancer risk and mortality of dermatomyositis and polymyositis in Taiwan: a nationwide population study. Br J Dermatol 2011;165(6):1273–9.
5. Regardt M, Welin Henriksson E, Alexanderson H, et al. Patients with polymyositis or dermatomyositis have reduced grip force and health-related quality of life in comparison with reference values: an observational study. Rheumatology (Oxford) 2011;50(3):578–85.
6. Quinter SD, Chiu YE, Lyon VB, et al. Inverse Gottron's papules: an unusual cutaneous manifestation of juvenile dermatomyositis. Pediatr Dermatol 2012;29(5):641–4. http://dx.doi.org/10.1111/j.1525-1470.2011.01585.x.

7. Schmeling H, Stephens S, Goia C, et al. Nailfold capillary density is importantly associated over time with muscle and skin disease activity in juvenile dermatomyositis. Rheumatology (Oxford) 2011;50(5):885–93.
8. Shirani Z, Kucenic MJ, Carroll CL, et al. Pruritus in adult dermatomyositis. Clin Exp Dermatol 2004;29:273–6.
9. Hundley JL, Carroll CL, Lang W, et al. Cutaneous symptoms of dermatomyositis significantly impact patients' quality of life. J Am Acad Dermatol 2006;54:217–20.
10. Bohan A, Peter JB. Polymyositis and dermatomyositis (first of two parts). N Engl J Med 1975;292(7):344–7.
11. Bohan A, Peter JB. Polymyositis and dermatomyositis (second of two parts). N Engl J Med 1975;292:403–7.
12. Targoff IN, Miller FW, Medsger TA, et al. Classification criteria for the idiopathic inflammatory myopathies. Curr Opin Rheumatol 1997;9(6):527–35.
13. Hoogendijk JE, Amato AA, Lecky BR, et al. 119th ENMC international workshop: trial design in adult idiopathic inflammatory myopathies, with the exception of inclusion body myositis, 10-12 October 2003, Naarden, The Netherlands. Neuromuscul Disord 2004;14(5):337–45.
14. Amato AA, Griggs RC. Unicorns, dragons, polymyositis and other mythical beasts. Neurol 2003;61:288–9.
15. Amato AA, Barohn RJ. Idiopathic inflammatory myopathies. Neurol Clin 1997;15: 615–48.
16. Dalakas MC, Hohlfeld R. Polymyositis and dermatomyositis. Lancet 2003;362: 971–82.
17. Pal S, Sanyal D. Jaw muscle weakness: a differential indicator of neuromuscular weakness–preliminary observations. Muscle Nerve 2011;43(6):807–11.
18. Ellis E, Ann Tan J, Lester S, et al. Necrotizing myopathy: clinicoserologic associations. Muscle Nerve 2012;45(2):189–94.
19. Suzuki S, Ohta M, Shimizu Y, et al. Anti-signal recognition particle myopathy in the first decade of life. Pediatr Neurol 2011;45(2):114–6.
20. Muzyka I, Barohn RJ, Dimachkie M, et al. Necrotizing autoimmune statin -associated myopathy. J Clin Neuromuscul Dis 2011;12(3):17.
21. Grable-Esposito P, Katzberg HD, Greenberg SA, et al. Immune-mediated necrotizing myopathy associated with statins. Muscle Nerve 2010;41(2):185–90.
22. Niewold TB, Wu SC, Smith M, et al. Familial aggregation of autoimmune disease in juvenile dermatomyositis. Pediatrics 2011;127(5):e1239–46.
23. Tymms KE, Webb J. Dermatopolymyositis and other connective tissue diseases: a review of 105 cases. J Rheumatol 1985;12(6):1140–8.
24. Marie I, Hatron PY, Dominique S, et al. Short-term and long-term outcomes of interstitial lung disease in polymyositis and dermatomyositis: a series of 107 patients. Arthritis Rheum 2011;63(11):3439–47.
25. Hochberg MC, Feldman D, Stevens MB, et al. Antibody to Jo-1 in polymyositis/dermatomyositis: association with interstitial pulmonary disease. J Rheumatol 1984;11(5):663–5.
26. Maoz CR, Langevitz P, Livneh A, et al. High incidence of malignancies in patients with dermatomyositis and polymyositis: an 11-year analysis. Semin Arthritis Rheum 1998;27(5):319–24.
27. Sigurgeirsson B, Lindelöf B, Edhag O, et al. Risk of cancer in patients with dermatomyositis or polymyositis. A population-based study. N Engl J Med 1992; 326(6):363–7.
28. Lakhanpal S, Bunch TW, Ilstrup DM, et al. Polymyositis-dermatomyositis and malignant lesions: does an association exist? Mayo Clin Proc 1986;61(8):645–53.

29. Scaling ST, Kaufman RH. Patten BM Dermatomyositis and female malignancy. Obstet Gynecol 1979;54(4):474–7.
30. Rider LG, Miller FW. Classification and treatment of the juvenile idiopathic inflammatory myopathies. Rheum Dis Clin North Am 1997;23(3):619–55.
31. Chen YJ, Wu CY, Huang YL, et al. Cancer risks of dermatomyositis and polymyositis: a nationwide cohort study in Taiwan. Arthritis Res Ther 2010;12(2):R70.
32. Needham M, Fabian V, Knezevic W, et al. Progressive myopathy with up-regulation of MHC-I associated with statin therapy. Neuromuscul Disord 2007; 17(2):194–200.
33. Wang Y, Barohn RJ, McVey AL, et al. Necrotizing myopathy: a unique immune-mediated myopathy. J Child Neurol 2004;19:207.
34. Miller T, Al-Lozi MT, Lopate G, et al. Myopathy with antibodies to the signal recognition particle: clinical and pathological features. J Neurol Neurosurg Psychiatry 2002;73(4):420–8.
35. Zöller B, Li X, Sundquist J, et al. Risk of subsequent coronary heart disease in patients hospitalized for immune-mediated diseases: a nationwide follow-up study from Sweden. PLoS One 2012;7(3):e33442.
36. Eimer MJ, Brickman WJ, Seshadri R, et al. Clinical status and cardiovascular risk profile of adults with a history of juvenile dermatomyositis. J Pediatr 2011; 159(5):795–801.
37. Hill CL, Zhang Y, Sigurgeirsson B, et al. Frequency of specific cancer types in dermatomyositis and polymyositis: a population-based study. Lancet 2001; 357(9250):96–100.
38. Marie I, Guillevin L, Menard JF, et al. Hematological malignancy associated with polymyositis and dermatomyositis. Autoimmun Rev 2012;11(9):615–20.
39. Sparsa A, Liozon E, Herrmann F, et al. Routine vs extensive malignancy search for adult dermatomyositis and polymyositis: a study of 40 patients. Arch Dermatol 2002;138(7):885–90.
40. Titulaer MJ, Soffietti R, Dalmau J, et al. European Federation of Neurological Societies. Screening for tumours in paraneoplastic syndromes: report of an EFNS task force. Eur J Neurol 2011;18(1):19-e3.
41. Marie I, Josse S, Hatron PY, et al. Interstitial lung disease in anti-Jo-1 patients with antisynthetase syndrome. Arthritis Care Res (Hoboken) 2013;65(5): 800–8.
42. Labirua A, Lundberg IE. Interstitial lung disease and idiopathic inflammatory myopathies: progress and pitfalls. Curr Opin Rheumatol 2010;22(6):633–8.
43. Marie I, Josse S, Decaux O, et al. Comparison of long-term outcome between anti-Jo1- and anti-PL7/PL12 positive patients with antisynthetase syndrome. Autoimmun Rev 2012;11(10):739–45.
44. Marie I, Josse S, Decaux O, et al. Outcome of anti-PL12 positive patients with antisynthetase syndrome. Presse Med 2013;42(6 Pt 1):e153–8.
45. Mimori T, Nakashima R, Hosono Y. Interstitial lung disease in myositis: clinical subsets, biomarkers, and treatment. Curr Rheumatol Rep 2012;14(3):264–74.
46. Hall JC, Casciola-Rosen L, Samedy LA, et al. Anti-melanoma differentiation-associated protein 5-associated dermatomyositis: expanding the clinical spectrum. Arthritis Care Res (Hoboken) 2013;65(8):1307–15.
47. Gono T, Kawaguchi Y, Sugiura T, et al. Interferon-induced helicase (IFIH1) polymorphism with systemic lupus erythematosus and dermatomyositis/polymyositis. Mod Rheumatol 2010;20(5):466–70.
48. Fathi M, Barbasso Helmers S, Lundberg IE. KL-6: a serological biomarker for interstitial lung disease in patients with polymyositis and dermatomyositis.

J Intern Med 2011;271(6):589–97. http://dx.doi.org/10.1111/j.1365-2796.2011.02459.x.

49. Gono T, Kawaguchi Y, Sugiura T, et al. Interleukin-18 is a key mediator in dermatomyositis: potential contribution to development of interstitial lung disease. Rheumatology (Oxford) 2010;49(10):1878–81.

50. Tanizawa K, Handa T, Nakashima R, et al. The prognostic value of HRCT in myositis-associated interstitial lung disease. Respir Med 2013;107(5):745–52.

51. López De Padilla CM, McNallan KT, Crowson CS, et al. BAFF expression correlates with idiopathic inflammatory myopathy disease activity measures and autoantibodies. J Rheumatol 2013;40(3):294–302.

52. Filková M, Senolt L, Vencovský J. The role of resistin in inflammatory myopathies. Curr Rheumatol Rep 2013;15(6):336.

53. Ichimura Y, Matsushita T, Hamaguchi Y, et al. Anti-NXP2 autoantibodies in adult patients with idiopathic inflammatory myopathies: possible association with malignancy. Ann Rheum Dis 2012;71(5):710–3.

54. Nakajima A, Yoshino K, Soejima M, et al. High Frequencies and co-existing of myositis-specific autoantibodies in patients with idiopathic inflammatory myopathies overlapped to rheumatoid arthritis. Rheumatol Int 2011;32(7):2057–61.

55. Vincze M, Molnár PA, Tumpek J, et al. An unusual association: anti-Jo1 and anti-SRP antibodies in the serum of a patient with polymyositis. Clin Rheumatol 2010;29(7):811–4.

56. Sugie K, Tonomura Y, Ueno S. Characterization of Dermatomyositis with Coexistence of Anti-Jo-1 and Anti-SRP Antibodies. Intern Med 2012;51(7):799–802.

57. Joffe MM, Love LA, Leff RL, et al. Drug therapy of the idiopathic inflammatory myopathies: predictors of response to prednisone, azathioprine, and methotrexate and a comparison of their efficacy. Am J Med 1993;94(4):379–87.

58. Kunimasa K, Arita M, Nakazawa T, et al. The clinical characteristics of two anti-OJ (anti-isoleucyl-tRNA synthetase) autoantibody-positive interstitial lung disease patients with polymyositis/dermatomyositis. Intern Med 2012;51(24):3405–10.

59. Kaji K, Fujimoto M, Hasegawa M, et al. Identification of a novel autoantibody reactive with 155 and 140 kDa nuclear proteins in patients with dermatomyositis: an association with malignancy. Rheumatology (Oxford) 2007;46:25–8.

60. Rider LG, Shah M, Mamyrova G, et al, Childhood Myositis Heterogeneity Collaborative Study Group. The myositis autoantibody phenotypes of the juvenile idiopathic inflammatory myopathies. Medicine (Baltimore) 2013;92(4):223–43.

61. Ikeda N, Takahashi K, Yamaguchi Y, et al. Analysis of dermatomyositis-specific autoantibodies and clinical characteristics in Japanese patients. J Dermatol 2011;38(10):973–9.

62. Tanizawa K, Handa T, Nakashima R, et al. HRCT features of interstitial lung disease in dermatomyositis with anti-CADM-140 antibody. Respir Med 2011;105(9):1380–7.

63. Kobayashi I, Okura Y, Yamada M, et al. Anti-melanoma differentiation-associated gene 5 antibody is a diagnostic and predictive marker for interstitial lung diseases associated with juvenile dermatomyositis. J Pediatr 2011;158(4):675–7.

64. Suzuki S. Anti-SRP myopathy. Rinsho Shinkeigaku 2011;51(11):961–3 [in Japanese].

65. Kao AH, Lacomis D, Lucas M, et al. Anti-signal recognition particle autoantibody in patients with and patients without idiopathic inflammatory myopathy. Arthritis Rheum 2004;50:209–15.

66. Hanisch F, Müller T, Stoltenburg G, et al. Unusual manifestations in two cases of necrotizing myopathy associated with SRP-antibodies. Clin Neurol Neurosurg 2012;114(7):1104–6.
67. Christopher-Stine L, Casciola-Rosen LA, Hong G, et al. A novel autoantibody recognizing 200-kd and 100-kd proteins is associated with an immune-mediated necrotizing myopathy. Arthritis Rheum 2010;62(9):2757–66.
68. Degardin A, Morillon D, Lacour A, et al. Morphologic imaging in muscular dystrophies and inflammatory myopathies. Skeletal Radiol 2010;39(12):1219–27.
69. Kissel JT, Mendell JR, Rammoha KW. Microvascular deposition of complement membrane attack complex in dermatomyositis. N Engl J Med 1986;314:329–34.
70. Emslie-Smith AM, Engel AG. Microvascular changes in early and advanced dermatomyositis: a quantitative study. Ann Neurol 1990;27:343–56.
71. Pestronk A, Schmidt RE, Choksi R. Vascular pathology in dermatomyositis and anatomic relations to myopathology. Muscle Nerve 2010;42(1):53–61.
72. Greenberg SA, Bradshaw EM, Pinkus JL, et al. Plasma cells in muscle in inclusion body myositis and polymyositis. Neurology 2005;65(11):1782–7.
73. Uchino M, Yamashita S, Uchino K, et al. Muscle biopsy findings predictive of malignancy in rare infiltrative dermatomyositis. Clin Neurol Neurosurg 2013; 115(5):603–6.
74. Nandakumar S, Miller CW, Kumaraguru U. T regulatory cells: an overview and intervention techniques to modulate allergy outcome. Clin Mol Allergy 2009;7:5.
75. Antiga E, Kretz CC, Klembt R, et al. Characterization of regulatory T cells in patients with dermatomyositis. J Autoimmun 2010;35(4):342–50.
76. Waschbisch A, Schwab N, Ruck T, et al. FOXP3+ T regulatory cells in idiopathic inflammatory myopathies. J Neuroimmunol 2010;225(1–2):137–42.
77. Gendek-Kubiak H, Gendek EG. Fascin-expressing dendritic cells dominate in polymyositis and dermatomyositis. J Rheumatol 2013;40(2):186–91.
78. De Visser M, Emslie-Smith AM, Engel AG. Early ultrastructural alterations in adult dermatomyositis. Capillary abnormalities precede other structural changes in muscle. J Neurol Sci 1989;94(1–3):181–92.
79. Zhou X, Dimachkie MM, Xiong M, et al. cDNA microarrays reveal distinct gene expression clusters in idiopathic inflammatory myopathies. Med Sci Monit 2004; 10(7):BR191–7.
80. Walsh RJ, Kong SW, Yao Y, et al. Type I interferon-inducible gene expression in blood is present and reflects disease activity in dermatomyositis and polymyositis. Arthritis Rheum 2007;56(11):3784–92.
81. Bilgic H, Ytterberg SR, Amin S, et al. Interleukin-6 and type I interferon-regulated genes and chemokines mark disease activity in dermatomyositis. Arthritis Rheum 2009;60(11):3436–46.
82. Liao AP, Salajegheh M, Nazareno R, et al. Interferon β is associated with type 1 interferon-inducible gene expression in dermatomyositis. Ann Rheum Dis 2011; 70(5):831–6.
83. Wong D, Kea B, Pesich R, et al. Interferon and biologic signatures in dermatomyositis skin: specificity and heterogeneity across diseases. PLoS One 2012; 7(1):e29161.
84. Salaroli R, Baldin E, Papa V, et al. Validity of internal expression of the major histocompatibility complex class I in the diagnosis of inflammatory myopathies. J Clin Pathol 2012;65(1):14–9.
85. Greenberg SA, Pinkus GS, Amato AA, et al. Myeloid dendritic cells in inclusion-body myositis and polymyositis. Muscle Nerve 2007;35(1):17–23.

86. Greenberg SA, Pinkus JL, Pinkus GS, et al. Interferon-alpha/beta-mediated innate immune mechanisms in dermatomyositis. Ann Neurol 2005;57(5):664–78.
87. Greenberg SA, Higgs BW, Morehouse C, et al. Relationship between disease activity and type 1 interferon- and other cytokine-inducible gene expression in blood in dermatomyositis and polymyositis. Genes Immun 2012;13(3):207–13. http://dx.doi.org/10.1038/gene.2011.61.
88. Emslie-Smith AM, Engel AG. Necrotizing myopathy with pipestem capillaries, microvascular deposition of complement membrane attack complex (MAC), and minimal cellular infiltration. Neurol 1991;41:936–9.
89. Bronner IM, Hoogendijk JE, Wintzen AR, et al. Necrotizing myopathy, an unusual presentation of a steroid-responsive myopathy. J Neurol 2003;250:480–5.
90. Mammen AL, Chung T, Christopher-Stine L, et al. Autoantibodies against 3-hydroxy-3-methylglutaryl-coenzyme A reductase in patients with statin-associated autoimmune myopathy. Arthritis Rheum 2011;63(3):713–21. http://dx.doi.org/10.1002/art.30156.
91. Amato AA, Barohn RJ. Inclusion body myositis: old and new concepts. J Neurol Neurosurg Psychiatry 2009;80(11):1186–93.
92. Bunch TW, Worthington JW, Combs JJ, et al. Azathioprine with prednisone for polymyositis. Ann Intern Med 1980;92(3):365–9.
93. Miller FW, Leitman SF, Cronin M, et al. Controlled trial of plasma exchange and leukapheresis in polymyositis and dermatomyositis. N Engl J Med 1992;326:1380–4.
94. Dalakas MC, Illa I, Dambrosia JM, et al. A controlled trial of high-dose intravenous immune globulin infusions as treatment for dermatomyositis. N Engl J Med 1993;329(27):1993–2000.
95. Miller J, Walsh Y, Saminaden S, et al. Randomised double blind controlled trial of methotrexate and steroids compared with azathioprine and steroids in the treatment of idiopathic inflammatory myopathy. J Neurol Sci 2002;199(Suppl 1):S53.
96. Vencovsky J, Jarosova K, Machacek S, et al. Cyclosporine A versus methotrexate in the treatment of polymyositis and dermatomyositis. Scand J Rheumatol 2000;29(2):95–102.
97. Villalba L, Hicks JE, Adams EM, et al. Treatment of refractory myositis: a randomized crossover study of two new cytotoxic regimens. Arthritis Rheum 1998;41(3):392–9.
98. Muscle Study Group. A randomized, pilot trial of etanercept in dermatomyositis. Ann Neurol 2011;70(3):427–36.
99. van de Vlekkert J, Hoogendijk JE, de Haan RJ, et al. Oral dexamethasone pulse therapy versus daily prednisolone in sub-acute onset myositis, a randomised clinical trial. Neuromuscul Disord 2010;20(6):382–9.
100. Rodd C, Lang B, Ramsay T, et al. Incident vertebral fractures among children with rheumatic disorders 12 months after glucocorticoid initiation: a national observational study. Arthritis Care Res (Hoboken) 2012;64(1):122–31.
101. Saad CG, Borba EF, Aikawa NE, et al. Immunogenicity and safety of the 2009 non-adjuvanted influenza A/H1N1 vaccine in a large cohort of autoimmune rheumatic diseases. Ann Rheum Dis 2011;70(6):1068–73.
102. Shinjo SK, de Moraes JC, Levy-Neto M, et al. Pandemic unadjuvanted influenza A (H1N1) vaccine in dermatomyositis and polymyositis: immunogenicity independent of therapy and no harmful effect in disease. Vaccine 2012;31(1):202–6.
103. Marie I, Ménard JF, Hachulla E, et al. Infectious complications in polymyositis and dermatomyositis: a series of 279 patients. Semin Arthritis Rheum 2011;41(1):48–60.

104. Efthimiou P, Pokharna H, Kukar M, et al. PCP chemoprophylaxis is essential for lymphopenic dermatomyositis patients treated with immunomodulators. Muscle Nerve 2011;43(6):918–9.

105. Evans WE, Hon YY, Bomgaars L, et al. Preponderance of thiopurine S-methyl-transferase deficiency and heterozygosity among patients intolerant to mercaptopurine or azathioprine. J Clin Oncol 2001;19(8):2293–301.

106. Booth RA, Ansari MT, Loit E, et al. Assessment of thiopurine S-methyltransferase activity in patients prescribed thiopurines: a systematic review. Ann Intern Med 2011;154(12):814–23.

107. Cherin P, Piette JC, Wechsler B, et al. Intravenous gamma globulin as first line therapy in polymyositis and dermatomyositis: an open study in 11 adult patients. J Rheumatol 1994;21:1092–7.

108. Danieli MG, Malcangi G, Palmieri C, et al. Cyclosporin A and intravenous immunoglobulin treatment in polymyositis/dermatomyositis. Ann Rheum Dis 2002;61: 37–41.

109. Patwa HS, Chaudhry V, Katzberg H, et al. Evidence-based guideline: intravenous immunoglobulin in the treatment of neuromuscular disorders: report of the Therapeutics and Technology Assessment Subcommittee of the American Academy of Neurology. Neurology 2012;78(13):1009–15.

110. Lam CG, Manlhiot C, Pullenayegum EM, et al. Efficacy of intravenous Ig therapy in juvenile dermatomyositis. Ann Rheum Dis 2011;70(12):2089–94.

111. Danieli MG, Pettinari L, Moretti R, et al. Subcutaneous immunoglobulin in polymyositis and dermatomyositis: a novel application. Autoimmun Rev 2011;10(3):144–9.

112. Rowin J, Amato AA, Deisher N, et al. Mycophenolate mofetil in dermatomyositis: is it safe? Neurology 2006;66(8):1245–7.

113. Levine TD. Rituximab in the treatment of dermatomyositis: an open-label pilot study. Arthritis Rheum 2005;52(2):601–7.

114. Noss EH, Hausner-Sypek DL, Weinblatt ME. Rituximab as therapy for refractory polymyositis and dermatomyositis. J Rheumatol 2006;33(5):1021–6.

115. Oddis CV, Sciurba FC, Elmagd KA, et al. Tacrolimus in refractory polymyositis with interstitial lung disease. Lancet 1999;353(9166):1762–3.

116. Cagnoli M, Marchesoni A, Tosi S. Combined steroid, methotrexate and chlorambucil therapy for steroid-resistant dermatomyositis. Clin Exp Rheumatol 1991; 9(6):658–9.

117. Oddis CV, Reed AM, Aggarwal R, et al. Rituximab in the Treatment of Refractory Adult and Juvenile Dermatomyositis and Adult Polymyositis: a randomized, placebo-phase trial. Arthritis Rheum 2013;65(2):314–24.

118. Valiyil R, Casciola-Rosen L, Hong G, et al. Rituximab therapy for myopathy associated with anti-signal recognition particle antibodies: a case series. Arthritis Care Res (Hoboken) 2010;62(9):1328–34.

119. Benveniste O, Drouot L, Jouen F, et al. Correlation of anti-signal recognition particle autoantibody levels with creatine kinase activity in patients with necrotizing myopathy. Arthritis Rheum 2011;63(7):1961–71.

120. Rouster-Stevens KA, Ferguson L, Morgan G, et al. Pilot study of etanercept in patients with refractory juvenile dermatomyositis. Arthritis Care Res (Hoboken) 2013. [Epub ahead of print]. http://dx.doi.org/10.1002/acr.22198.

121. Park JK, Yoo HG, Ahn DS, et al. Successful treatment for conventional treatment-resistant dermatomyositis-associated interstitial lung disease with adalimumab. Rheumatol Int 2012;32(11):3587–90.

122. Brunasso AM, Scocco GL, Massone C. Dermatomyositis during adalimumab therapy for rheumatoid arthritis. J Rheumatol 2010;37(7):1549–50.

123. Morganroth PA, Kreider ME, Werth VP. Mycophenolate mofetil for interstitial lung disease in dermatomyositis. Arthritis Care Res (Hoboken) 2010;62(10): 1496–501.
124. Kotani T, Takeuchi T, Makino S, et al. Combination with corticosteroids and cyclosporin-A improves pulmonary function test results and chest HRCT findings in dermatomyositis patients with acute/subacute interstitial pneumonia. Clin Rheumatol 2011;30(8):1021–8.
125. Cavagna L, Caporali R, Abdì-Alì L, et al. Cyclosporine in anti-Jo1-positive patients with corticosteroid-refractory interstitial lung disease. J Rheumatol 2013; 40(4):484–92.
126. Ogata A, Tanaka T. Tocilizumab for the treatment of rheumatoid arthritis and other systemic autoimmune diseases: current perspectives and future directions. Int J Rheumatol 2012;2012:946048.
127. Arabshahi B, Silverman RA, Jones OY, et al. Abatacept and sodium thiosulfate for treatment of recalcitrant juvenile dermatomyositis complicated by ulceration and calcinosis. J Pediatr 2012;160(3):520–2.
128. Musuruana JL, Cavallasca JA. Abatacept for treatment of refractory polymyositis. Joint Bone Spine 2011;78(4):431–2.
129. Thompson B, Corris P, Miller JA, et al. Alemtuzumab (Campath-1H) for treatment of refractory polymyositis. J Rheumatol 2008;35(10):2080–2.
130. Reiff A, Shaham B, Weinberg KI, et al. Anti-CD52 antibody-mediated immune ablation with autologous immune recovery for the treatment of refractory juvenile polymyositis. J Clin Immunol 2011;31(4):615–22.
131. Cooles FA, Jackson GH, Menon G, et al. Epstein-Barr virus-driven lymphoproliferative disorder post-CAMPATH-1H (alemtuzumab) in refractory polymyositis. Rheumatology (Oxford) 2011;50(4):810–2.
132. Wang D, Zhang H, Cao M, et al. Efficacy of allogeneic mesenchymal stem cell transplantation in patients with drug-resistant polymyositis and dermatomyositis. Ann Rheum Dis 2011;70(7):1285–8.
133. Varjú C, Pethö E, Kutas R, et al. The effect of physical exercise following acute disease exacerbation in patients with dermato/polymyositis. Clin Rehabil 2003; 17(1):83–7.
134. Mathiesen PR, Ørngreen MC, Vissing J, et al. Aerobic fitness after JDM–a long-term follow-up study. Rheumatology (Oxford) 2013;52(2):287–95.
135. Alexanderson H, Stenström CH, Jenner G, et al. The safety of a resistive home exercise program in patients with recent onset active polymyositis or dermatomyositis. Scand J Rheumatol 2000;29(5):295–301.
136. Alexanderson H. Exercise effects in patients with adult idiopathic inflammatory myopathies. Curr Opin Rheumatol 2009;21(2):158–63.
137. Nader GA, Dastmalchi M, Alexanderson H, et al. A longitudinal, integrated, clinical, histological and mRNA profiling study of resistance exercise in myositis. Mol Med 2010;16(11–12):455–64.
138. Chung YL, Alexanderson H, Pipitone N, et al. Creatine supplements in patients with idiopathic inflammatory myopathies who are clinically weak after conventional pharmacologic treatment: six-month, double-blind, randomized, placebo-controlled trial. Arthritis Rheum 2007;57(4):694–702.
139. Marie I, Hachulla E, Hatron PY, et al. Polymyositis and dermatomyositis: short term and longterm outcome, and predictive factors. J Rheumatol 2001;28: 2230–7.
140. Bronner IM, van der Meulen MF, de Visser M, et al. Long-term outcome in polymyositis and dermatomyositis. Ann Rheum Dis 2006;65:1456–61.

141. Ponyi A, Borgulya G, Constantin T, et al. Functional outcome and quality of life in adult patients with idiopathic inflammatory myositis. Rheumatology (Oxford) 2005;44:83–8.
142. Limaye V, Hakendorf P, Woodman RJ, et al. Mortality and its predominant causes in a large cohort of patients with biopsy-determined inflammatory myositis. Intern Med J 2012;42(2):191–8.
143. Airio A, Kautiainen H, Hakala M. Prognosis and mortality of polymyositis and dermatomyositis patients. Clin Rheumatol 2006;25:234–9.
144. Marie I, Hatron PY, Levesque H, et al. Influence of age on characteristics of polymyositis and dermatomyositis in adults. Medicine (Baltimore) 1999;78: 139–47.
145. Yamasaki Y, Yamada H, Ohkubo M, et al. Longterm survival and associated risk factors in patients with adult-onset idiopathic inflammatory myopathies and amyopathic dermatomyositis: experience in a single institute in Japan. J Rheumatol 2011;38:1636–43.
146. Danko K, Ponyi A, Constantin T, et al. Long-term survival of patients with idiopathic inflammatory myopathies according to clinical features: a longitudinal study of 162 cases. Medicine (Baltimore) 2004;83:35–42.
147. Marie I, Hatron PY, Dominique S, et al. Short-term and long-term outcome of anti-Jo1-positive patients with Anti-Ro52 antibody. Semin Arthritis Rheum 2011;41(6):890–9.
148. Griggs RC, Askanas V, DiMauro S, et al. Inclusion body myositis and myopathies. Ann Neurol 1995;38:705–13.

Inclusion Body Myositis

Mazen M. Dimachkie, MD[a],*, Richard J. Barohn, MD[b]

KEYWORDS

- Inclusion body myositis • Idiopathic inflammatory myopathies • Polymyositis
- Diagnosis • Pathology • Pathophysiology • Treatment • Prognosis

KEY POINTS

- Inclusion body myositis (IBM) is the most common inflammatory myopathy after age 50 years.
- Despite similarities with polymyositis (PM) inflammatory disorders, IBM histopathology shows marked degeneration and protein aggregation.
- The clinical phenotype of typical IBM is distinctive, manifesting as proximal leg or distal arm weakness, although in our experience there are several phenotypic variants.
- IBM is refractory to all known immunosuppressive therapies.
- Low-intensity exercise may slow the rate of functional decline.
- Patients with IBM are highly motivated and should be encouraged to participate in clinical trials.

EPIDEMIOLOGY

Inclusion body myositis (IBM) is a rare sporadic disorder with a male/female ratio of 2:1 to 3:1. Data on prevalence and incidence of IBM vary depending on methodology, countries, and regions. In Western Australia, the overall prevalence was 9.3 per million, whereas the age-adjusted prevalence of IBM in people more than the age of 50 years is 3.5 per 100,000, making it the most common idiopathic inflammatory myopathy (IIM) in this age group.[1] A recent study from South Australia yielded a higher overall prevalence rate of 51 per million, with an incidence of 2.9 per million.[2] The latter is comparable with the incidence observed in Sweden (2.2 per million)[3] but lower than the 7.9 per million recorded in Olmstead County, Minnesota, adjusted for sex and age to the

This work was supported by an Institutional Clinical and Translational Science Award, NIH/National Center for Advancing Translational Sciences grant number UL1TR000001. The contents of this article are solely the responsibility of the authors and do not necessarily represent the official views of the NIH.

a Neuromuscular Section, Neurophysiology Division, Department of Neurology, University of Kansas Medical Center, 3901 Rainbow Boulevard, Mail Stop 2012, Kansas City, KS 66160, USA; b Department of Neurology, University of Kansas Medical Center, 3901 Rainbow Boulevard, Mail Stop 2012, Kansas City, KS 66160, USA
* Corresponding author.
E-mail address: mdimachkie@kumc.edu

Neurol Clin 32 (2014) 629–646
http://dx.doi.org/10.1016/j.ncl.2014.04.001
0733-8619/14/$ – see front matter © 2014 Elsevier Inc. All rights reserved.

neurologic.theclinics.com

2000 US Census population.[4] The highest reported prevalence is 71 per million inhabitants of Olmsted County, Minnesota, whereas it is lowest in the Netherlands at 4.9 per million and, when age-adjusted to those older than 50 years, it is 16 per million Dutch inhabitants.[3] IBM is rare in African Americans and in nonwhite people. IBM should be considered in patients with appropriate symptoms who are older than 30 years. Symptom onset before age 60 years occurs in 18% to 20% of patients.[5,6]

Clinical Presentation

In most cases, IBM classically presents with insidious weakness in the proximal leg and/or distal arm.[7,8] There is typically a 5-year to 8-year delay in presentation and diagnosis.[3,5,7,9–11] In the University of Kansas Medical Center (KUMC) IBM series fulfilling pathologic criteria for probable IBM (**Table 1**), delay to diagnosis in 51 cases ranged from 1 to 15 years (mean, 5.1 years).[12] IBM typically manifests as slowly

Table 1	
Retrospective chart review of IBM from 2000 to 2010 at KUMC	
Male/female ratio	1.7:1
Ethnicity (n = 51)	49 white; 2 Hispanic
Mean age at onset (y)	61 (45–80)
Symptom onset before age 50 y (%)	12
Mean time to diagnosis (y)	5.1 (1–15)
Mean follow-up period (y)	2.5 (0.5–8)
CK (IU/L)	609 (59–3000)
Nerve conductions with axon loss neuropathy (%)	32
Electromyography (%)	60 irritative myopathy 12 nonirritative myopathy 28 mixed neuropathic/myopathic pattern
Asymmetry (%)	90
Nondominant side weaker (%)	85
Typical phenotype: FF and (quads)	39/51 (76%): 13: classic phenotype (FF and quads weakest) 11: classic FF, no preferential quads weakness 6: classic quads, no preferential FF weakness 9: FF and quads weak but not weakest
Atypical phenotype	12/51 (24%): 5/12: classic FF with leg weakness sparing quads 4/12: limb-girdle weakness 3/12: other atypical phenotypes (FF arm only, hip flexion/ankle dorsiflexion, facioscapulohumeral)
Muscle pathology	43: inflammation and rimmed vacuoles 8: phenotypic IBM with inflammation
Mobility outcome	75%: recurrent falls 56%: assistive device use at mean 7.5 y 20%: wheelchair or scooter
Bulbar dysfunction (%)	51 dysphagia 55 facial weakness

Abbreviations: CK, creatine kinase; FF, finger flexor; quads, quadriceps.

Adapted from Estephan B, Barohn RJ, Dimachkie MM, et al. Sporadic IBM: a case cohort. J Clin Neuromuscul Dis 2011;12(3):18–9; with permission.

progressive quadriceps muscle more than hip flexor weakness leading to falls or difficulty standing, and the next most common is finger flexor weakness leading to loss of dexterity (**Fig. 1**).[11] Falls were reported by 98% of questionnaire respondents, with 60% (37 of 62) falling frequently.[13] In most cases weakness is markedly asymmetric by at least 1 Medical Research Council (MRC) grade and preferentially affects the distal phalangeal flexors in the nondominant hand (see **Table 1**). Sparing of thenar, hypothenar, and finger extensor muscles sets IBM apart from a myotomal disease such as amyotrophic lateral sclerosis or focal peripheral nerve disorders such as multifocal motor neuropathy. In general, it is anticipated that wrist and finger flexors are weaker than the corresponding extensors, and wrist and finger flexors are more affected than shoulder abductors.

In our case series, 82% of subjects presented with limb weakness symptoms, most commonly restricted to the legs (34 of 51).[12] Arm presentation was less common, affecting 6 of 51 cases. Although it is reportedly a less frequent initial symptom, 8 cases (16%) presented with dysphagia. Less typical initial complaints include foot drop, as in 2 of our cases. Other rare presentations include sparing of the quadriceps muscles with prominent forearm muscle weakness, camptocormia,[14] or even asymptomatic hyperCKemia.[15] There has been a reported case of primary respiratory failure in IBM.[16] On examination, all patients in the KUMC case series (39) with typical phenotype and most cases (10 of 12) with atypical phenotype had evidence of arm and leg weakness (see **Table 1**).[12] However, 71% (36 of 51) showed a typical IBM weakness pattern in the arm or leg muscles. In 9 cases, finger flexors and knee extensors were not weaker than finger extensors and hip flexors, and 4 cases displayed a limb-girdle pattern of weakness.

Dysphagia is a significant problem because it affects 50% to 70% of patients.[5,17] In our case series (see **Table 1**), 8 subjects had dysphagia as the initial symptoms and in 7 of 8 cases dysphagia was the only presenting symptom of IBM for up to 10 years.[12] Fifty-one percent of our cases eventually experienced dysphagia. Mild to moderate facial weakness is frequently shown (55%) and was the earliest IBM symptom for 20 years in 1 of 51 cases. Others have recently reported facial diplegia as a presenting manifestation of IBM.[18] The tibialis anterior muscle was involved in 70% of our patients with IBM but, in 12%, ankle dorsiflexors were weaker than knee extensors. Scapular winging affected 8% of KUMC cases. Although mostly asymptomatic, a third of patients harbor a distal sensory loss gradient and/or electrophysiologic evidence of a mild distal sensory axon loss peripheral polyneuropathy.

Associated Conditions

Although IBM is thought to be a neurodegenerative disorder, there is some association with autoimmune disorders in up to 15% of cases. Systemic lupus erythematosus,

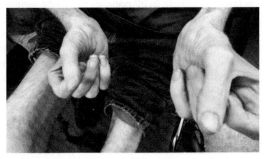

Fig. 1. Finger flexor weakness and severe thigh muscle atrophy in IBM.

Sjögren syndrome, thrombocytopenia, and sarcoidosis have been reported with IBM. The HLA-DRB1*03:01/*01:01 genotype confers the highest disease risk in IBM.[19,20] There is no increased risk of myocarditis, interstitial lung disease, or malignancy in IBM.[21]

Laboratory and Electrophysiologic Testing

Serum creatine kinase (CK) level may be normal or increased, up to 12 to 15 times the upper normal limit. On occasion, it may be as high as 20 times the normal limit. Anti-nuclear antibody is positive in 20% of patients with IBM and, in some, sjogren antibody may be increased.

Needle electromyography typically shows an irritative myopathy that is associated with fibrillation potentials. In our series, 60% of subjects showed an irritative myopathy pattern and 12% had a nonirritative myopathy.[12] In 28% of our IBM cases, the motor unit action potentials were mixed myopathic and neuropathic, with the latter being caused by reinnervation of denervated and split muscle fibers. In some cases, the neurogenic motor unit action potentials in IBM may be sufficiently dense to over-shadow the myopathic changes, leading to a misdiagnosis of motor neuron disease. However, the clinical pattern of selective finger flexor weakness is helpful clinically in making that distinction. In our series, nerve conduction studies revealed a mild sensory axonal peripheral polyneuropathy in nearly a third of patients (see **Table 1**).

Muscle Imaging

The role of magnetic resonance imaging (MRI) in neuromuscular diseases is expand-ing.[22] Specific patterns of muscular involvement can be identified on qualitative MRI of the lower limbs in patients with IBM.[23–25] Beyond diagnosis, quantitative MRI pro-vides potentially very sensitive outcome measures, and has been used in clinical trials in other neuromuscular diseases.[26] In IBM, targets for quantification include markers of both chronic and acute muscle disorders. Chronic muscle damage results in the infil-tration of muscle tissue with fat and reduction in muscle size. Fatty infiltration is quantifi-able using several MRI methods, notably the Dixon fat-water separation technique,[27,28] whereas atrophy can be quantified with any anatomic MRI sequence. Acute muscle disorder in IBM is qualitatively identifiable as hyperintensity on T2-weighted sequences with fat suppression. This condition can be quantified by measurement of the prolon-gation of the T2-relaxation time, as has been applied to juvenile dermatomyositis.[29]

Degardin and colleagues[23] performed MRI studies on 4 patients with IBM, 2 of whom had predominantly distal muscle involvement and 2 who had asymmetric fat deposition. Muscle involvement was typically found in the quadriceps, medial head of the gastrocnemius, and often in the soleus and tibialis anterior muscles. T2 hyper-intensities were identified on short tau inversion recovery images and were associated with adjacent muscle fatty infiltration. In 32 patients with IBM evaluated in 68 muscles of the upper and lower extremities for muscle atrophy, fatty infiltration, and inflamma-tion, fatty infiltration was far more common than inflammation. Fatty replacement most frequently affected the long finger flexors, anterior thigh muscles (sparing the rectus femoris), and all muscles of the lower leg, preferentially affecting the medial gastroc-nemius muscle.[24] Inflammation was present in 78% of the patients, with a median of 2 inflamed muscles per patient. However, the amount of fatty infiltration correlated significantly with disease severity, disease duration, and CK levels.

In a study of whole-body positron emission tomography using Pittsburgh com-pound B (PIB), an in vivo marker of amyloid-β in the brains of patients with Alzheimer disease, 6 of 7 patients with IBM showed increased PIB levels in at least one gastroc-nemius muscle.[30] The median gastrocnemius muscle PIB was significantly higher in patients with IBM than in 6 patients without IBM. In 2 patients with IBM with radiographically increased PIB uptake, gastrocnemius muscle biopsy showed several fibers with dense amyloid-β and PIB-positive inclusions. However, another patient with IBM with normal deltoid muscle PIB uptake was pathologically positive for amyloid-β without any detectable PIB-positive inclusions.

Muscle Histopathology

IBM pathology shows combined evidence of an inflammatory process with marked degenerative changes. Besides endomysial inflammation invading nonnecrotic fibers (**Fig. 2**A), the presence of small groups of atrophic fibers; eosinophilic cytoplasmic inclusions; and, importantly, multiple myofibers with 1 or more rimmed vacuoles lined with granular material strongly supports the diagnosis of IBM (see **Fig. 2**B). Twenty percent of IBM cases are mislabeled as polymyositis (PM) when no vacuoles are found even though they have classic IBM clinical phenotype.[31] Repeat muscle biopsies may be necessary to detect vacuoles in treatment-refractory patients with the phenotype of IBM and histopathology of PM.[5,7] To add to the complexity, patients who have steroid-responsive PM may have a few rimmed vacuoles.[32] Although better visualized on immunostaining of phosphorylated tau (with SMI-31), eosinophilic cytoplasmic inclusions are rarely seen in IBM.

The Congo red method occasionally shows positive material in vacuolated fibers that is likely to represent amyloid deposits. Ubiquitin-positive multiprotein aggregates contain misfolded proteins in the β-pleated sheet conformation of amyloid, especially amyloid composed of proteolytic Aβ42 within and next to the vacuoles. Fluorescent methods for detecting amyloid material are more sensitive than the Congo red. There is evidence for mitochondrial stress, as shown by abnormally increased numbers of ragged red fibers or of cyclooxygenase-negative/succinate dehydrogenase-positive fibers. Some nuclei containing eosinophilic inclusions seem to be enlarged within or at the edge of the vacuoles. There is an increased likelihood of finding 15-nm to 18-nm tubulofilamentous cytoplasmic and intranuclear inclusions on electron microscopy (EM) when at least 3 vacuolated fibers are examined. The eosinophilic cytoplasmic inclusions correspond with the tubulofilamentous inclusions. Identifying more than 1 rimmed vacuole, more than 1 group of atrophic fibers per high-power field, and endomysial inflammation is 95% predictive of finding the filamentous inclusions on EM.[5]

There are several histopathologic similarities between PM and IBM.[33] In both, intact myofibers are surrounded and invaded by endomysial inflammatory cells that consist

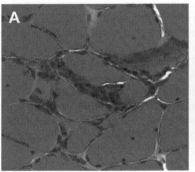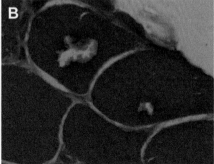

Fig. 2. (A) Polymyositis: inflammatory infiltrates invading nonnecrotic fibers (20×; hematoxylin and eosin stain). (B) IBM muscle: muscle fibers with rimmed vacuoles (40×; modified Gomori trichrome stain).

of macrophages and cytotoxic CD8+ T cells with major histocompatibility complex 1 (MHC-1) expression on the surface of necrotic and nonnecrotic myofibers. In addition, myeloid dendritic cells surround nonnecrotic fibers and present antigen to CD8+ lymphocytes. However, mononuclear cells invade nonnecrotic muscle fibers more frequently in IBM than in PM.[31]

Patients who have typical IBM clinical features but few inflammatory cells or few rimmed vacuoles can be difficult to diagnose.[7] Both of the 1995 Griggs IBM diagnostic categories (definite and possible IBM) require inflammation with invasion of nonnecrotic muscle fibers by mononuclear cells (discussed later).[34] In addition to an endomysial inflammatory exudate, definite IBM histopathology includes the identification of vacuolated muscle fibers and either intracellular amyloid deposits or 15-nm to 18-nm tubulofilaments on EM. According to the 2010 IBM diagnostic criteria,[35] the pathologic features of clinically defined IBM and of possible IBM require at least 1 of the following: invasion of nonnecrotic fibers by mononuclear cells, rimmed vacuoles, or increased MHC-1 expression on the surface of intact muscle fibers. Since then, it has been suggested that sarcoplasmic redistribution of Tar DNA binding protein 43 (TDP-43) is highly sensitive and specific in IBM.[36] Based on conventional stains in 36 patients with characteristic clinical features of IBM, 17 had Griggs definite IBM and 19 had possible IBM. On immunohistochemistry, TDP-43 and p62 were the most sensitive markers, accumulating in all definite IBM and in 31% and 37%, respectively, of possible IBM cases.[37] Hence, the European Neuromuscular Centre (ENMC) 2011 criteria introduce 3 additional alternative pathologic findings for the diagnosis of clinically defined IBM and probable IBM (**Table 2**), including 15-nm to 18-nm filaments, accumulation of amyloid (as shown on Congo red, crystal violet, or thioflavine T/S), or increase in other proteins (as evident on immunostains with antibodies to p62, SMI-31, or TDP-43).

Pathogenesis

Based on endomysial inflammation, IBM was originally thought to be a primary inflammatory myopathy. However, there is a significant body of evidence in support of a neurodegenerative cause including the deposition of p62 and redistribution of TDP-43. The exact contribution of these two pathways to the pathogenesis of IBM remains unknown.

Autoimmune modes of injury in IBM are supported by the identification of cytotoxic T cells, myeloid dendritic cells (mDCs), B cells, and the recently discovered IBM autoantibody.[38,39] As in PM, clonally restricted cytotoxic T cells invade nonnecrotic muscle fibers and destroy them through perforin, granzyme A, and granulysin pathways. The frequency of intact muscle fiber invasion in IBM is higher than that observed for vacuolated fibers or fibers with amyloid deposits. In addition, myeloid dendritic cells serve as antigen-presenting cells.[33] These mDCs help the maturation of naive CD8+ T cells into cytotoxic autoaggressive T cells that surround and invade nonnecrotic muscle fibers. Microarray studies showed an abundance of immunoglobulin transcripts in IBM muscle[40] and led to the recognition of antigen-directed and clonally expanded plasma cells in IBM muscle.[41] As in PM, type 1 interferon genes are modestly upregulated in IBM muscle but, unlike PM, blood derived from patients with IBM does not show this increase. Salajegheh and colleagues[39] recently reported on plasma autoantibodies from 65 people, including 25 with IBM. Immunoblots against normal human muscle show that 13 of 25 (52%) samples from patients with IBM recognized a 43-kDa muscle protein. None of the other disease (N = 25) or healthy volunteer (N = 15) samples recognized this protein. Since then, 2 separate groups confirmed the identity of the antigen to be cytosolic 5'-nucleotidase 1A

Table 2
Proposed diagnostic criteria following ENMC Workshop 2011

Clinical and Laboratory Features	Classification	Pathologic Features
Duration >12 mo Age at onset >45 y Quads weakness ≥ hip flex And/or FF weakness > should abd sCK not >15 × ULN	Clinicopathologically defined IBM	Endomysial inflammation And Rimmed vacuoles And Protein accumulation (amyloid or other proteins)[a] Or Filaments 15–18 nm
Duration >12 mo Age at onset >45 y Quads weakness ≥ hip flex And FF weakness > should abd sCK not >15 × ULN	Clinically defined IBM	One or more of: Endomysial inflammation Or ↑ MHC-1 Or Rimmed vacuoles Or Protein accumulation (amyloid or other proteins)[a] Or Filaments 15–18 nm
Duration >12 mo Age at onset >45 y Quads weakness ≥ hip flex or FF weakness > should abd sCK not >15 × ULN	Probable IBM	One or more of: Endomysial exudate Or ↑ MHC-1 Or Rimmed vacuoles Or Protein accumulation (amyloid or other proteins)[a] Or Filaments 15–18 nm

Abbreviations: abd, abdominals; flex, flexors; MHC-1, major histocompatibility complex 1; sCK, serum CK; should, shoulders; ULN upper limit of normal.

[a] Amyloid or other protein accumulation by established methods: for amyloid Congo red, crystal violet, thioflavine T/S, and for other proteins p62, SMI-31, TDP-43.

Adapted from Machado P, Brady S, Hanna MG. Update in inclusion body myositis. Curr Opin Rheumatol 2013;25(6):763–71; with permission.

(cN1A).[42,43] Moderate reactivity of anti-cN1A autoantibodies was 70% sensitive and 92% specific, and high reactivity was 34% sensitive and 98% specific for the diagnosis of IBM.[42] cN1A reactivity by immunohistochemistry accumulated in perinuclear regions and rimmed vacuoles in IBM muscle, localizing to areas of myonuclear degeneration. In the Dutch study, high concentrations of cN1A autoantibodies were confirmed in 33% of sera from patients with IBM, whereas their prevalence in dermatomyositis, PM, and other neuromuscular disorders was rare (4.2%, 4.5%, and 3.2%, respectively).[43]

Support for a degenerative pathophysiology originated from the lack of IBM response to immunomodulatory therapies. Immunohistochemical evidence backing the degenerative pathogenesis model of IBM stems from the identification in vacuolated muscle fibers of protein aggregates often associated with other neurodegenerative diseases. These aggregates include amyloid-β, hyperphosphorylated tau, ubiquitin, neurofilament heavy chain, presenilin, and parkin and are postulated to occur because of aberrant protein misfolding and accumulation.[44] Mechanisms contributing to this defect include the inhibition of the 26S proteasome system, over-expression of various heat shock proteins such as alpha B-crystallin (induced by the β-amyloid precursor protein),[45] and impairment of autophagy.[46] Until recently, propo-nents of the autoimmune theory of IBM have countered about the lack of critically sup-ported data showing the presence of amyloid proteins deposits on muscle Western blot. In addition, amyloid precursor protein that is secreted by inflammatory cells has also been shown in PM tissues. Besides its presence in 10 IBM samples, tau immunoreactivity was shown in myonuclei of 10 normal subjects and 10 cases of PM/dermatomyositis, suggesting a lack of specificity to tau of standard so-called antitau antibodies including those directed at SMI-31.[47] Nogalska and colleagues[48] reported in 2010 that IBM muscle samples had accumulations of toxic low-molecular-weight amyloid-β oligomers on dot immunoblots with a variety of molecular weights and intensities but none of the control muscle biopsies had amyloid-β oligo-mers. Nonfibrillar cytotoxic Aβ-derived diffusible ligands originally derived from Aβ42 are prominently increased on dot immunoblots, being consistent with the concept that intracellular toxicity of Aβ42 oligomers is likely an important aspect of IBM pathogen-esis. In addition, they showed in cultured human muscle fibers that inhibition of autophagy is a novel cause of Aβ oligomerization.[48] A recent positron emission tomo-graphy study using PIB, a marker of amyloid-β, confirmed increased PIB uptake in the gastrocnemius muscle of patients with IBM.[30]

There is also myonuclear degeneration early in IBM because most rimmed vacuoles are lined with nuclear membrane proteins. IBM myonuclei are often abnormally filled with neurofilaments and this may be the earliest detectable pathologic change in IBM.[21] TDP-43, which acts as a scaffold for nuclear bodies through an interaction with survival motor neuron protein, is redistributed from nuclei to sarcoplasm in a large percentage of IBM myofibers, reflecting a defect in nucleocytoplasmic shuttling.[36] The extranuclear accumulation of TDP-43 is toxic to cells through RNA binding. p62, also known as sequestosome 1, is a shuttle protein transporting polyubiquitinated proteins for their degradation by the proteasome and lysosome and is a component of the inclusions in several neurodegenerative disorders. TDP-43 and p62 accumulate in all definite IBM and in a third of possible IBM cases.[37] Thus, IBM muscle accumu-lates multiple toxic protein aggregates, suggesting a disorder of protein homeostasis.

DIAGNOSTIC AND RESEARCH CRITERIA

A multitude of IBM criteria have been proposed based on a variety of clinical and his-topathologic features. Although these have been advanced for research use, they have permeated into the clinical realm. This article limits discussion to the 4 most prominent criteria sets, namely those by Griggs, the ENMC 2000, MRC 2010, and ENMC 2011. The 1995 Griggs IBM criteria represent the first major effort to define diagnostic criteria for IBM and are heavily weighted toward muscle pathology because cases classified as definite IBM only need to show histopathologic findings of inflam-matory myopathy with mononuclear cell invasion of nonnecrotic muscle fibers, vacu-olated muscle fibers, and either intracellular amyloid deposits or 15-nm to 18-nm tubulofilaments by EM. The original 1995 criteria also included the category of possible IBM in patients with only inflammation on muscle biopsy but with some spe-cific clinical features: age at onset exceeding 30 years, illness duration greater than 6 months, CK less than 12 times the upper normal limit, and electromyogram consis-tent with inflammatory myopathy (long-duration potentials are acceptable).[34] In possible IBM, muscle weakness must be in proximal and distal arm and leg muscles and must endorse at least 1 of the following patterns: finger flexor weakness, wrist flexor greater than wrist extensor weakness, and quadriceps muscle weakness (MRC≤4). In 2002, Tawil and Griggs[49] added the category of probable IBM in patients fulfilling possible IBM criteria but with additional histopathologic evidence of rimmed vacuoles. Issues with the Griggs criteria include the low sensitivity of definite IBM, being heavily weighted toward inflammation and difficulty in admitting possible IBM in clinical trials.

ENMC 2000

In 2000, and to improve sensitivity, Badrising and colleagues[9] described the ENMC criteria for definite and probable IBM in cases of slowly progressive sporadic muscle weakness with mononuclear inflammatory infiltrates and invasion of nonnecrotic muscle fibers. Probable IBM also requires either a weakness pattern (finger flexors or wrist flexors more than wrist extensors) or rimmed vacuoles. In ENMC 2000, definite IBM requires both features or, in the absence of typical weakness pattern, presence of both rimmed vacuoles on modified Gomori trichrome and tubulofilaments on EM. In this Dutch series, the sensitivity of Griggs definite IBM was 16%, whereas that of ENMC 2000 definite IBM was 70% and this increase in sensitivity was caused by including Griggs probable IBM under ENMC definite IBM. An issue with the ENMC 2000 set of criteria is that definite IBM required the presence of rimmed vacuoles. The absence of rimmed vacuoles despite inflammation and typical weakness pattern was seen in 20% (16 of 80) of the Mayo Clinic IBM cases.[31] This finding led to the next set of criteria in order to facilitate the diagnosis of patients with IBM who fulfill clinical criteria for IBM but do not have strict pathologic features.

MRC 2010

As a result of the 2008 MRC Center for Neuromuscular Diseases IBM workshop, the MRC 2010 IBM diagnostic criteria were published.[35] Besides pathologically defined IBM (identical with Griggs definite IBM) and for suspected patients presenting with weakness onset after 35 years of age and lasting at least for 12 months, the 2 other categories are clinically defined IBM and possible IBM (essentially the same as defined by the Griggs definite criteria). In clinically defined IBM, weakness involves finger flexion more than shoulder abduction as well as knee extension more than hip flexion. Possible IBM is when weakness follows either of the preceding 2 patterns. The pathologic criteria are identical for possible and clinically defined IBM and require 1 of the following: invasion of nonnecrotic fibers by mononuclear cells or rimmed vacuoles or increased MHC-1 expression on intact muscle fibers.

ENMC 2011

In addition, in 2011, 24 representatives from Europe, Australia, and the United States, including neurologists, rheumatologists, physiotherapists, industry representatives, and patient representatives, convened in Naarden, in the Netherlands. The MRC IBM criteria were further discussed and refined and this led to the newly proposed ENMC 2011 criteria, which are yet to be validated.[50] No longer is definite IBM diagnosis possible based on only pathologic features because the 3 new categories are clinicopathologically defined IBM, clinically defined IBM, and probable IBM (see **Table 2**). All three diagnostic categories require weakness duration greater than 12 months, age at onset more than 45 years, and CK increased up to 15 times. Although weakness in clinicopathologically defined IBM and probable IBM is in the quadriceps muscles more than hip flexors or in finger flexors more than shoulder abductors, both weakness patterns must coexist in clinically defined IBM. Required pathologic features for clinically defined IBM and probable IBM have been relaxed to include at least 1 of the following: endomysial inflammation, rimmed vacuoles, increased MHC-1, 15-nm to 18-nm filaments, or accumulation of amyloid or other proteins (see **Table 2**). Hence, MRC 2010 possible IBM becomes ENMC 2011 probable IBM. Clinicopathologically defined IBM is based on pathologic demonstration of endomysial inflammation, rimmed vacuoles, and 1 of the following: 15-nm to 18-nm filaments on EM, accumulation of amyloid (clarified on Congo red, crystal violet, or thioflavine T/S), or buildup of other proteins (specified on p62, SMI-31, or TDP-43). The relative sensitivity and specificity of all of these methods in IBM remains unproved and requires prospective validation.

Therapy

IBM is refractory to all treatments known to be effective in the IIMs, including prednisone.[5,17] On occasion, there may be a transient and mild improvement in response to corticosteroids (CS) early in the course of the disease[3] or the initial response to CS may be more dramatic in some cases, but it is followed by progressive resistance to therapy over 3 to 6 years.[51] Furthermore, in a long-term observational study of 136 patients, those who received immunosuppressive treatments (52%) were more severely affected on disability scales and on the sporadic IBM (sIBM) weakness composite index compared with those who did not.[52] Progression toward walking handicap was more rapid among patients receiving immunosuppressive treatments. Because immunosuppressive treatments do not ameliorate the natural course of IBM, it has become more controversial whether to offer CS early in the course of IBM.[9] Despite an earlier encouraging report,[5] randomized controlled trials of intravenous immunoglobulin (IVIG) without CS[25,53] and with CS[54] did not show any benefit. IVIG and prednisone reduce some inflammatory and degenerative molecules in the muscles of patients with IBM and in vitro, but do not sufficiently suppress myotoxic and cell stress mediators such as inducible nitric oxide synthase,[55] which may in part explain resistance of sIBM to immunotherapy.

Two Muscle Study Group[56,57] randomized controlled studies of interferon beta-1a at standard or high doses did not reveal any efficacy in IBM. A 48-week randomized controlled trial of methotrexate (MTX) in 44 IBM cases was also negative despite a decrease in serum CK in the MTX group.[58] A 12-month small pilot trial comparing the effect of MTX combined with antithymocyte globulin (n = 6) with that of MTX in 5 patients suggested a mild benefit on muscle myometry in the group taking antithymocyte globulin.[59] A small randomized crossover pilot trial of placebo versus oxandrolone (an androgen receptor agonist) for 12 weeks did not reveal a statistically significant difference in the primary outcome measure of whole-body maximal voluntary isometric contraction (MVICT). However, a significant benefit in upper extremity MVICT was identified.[60] In a small pilot trial, there was no clinically meaningful improvement in handgrip after 12 months of etanercept administration.[61] A small open-label proof-of-principle study of alemtuzumab in IBM showed a reduction in muscle CD3+ lymphocytes but no significant improvement in strength or function.[62] An open-label pilot trial of 12 months of oral simvastatin 40 mg daily confirmed its safety but none of the 10 patients with IBM had a significant clinical improvement.[63] Interleukin (IL)-1β is upregulated in sIBM myofibers, colocalizes with amyloid precursor protein (APP) and promotes the production of APP and amyloid deposits. In a small pilot study to examine whether anakinra, an IL1 receptor antagonist, could benefit patients with sIBM, 4 patients with biopsy-proven sIBM received this drug for a mean period of 7.7 months. No improvement in muscle strength or stabilization was noted in any of the patients based on grip strength and MRC measurements. This treatment failure was thought to be caused by insufficiency of anakinra to suppress the intramuscular IL1, short study duration, or irrelevance of IL1 in the disease process.[64]

Balloon dilation is often performed in IBM and dysphagia with variable response and often transient benefit.[65] Caution is suggested in recommending cricopharyngeal myotomy because there is a report of worsening after that procedure in a patient who also had a hiatal hernia.[66]

Ongoing Research

We developed the IBM functional rating scale (IBMFRS), which is 10-point functional rating scale for patients with IBM (**Box 1**). Based on analysis of 6-month data obtained in the high-dose interferon beta-1a trial,[57,67] the IBMFRS showed statistically significant correlations ($P<.001$) with maximal voluntary isometric contraction, manual muscle testing, and handgrip dynamometry. Compared with these other outcome measures, the IBMFRS was also the most sensitive measure of change.

A 12-month trial of lithium chloride was completed, designed to decrease the activity of glycogen synthase kinase (GSK), an enzyme that has a key role in the development of phosphorylated tau.[68] In addition, lithium in low doses is a well-known autophagy inducer that clears misfolded proteins and altered mitochondria from motor neurons.[69] Fifteen subjects were enrolled; 4 withdrew because of side effects and 9 completed the 12-month study. One year of lithium treatment produced no benefit. Despite a nonsignificant trend on quantitative muscle testing, the average MRC and IBMFRS scores did not improve significantly. Muscle GSK levels did not significantly change. Several experimental agents are being evaluated in ongoing clinical trials, including arimoclomol, BYM338, and follistatin gene transfer therapy, as listed on clinicaltrials.gov. Given the putative role of heat shock protein abnormalities in the pathogenesis of IBM, we conducted a 2-center trial of arimoclomol, a heat shock protein 70 inducer that may therefore prevent protein misfolding. We completed this randomized controlled pilot study in 24 subjects with IBM, 18 of whom received arimoclomol for 4 months and 8 who were on placebo. Preliminary data analysis indicates that arimoclomol is well tolerated and safe in IBM.[70] We identified encouraging trends in some of the secondary outcome measures, including the IBMFRS.[71] These encouraging preliminary signals support moving forward with a large multicenter study of arimoclomol in IBM.

The other 2 ongoing studies are intended to increase muscle size, strength, and function using different approaches, and for more details the reader is referred to clinicaltrials.gov. In the follistatin gene transfer therapy, follistatin gene carried by adeno-associated virus is injected into the thigh muscles of patients with IBM and Becker muscular dystrophy. Using a different approach, Novartis is investigating the efficacy, safety, and tolerability of BYM338 in patients with IBM, as listed on clinicaltrials.gov.

Prognosis

IBM usually progresses to disability without affecting life expectancy. An earlier study had shown that, at 5 years, 10 of 14 cases required a cane or support, and, at 10 years, most cases (3 of 5) were wheelchair confined.[72] After mean disease duration of 7 years,[12] 56% of our cases required an assistive device, with 20% requiring a wheelchair or motorized scooter (see **Table 1**). More recently, 2 long-term observational studies have provided more data on the rate of disease progression of IBM to disability.[52,73] After a mean disease duration of 20 years, the mean yearly decline in strength of 15 surviving patients with IBM ranged from 3.5% to 5.4% as assessed by manual muscle testing and quantitative muscle testing, respectively.[74] This decline

Box 1
IBMFRS

1. Swallowing
   - 4, Normal
   - 3, Early eating problems; occasional choking
   - 2, Dietary consistency changes
   - 1, Frequent choking
   - 0, Needs tube feeding
2. Handwriting (with dominant hand before IBM onset)
   - 4, Normal
   - 3, Slow or sloppy; all words are legible
   - 2, Not all words are legible
   - 1, Able to grip pen but unable to write
   - 0, Unable to grip pen
3. Cutting food and handling utensils
   - 4, Normal
   - 3, Somewhat slow and clumsy, but no help needed
   - 2, Can cut most foods, although clumsy and slow; some help needed
   - 1, Food must be cut by someone, but can still feed slowly
   - 0, Needs to be fed
4. Fine motor tasks (opening doors, using keys, picking up small objects)
   - 4, Independent
   - 3, Slow or clumsy in completing task
   - 2, Independent but requires modified techniques or assistive devices
   - 1, Frequently requires assistance from caregiver
   - 0, Unable to complete task
5. Dressing
   - 4, Normal
   - 3, Independent but with increased effort or decreased efficiency
   - 2, Independent but requires assistive devices or modified techniques (Velcro snaps, shirts without buttons, and so forth)
   - 1, Requires assistance from caregiver for some clothing items
   - 0, Total dependence
6. Hygiene (bathing and toileting)
   - 4, Normal
   - 3, Independent but with increased effort or decreased activity
   - 2, Independent but requires use of assistive devices (shower chair, raised toilet seat, and so forth)
   - 1, Requires occasional assistance from caregiver
   - 0, Completely dependent

7. Turning in bed and adjusting covers

- 4, Normal
- 3, Somewhat slow and clumsy but no help needed
- 2, Can turn alone or adjust sheets, but with great difficulty
- 1, Can initiate, but not turn or adjust sheets alone
- 0, Incapable or requires total assistance

8. Sit to stand

- 4, Independent (without use of arms)
- 3, Performs with substitute motions (leaning forward, rocking) but without use of arms
- 2, Requires use of arms
- 1, Requires assistance from a device or person
- 0, Unable to stand

9. Walking

- 4, Normal
- 3, Slow or mild unsteadiness
- 2, Intermittent use of an assistive device (eg, ankle-foot orthosis, cane, walker)
- 1, Dependent on assistive device
- 0, Wheelchair dependent

10. Climbing stairs

- 4, Normal
- 3, Slow with hesitation or increased effort; uses hand rail intermittently
- 2, Dependent on hand rail
- 1, Dependent on hand rail and additional support (cane or person)
- 0, Cannot climb stairs

Adapted from Jackson CE, Barohn RJ, Gronseth G, et al, Muscle Study Group. Inclusion body myositis functional rating scale: a reliable and valid measure of disease severity. Muscle Nerve 2008;37(4):473–6; with permission.

resulted in progressive impairment in activities of daily living and all 15 patients with IBM were using wheelchairs after a mean disease duration of 20 years, with 7 of the patients (47%) being completely wheelchair bound. In another study of 136 cases followed in clinics in Paris, France, and Oxford, United Kingdom, between 1990 and 2008, 75% of patients had significant walking difficulties.[52] Thirty-seven percent used a wheelchair after a median duration from onset of 14 years, the 95% confidence interval being 13 to 18 years. Disease progression toward walking handicap was more rapid among men, patients older at first symptoms, and (as noted earlier) patients receiving immunosuppressive treatments.[52] At 1-year follow-up of 23 IBM cases, manual muscle testing, quadriceps quantitative muscle testing (QMT), and IBMFRS significantly declined by 5.2%, 27.9%, and 13.8%, respectively.[74] QMT of the quadriceps muscle and IBMFRS were the most sensitive measures of disease progression. After a median time of 7 years of disease duration, 63% of patients had lost independent ambulation. Disease onset after 55 years of age, but not sex or treatment, predicted a shorter time to requirement of a cane.

Exercise

There is a role for physical therapy, orthotic devices, occupational therapy, a healthy well-balanced diet, and exercise in IBM. Despite falls being a common occurrence for people with IBM, falls guidelines are not being followed, and referral rates to physiotherapy need to improve.[13] A tailored 12-week home exercise program, 5 days a week for 12 weeks, in combination with stationary biking or walks was safe in 7 patients.[75] There was no strength deterioration, no change in serum CK, and no increase in muscle inflammation on biopsy. However, the study was not able to show improved muscle strength or function.

Other investigators recently reported the benefits of a 16-week home exercise program performed twice per day in 7 patients with IBM, 2 of whom used a cane and another 2 a motorized scooter.[76] The exercises consisted of whole-body sit-to-stand exercises, biceps curl, shoulder press, heel lifts, isometric vastus medialis exercises, and ankle dorsiflexion. Patients improved in all muscle groups, including hip flexion, elbow extension, knee flexion and extension, and grip strength. Timed functional tests (to climb 1 flight of stairs and to walk 30 m) were also improved. In another report, the same group of investigators described the effects of an aerobic exercise program using a stationary cycle ergometer at 80% of the initial maximal heart rate combined with the resistance isometric and isotonic exercises of the upper and lower limbs mentioned earlier in a group of 7 IBM cases.[77] Besides showing safety, this exercise routine improved aerobic capacity and muscle strength in shoulder abduction, hip flexion, hip abduction, and knee flexion. However, no changes were noted in knee extension and grip strength and there were no significant changes in stair time or 30-m walk test.

Given the encouraging safety data, we recommend to our patients with IBM nonfatiguing exercises of mild to moderate-intensity. There is a suggestion that exercise might lead to modestly improved or sustained muscle strength in some patients. However, there are conflicting data on the effect of exercise on the 2 muscle groups most severely affected in IBM (finger flexors and knee extensors) and on the potential for functional mobility benefit. Large multicenter controlled trials are needed to clarify any potential gains from exercise in people with IBM.

SUMMARY

IBM is the most common inflammatory myopathy after age 50 years. Despite similarities with PM inflammatory disorders, IBM histopathology shows marked degeneration and protein aggregation. The clinical phenotype of typical IBM is distinctive, manifesting as proximal leg or distal arm weakness, although in our experience there are several phenotypic variants. IBM is refractory to all known immunosuppressive therapies. Low-intensity exercise may slow the rate of functional decline. Patients with IBM are highly motivated and should be encouraged to participate in clinical trials.

REFERENCES

1. Phillips BA, Zilko PJ, Mastaglia FL. Prevalence of sporadic inclusion body myositis in Western Australia. Muscle Nerve 2000;23(6):970–2.
2. Tan JA, Roberts-Thomson PJ, Blumbergs P, et al. Incidence and prevalence of idiopathic inflammatory myopathies in South Australia: a 30-year epidemiologic study of histology-proven cases. Int J Rheum Dis 2013;16(3):331–8.
3. Lindberg C, Persson LI, Bjorkander J, et al. Inclusion body myositis: clinical, morphological, physiological and laboratory findings in 18 cases. Acta Neurol Scand 1994;89:123–31.

4. Wilson FC, Ytterberg SR, St Sauver JL, et al. Epidemiology of sporadic inclusion body myositis and polymyositis in Olmsted County, Minnesota. J Rheumatol 2008;35(3):445–7.
5. Lotz BP, Engel AG, Nishino H, et al. Inclusion body myositis. Observations in 40 patients. Brain 1989;112(Pt 3):727–47.
6. Badrising UA, Maat-Schieman ML, van Houwelingen JC, et al. Inclusion body myositis. Clinical features and clinical course of the disease in 64 patients. Neurology 2005;252(12):1448–54.
7. Amato AA, Gronseth GS, Jackson CE, et al. Inclusion body myositis: clinical and pathological boundaries. Ann Neurol 1995;40:581–6.
8. Barohn RJ, Amato AA. Inclusion body myositis. Curr Treat Options Neurol 2000; 2:7–12.
9. Badrising UA, Maat-Schieman M, van Duinen SG, et al. Epidemiology of inclusion body myositis in the Netherlands: a nationwide study. Neurology 2000;55: 1385–7.
10. Sayers ME, Chou SM, Calabrese LH. Inclusion body myositis: analysis of 32 cases. J Rheumatol 1992;19:1385–9.
11. Needham M, James I, Corbett A, et al. Sporadic inclusion body myositis: phenotypic variability and influence of HLA-DR3 in a cohort of 57 Australian cases. J Neurol Neurosurg Psychiatry 2008;79(9):1056–60.
12. Estephan B, Barohn RJ, Dimachkie MM, et al. Sporadic IBM: a case cohort. J Clin Neuromuscul Dis 2011;12(3):18–9.
13. Hiscock A, Dewar L, Parton M, et al. Frequency and circumstances of falls in people with inclusion body myositis: a questionnaire survey to explore falls management and physiotherapy provision. Physiotherapy 2013;100:61–5 pii: S0031-9406(13) 00073–4.
14. Goodman BP, Liewluck T, Crum BA, et al. Camptocormia due to inclusion body myositis. J Clin Neuromuscul Dis 2012;14(2):78–81.
15. Finsterer J, Stöllberger C, Kovacs GG. Asymptomatic hyper-creatine-kinase-emia as sole manifestation of inclusion body myositis. Neurol Int 2013;5(2):34–6.
16. Jethava A, Ali S, Dasanu CA. Primary respiratory failure due to inclusion body myositis: think outside the box. Conn Med 2013;77(3):155–8.
17. Barohn RJ, Amato AA, Sahenk Z, et al. Inclusion body myositis: explanation for poor response to immunosuppressive therapy. Neurology 1995;45(7):1302–4.
18. Ghosh PS, Laughlin RS, Engel AE. Inclusion body myositis presenting with facial diplegia. Muscle Nerve 2013;49:287–9. http://dx.doi.org/10.1002/mus.24060.
19. Garlepp MJ, Laing B, Zilko PJ, et al. HLA associations with inclusion body myositis. Clin Exp Immunol 1994;98:40–5.
20. Rothwell S, Cooper RG, Lamb JA, et al. Entering a new phase of immunogenetics in the idiopathic inflammatory myopathies. Curr Opin Rheumatol 2013;25(6):735–41.
21. Amato AA, Barohn RJ. Inclusion body myositis: old and new concepts. J Neurol Neurosurg Psychiatry 2009;80(11):1186–93.
22. Mercuri E, Pichiecchio A, Allsop J, et al. Muscle MRI in inherited neuromuscular disorders: past, present, and future. J Magn Reson Imaging 2007;25(2):433–40.
23. Degardin A, Morillon D, Lacour A, et al. Morphologic imaging in muscular dystrophies and inflammatory myopathies. Skeletal Radiol 2010;39(12):1219–27.
24. Cox FM, Reijnierse M, van Rijswijk CS, et al. Magnetic resonance imaging of skeletal muscles in sporadic inclusion body myositis. Rheumatology 2011; 50(6):1153–61.
25. Amato AA, Barohn RJ, Jackson CE, et al. Inclusion body myositis: treatment with intravenous immunoglobulin. Neurology 1994;44(8):1516–8.

26. Wagner KR, Fleckenstein JL, Amato AA, et al. A phase I/II trial of MYO-029 in adult subjects with muscular dystrophy. Ann Neurol 2008;63(5):561–71.

27. Glover GH, Schneider E. Three-point Dixon technique for true water/fat decomposition with B0 inhomogeneity correction. Magn Reson Med 1991;18(2):371–83.

28. Hiba B, Richard N, Hébert LJ, et al. Quantitative assessment of skeletal muscle degeneration in patients with myotonic dystrophy type 1 using MRI. J Magn Reson Imaging 2012;35(3):678–85.

29. Maillard SM, Jones R, Owens C, et al. Quantitative assessment of MRI T2 relaxation time of thigh muscles in juvenile dermatomyositis. Rheumatology (Oxford) 2004;43(5):603–8.

30. Maetzler W, Reimold M, Schittenhelm J, et al. Increased [11C]PIB-PET levels in inclusion body myositis are indicative of amyloid beta deposition. J Neurol Neurosurg Psychiatry 2011;82(9):1060–2.

31. Chahin N, Engel AG. Correlation of muscle biopsy, clinical course, and outcome in PM and sporadic IBM. Neurology 2008;70(6):418–24.

32. Van der Meulen MF, Hoogendijk JE, Moons KG, et al. Rimmed vacuoles and the added value of SMI-31 staining in diagnosing sporadic inclusion body myositis. Neuromuscul Disord 2001;11:447–51.

33. Greenberg SA, Pinkus GS, Amato AA, et al. Myeloid dendritic cells in inclusion-body myositis and polymyositis. Muscle Nerve 2007;35(1):17–23.

34. Griggs RC, Askanas V, DiMauro S, et al. Inclusion body myositis and myopathies. Ann Neurol 1995;38(5):705–13.

35. Hilton-Jones D, Miller A, Parton M, et al. Inclusion body myositis: MRC centre for neuromuscular diseases, IBM workshop, London, 13 June 2008. Neuromuscul Disord 2010;20(2):142–7.

36. Salajegheh M, Pinkus JL, Taylor JP, et al. Sarcoplasmic redistribution of nuclear TDP-43 in inclusion body myositis. Muscle Nerve 2009;40:19–31.

37. Dubourg O, Wanschitz J, Maisonobe T, et al. Diagnostic value of markers of muscle degeneration in sporadic inclusion body myositis. Acta Myol 2011; 30(2):103–8.

38. Greenberg SA. Inclusion body myositis. Curr Opin Rheumatol 2011;23(6): 574–8.

39. Salajegheh M, Lam T, Greenberg SA. Autoantibodies against a 43 kDa muscle protein in inclusion body myositis. PLoS One 2011;6:e20266.

40. Greenberg SA, Sanoudou D, Haslett JN, et al. Molecular profiles of inflammatory myopathies. Neurology 2002;59(8):1170–82.

41. Greenberg SA, Bradshaw EM, Pinkus JL, et al. Plasma cells in muscle in inclusion body myositis and polymyositis. Neurology 2005;65(11):1782–7.

42. Larman HB, Salajegheh M, Nazareno R, et al. Cytosolic 5'-nucleotidase 1A autoimmunity in sporadic inclusion body myositis. Ann Neurol 2013;73(3):408–18.

43. Pluk H, van Hoeve BJ, van Dooren SH, et al. Autoantibodies to cytosolic 5'-nucleotidase 1A in inclusion body myositis. Ann Neurol 2013;73(3):397–407.

44. Askanas V, Engel WK. Inclusion-body myositis: a myodegenerative conformational disorder associated with Abeta, protein misfolding, and proteasome inhibition. Neurology 2006;66(2 Suppl 1):S39–48.

45. Wojcik S, Engel WK, McFerrin J, et al. Overexpression and proteasome inhibition increase alpha B-crystallin in cultured human muscle: relevance to inclusion-body myositis. Neuromuscul Disord 2006;16(12):839–44.

46. Askanas V, Engel WK. Sporadic inclusion-body myositis: conformational multifactorial ageing-related degenerative muscle disease associated with proteasomal and lysosomal inhibition, endoplasmic reticulum stress, and accumulation

of amyloid-β42 oligomers and phosphorylated tau. Presse Med 2011;40(4 Pt 2): e219–35.

47. Salajegheh M, Pinkus JL, Nazareno R, et al. Nature of "Tau" immunoreactivity in normal myonuclei and inclusion body myositis. Muscle Nerve 2009;40(4): 520–8.

48. Nogalska A, D'Agostino C, Engel WK, et al. Novel demonstration of amyloid-β oligomers in sporadic inclusion-body myositis muscle fibers. Acta Neuropathol 2010;120(5):661–6.

49. Tawil R, Griggs RC. Inclusion body myositis. Curr Opin Rheumatol 2002;14: 653–7.

50. Machado P, Brady S, Hanna MG. Update in inclusion body myositis. Curr Opin Rheumatol 2013;25(6):763–71.

51. Verma A, Bradley WG, Ringel SP. Treatment-responsive polymyositis transforming into inclusion body myositis. Neurology 2008;P060:19.

52. Benveniste O, Guiguet M, Freebody J, et al. Long-term observational study of sporadic inclusion body myositis. Brain 2011;134(Pt 11):3176–84.

53. Dalakas MC, Sonies B, Dambrosia J, et al. Treatment of inclusion-body myositis with IVIg: a double-blind, placebo-controlled study. Neurology 1997;48:712–6.

54. Dalakas MC, Koffman B, Fujii M, et al. A controlled study of intravenous immunoglobulin combined with prednisone in the treatment of IBM. Neurology 2001; 56:323–7.

55. Zschüntzsch J, Voss J, Creus K, et al. Provision of an explanation for the inefficacy of immunotherapy in sporadic inclusion body myositis: quantitative assessment of inflammation and β-amyloid in the muscle. Arthritis Rheum 2012; 64(12):4094–103.

56. Muscle Study Group. Randomized pilot trial of betaINF1a (Avonex) in patients with inclusion body myositis. Neurology 2001;57:1566–70.

57. Muscle Study Group. Randomized pilot trial of high-dose betaINF-1a in patients with inclusion body myositis. Neurology 2004;63:718–20.

58. Badrising UA, Maat-Schieman ML, Ferrari MD, et al. Comparison of weakness progression in inclusion body myositis during treatment with methotrexate or placebo. Ann Neurol 2002;51:369–72.

59. Lindberg C, Trysberg E, Tarkowski A, et al. Anti-T-lymphocyte globulin treatment in inclusion body myositis: a randomized pilot study. Neurology 2003;61:260–2.

60. Rutkove SB, Parker RA, Nardin RA, et al. A pilot randomized trial of oxandrolone in inclusion body myositis. Neurology 2002;58(7):1081–7.

61. Barohn RJ, Herbelin L, Kissel JT, et al. Pilot trial of etanercept in the treatment of inclusion-body myositis. Neurology 2006;66(2 Suppl 1):S123–4.

62. Dalakas MC, Rakocevic G, Schmidt J, et al. Effect of Alemtuzumab (CAMPATH 1-H) in patients with inclusion-body myositis. Brain 2009;132(Pt 6):1536–44.

63. Sancricca C, Mora M, Ricci E, et al. Pilot trial of simvastatin in the treatment of sporadic inclusion-body myositis. Neurol Sci 2011;32(5):841–7.

64. Kosmidis ML, Alexopoulos H, Tzioufas AG, et al. The effect of anakinra, an IL1 receptor antagonist, in patients with sporadic inclusion body myositis (sIBM): a small pilot study. J Neurol Sci 2013;334:123–5 pii:S0022–510X(13)02856-6.

65. Murata KY, Kouda K, Tajima F, et al. Balloon dilation in sporadic inclusion body myositis patients with dysphagia. Clin Med Insights Case Rep 2013;6:1–7.

66. Sanei-Moghaddam A, Kumar S, Jani P, et al. Cricopharyngeal myotomy for cricopharyngeus stricture in an inclusion body myositis patient with hiatus hernia: a learning experience. BMJ Case Rep 2013;22:2013 pii:bcr2012008058.

67. Jackson CE, Barohn RJ, Gronseth G, et al, Muscle Study Group. Inclusion body myositis functional rating scale: a reliable and valid measure of disease severity. Muscle Nerve 2008;37(4):473–6.

68. Saperstein DS, Levine T, Hank N, et al. Pilot trial of lithium treatment in inclusion body myositis. Neurology 2011;76(Suppl 4):A106.

69. Pasquali L, Longone P, Isidoro C, et al. Autophagy, lithium, and amyotrophic lateral sclerosis. Muscle Nerve 2009;40(2):173–94.

70. Wang Y, He J, McVey AL, et al. Twelve-month change of IBMFRS in the arimo-colomol inclusion body myositis pilot study. Poster 7.255 at the American Academy of Neurology Annual Meeting. New Orleans, April 26, 2012.

71. Wang Y, He J, McVey AL, et al. Twelve-month change of IBMFRS in the Arimo-colomol Inclusion Body Myositis Pilot Study. Ann Neurol 2013;74(Suppl 17): S95–6.

72. Sekul EA, Dalakas MC. Inclusion body myositis: new concepts. Semin Neurol 1993;13(3):256–63.

73. Cox FM, Titulaer MJ, Sont JK, et al. A 12-year follow-up in sporadic inclusion body myositis: an end stage with major disabilities. Brain 2011;134(Pt 11): 3167–75.

74. Cortese A, Machado P, Morrow J, et al. Longitudinal observational study of sporadic inclusion body myositis: implications for clinical trials. Neuromuscul Disord 2013;23(5):404–12.

75. Arnardottir S, Alexanderson H, Lundberg IE, et al. Sporadic inclusion body myositis: pilot study on the effects of a home exercise program on muscle function, histopathology and inflammatory reaction. J Rehabil Med 2003;35(1):31–5.

76. Johnson LG, Edwards DJ, Walters SB, et al. The effectiveness of an individualized, home-based functional exercise program for patients with sporadic inclusion body myositis. J Clin Neuromuscul Dis 2007;8:187–94.

77. Johnson LG, Collier KE, Edwards DJ, et al. Improvement in aerobic capacity after an exercise program in sporadic inclusion body myositis. J Clin Neuromuscul Dis 2009;10(4):178–84.

Toxic Myopathies

Mamatha Pasnoor, MD*, Richard J. Barohn, MD,
Mazen M. Dimachkie, MD

KEYWORDS

- Toxic myopathies • Muscle tissue • Statins • Myopathy

KEY POINTS

- Many drugs have potential to cause muscle damage, including commonly prescribed medications, such as statins.
- A good medical history, including current and previous medication history, should be obtained; stopping the offending agent usually leads to improvement of myopathy because muscle cells have the capacity to regenerate.
- Continued use, however, and immune-mediated myopathies can be associated with significant morbidity and mortality.

INTRODUCTION

Many substances, including commonly prescribed medications, can produce adverse effects on muscle.[1–4] Alcohol, one of the oldest substances known, has an ability to cause muscle weakness that has been recognized since the middle of nineteenth century.[5] Adverse effects of pharmaceuticals on muscles have been described mostly within the past 50 years. Cholesterol-lowering medications, in particular the statins,[3,6–9] have been the most commonly prescribed drugs that have been described to cause a myopathy in recent years, and autoimmune mechanisms are discussed in the idiopathic inflammatory myopathy article in this issue by Dimachkie. Medications can have a direct or indirect adverse effect on the muscle. Direct effect can be focal, as might occur secondary to drug injected into tissue, or generalized. Indirect toxic effects may result from the agent creating an electrolyte imbalance or inducing an immunologic reaction. Clinical manifestations of toxic myopathies range from muscle pain to more serious muscle damage, leading to rhabdomyolysis.[1,10] Although some categories of drugs are associated with specific forms of myopathies,

This publication was supported by an Institutional Clinical and Translational Science Award, NIH/National Center for Advancing Translational Sciences Grant Number UL1TR000001. Its contents are solely the responsibility of the authors and do not necessarily represent the official views of the NIH.

Department of Neurology, University of Kansas Medical Center, 3901 Rainbow Boulevard, Kansas City, KS 66160, USA
* Corresponding author.
E-mail address: mpasnoor@kumc.edu

a drug can cause more than one type of myopathy. History of drug use is important in the evaluation of patients presenting with various muscle disorders, and an understanding of the pathophysiology of drug-induced myopathy is useful in the management of these patients.

Clinical presentation

Clinical manifestations of drug-induced myopathy are often indistinguishable from those of myopathies due to other causes, as well as from idiopathic forms. Clinical manifestations can be varied and with combination of various symptoms including diffuse myalgia (muscle pain and stiffness) without any other neurologic signs, painless proximal myopathy (weakness), painful myopathies, focal myopathy with focal area of damage due to injections, myokymia or rhythmic rippling of muscles, mitochondrial myopathy associated with inhibition of mitochondrial DNA and characterized by ragged red fibers, rhabdomyolysis with myoglobinuria, malignant hyperthermia, and secondary effects of myopathies.

PATHOPHYSIOLOGY/PATHOGENESIS

Based on pathogenic mechanisms, 7 main categories of toxic myopathies are recognized[3,4]: (1) necrotizing myopathy, (2) amphiphillic myopathies, (3) antimicrotubular myopathy, (4) mitochondrial myopathy, (5) inflammatory myopathy, (6) hypokalemic myopathy, and (7) steroid myopathy/critical illness myopathy (**Table 1**).

NECROTIZING MYOPATHY
Introduction

Several drugs can cause a generalized necrotizing myopathy, with cholesterol-lowering drugs the major cause of this type of myopathy.[11,12] Other agents include the immunophilins (cyclosporine and tacrolimus); rarely, the antihypertensive agent labetalol; and propofol. With statins, besides toxic necrotizing myopathy, which stops with discontinuation of the medication, recent evidence suggests that they also trigger an autoimmune myopathy that progresses for months after statin discontinuation, referred to as statin-associated necrotizing autoimmune myopathy (SANAM) (see idiopathic inflammatory myopathy article in this issue by Dimachkie).

Statins

Clinical presentation
Although myalgias, weakness, or asymptomatic elevation of creatine kinase (CK) levels[6] occur with statin exposure, severe necrotizing myopathy may be complicated by myoglobinuria and renal failure. The degree of serum CK elevation is proportionate to the amount of muscle damage. Proximal weakness develops after periods of statin exposure, ranging from weeks to years in SANAM. The weakness usually progresses beyond 2 months after statin cessation in the autoimmune variant whereas patients with toxic necrotizing myopathy stabilize in strength and markedly improve within 2 to 3 months of statin cessation. The CK levels are markedly elevated. A retrospective chart review performed at the University of Kansas Medical Center showed 11 of 18 (61%) patients on statins having SANAM and 7 of 18 (39%) with toxic necrotizing myopathy (**Table 2**). Mean age of onset was 55, with more women than men, and disease duration on presentation was 2 to 12 months (see **Table 2**). Proximal leg weakness was the most common presentation with SANAM; few had proximal arm weakness and neck flexor weakness. Respiratory or bulbar dysfunction was not seen in the authors' patients.[13]

Table 1
Toxic myopathies

Pathogenic Classification	Drugs
Necrotizing myopathy	Cholesterol-lowering agents Cyclosporine Labetolol Proprofol Alcohol
Amphiphillic	Chloroquine Hydroxycholoroquine Amiodarone
Antimicrotubular	Cochicine Vincristine
Mitochondrial myopathy	Zidovudine Other HIV-related antiretrovirals
Inflammatory myopathy	L-tryptophan D-Penicillamine Cimetidine Phenytoin Lamotrigine Interferon alfa Hydroxyurea Imatinib
Hypokalemic myopathy	Diuretics Laxatives Amphotericin Toluene abuse Licorice Corticosteroids Alcohol abuse
Critical illness myopathy	Corticosteroids Nondepolarizing neuromuscular blocking agents
Others	Omeprazole Isotretinoin Finasteride Emetine

Table 2
Comparison of KU SANAM group with prior literature

	Grable-Esposito et al,[17] 2010	KU
Cases	25	11
Mean age of onset (y)	64.7	55
Female/male ratio	1.1/1	2.6/1
Phenotype	Proximal arm and leg	Proximal leg mainly
Bulbar symptoms	3	2
Poststatin D/C weakness for	>1 mo	>2 mo
Mean CK	8203	5700
Autoimmune d/o and abnormal labs	Hashimoto thyroiditis ANA (2)	— Jo1 (1), ANA (1), and RF
# RX with immunosupressants	22	10

Abbreviations: D/C, discontinuation; d/o, disorder; #RX, no. of patients on treatment.

Laboratory features and electrophysiology

Myositis autoantibody panel is usually negative in these patients but a novel antibody is present in most cases (discussed later). In the authors' SANAM group, 1 patient was antinuclear antigen (ANA) positive and rheumatoid factor positive. One patient also was Jo-1 positive without any evidence for interstitial lung disease. Erythrocyte sedimentation rate (ESR) is usually normal. Electromyography (EMG) showed myopathic units in all SANAM cases, with fibrillation potentials seen in 9 patients and myotonia seen in 5.

Histopathology

Muscle biopsies reveal muscle fiber necrosis with prominent phagocytosis and small basophilic regenerating fibers in patients with elevated serum CK and weakness or myalgias. Lipid-filled vacuoles within myofibers and cytochrome oxidase-negative myofibers are rarely appreciated, but these are not consistent findings.[14] Scattered myofiber necrosis; myophagocytosis, with at times mild perivascular inflammation; and some regenerating myofibers are seen in SANAM.

Pathogenesis

Needham and colleagues in 2007[15] reported an up-regulation of major histocompatibility complex (MHC)-I expression even in non-necrotic fibers of patients presenting with progressive necrotizing myopathy after statin use. Later, Mammen and colleagues, in 2011,[16] showed that statins induce antibody to 200- and 100-kD autoantigens. Statins also up-regulate expression of 3-hydroxy-3-methylglutaryl coenzyme A reductase (HMGCR), which is the main autoantibody target in SANAM. Neural cell adhesion molecule–positive regenerating muscle cells express high levels of HMGCR. This may sustain the immune response even after statin discontinuation.[14,16–19]

Treatment

Multiple long-term immunosuppressive agents are required in most SANAM cases, as described in the idiopathic inflammatory myopathies article in this issue by Dimachkie.

Cholesterol-Lowering Drugs (Excluding Statins)

Niacin, ezetimibe (Zetia), colevesam (Welchol), and fibric acid derivatives, such as fenofibrate and gemfibrozil, are other cholesterol-lowering agents. Although monotherapy with each of these has been reported to cause myopathy in few case reports and review articles,[20] the link between exposure to these drugs and development of myopathy is best established for gemfibrozil. With each agent, the risk of myopathy seems to increase with concomitant statin therapy. Gemfibrozil interferes with statin metabolism, increases statin plasma concentrations, and is associated with increased risk of rhabdomyolysis compared with fenofibrate when coadministered with a statin.[21] Patients may present with myalgias, CK elevations, or weakness that may start a few weeks after starting the medications and sometimes may develop several years after drug initiation.

Immunophilins

The immunophilins (ie, cyclosporine and tacrolimus) are commonly used as immunosuppressive agents, especially in patients requiring transplantation and, rarely, in some autoimmune diseases.

Clinical features
The immunophilins cause generalized myalgias, and proximal muscle weakness develops within months after starting these medications.[22] Myoglobinuria can also occur. Tacrolimus has also been associated with hypertrophic cardiomyopathy and congestive heart failure.[23] In a comprehensive review, including 34 patients who developed myopathy on cyclosporine, only 2 received cyclosporine monotherapy.[24] In remaining cases, cyclosporine was administered along with other potential myotoxins, such as a statin or colchicine, making it difficult to determine whether cyclosporine alone can cause myopathy.

Laboratory features and electrophysiology
Serum CK is usually elevated and nerve conduction studies (NCSs) are usually normal. EMG is remarkable for evidence of increased muscle membrane instability with fibrillation potentials, positive sharp waves, and occasional myotonic potentials. Early recruitment of small-amplitude, short-duration motor unit action potentials (MUAPs) may be demonstrated in weak muscle groups.

Histopathology
Muscle biopsies demonstrate necrosis and nonspecific type 2 muscle fiber atrophy. Sometimes there is evidence of mitochondrial damage, including ragged red fibers and lipid vacuoles.

Pathogenesis
Pathogenic basis is not known. Perhaps these agents destabilize the lipophilic muscle membrane leading to muscle fiber degeneration, due to their cholesterol-lowering effect. This may explain the increased risk of myopathy in patients receiving cyclosporine and the more classic lipid-lowering agents (eg, fibric acid derivatives and statins).[24]

Treatment
Myalgias, muscle strength, and cardiac function improve with reduction or discontinuation of the offending cyclophillin.

Labetolol

Clinical features
Labetolol results rarely in myotoxocity, manifesting as acute or insidious onset proximal weakness or myalgias.[25,26]

Laboratory features and electrophysiology
Serum CK can be markedly elevated. EMG demonstrates increased insertional and spontaneous activity with short duration and small amplitude; polyphasic MUAPs, which recruit early, are evident.

Histopathology
Routine light microscopy can be normal or can reveal necrotic and regenerating fibers. Electron microscopy revealed subsarcolemmal vacuoles in 1 case.[25]

Pathogenesis
Etiology of the muscle necrosis is not known.

Propofol

Clinical features
Propofol is an anesthetic agent that is frequently used for sedation in mechanically ventilated patients and sometimes used for treatment of status epilepticus. Propofol

infusion syndrome is associated with myoglobinuria, metabolic acidosis, acute cardio-myopathy, and skeletal myopathy. This is usually seen with infusion rates of 5 mg/kg/h and greater for more than 48 hours.[27,28] Acute quadriplegic myopathy (AQM) in ICUs has also developed in patients treated with propofol in combination with high-dose intravenous corticosteroids.[28] It remains to be determined, however, if propofol is an independent risk factor for the development of AQM.[29]

Laboratory features
Serum CK levels are markedly elevated. Electrophysiologic findings are not known in children. In adults, however, AQM patients have low-amplitude CMAPs, profuse fibril-lation potentials, positive sharp waves, and early recruitment of short-duration, small-amplitude polyphasic MUAPs.[28]

Histopathology
Muscle biopsies reveal necrosis of skeletal and cardiac muscle.[30] Patients with AQM may have prominent necrosis and loss of thick filaments.[28]

Pathogenesis
Mechanism is unknown. The propofol infusion syndrome, however, is thought to be a failure of free fatty acid metabolism due to inhibition of free fatty acid entry into the mitochondria and to specific sites in the mitochondrial respiratory chain.[27]

Treatment
Propofol should be discontinued and supportive therapy instituted for myoglobinuria, metabolic acidosis, hyperkalemia, and renal failure.

Snake Venom

Clinical features
Some of the snake venoms contain potent myotoxins. For example, venom from the South American rattlesnake (*Crotalus durissus*) causes severe weakness. Snake venom poisoning often involves multiple organ systems.

Histopathology and pathogeneisis
The mechanism depends on the snake venom. The South American rattlesnake venom contains crotamine and other peptides that interact with sodium channels in the sarcolemma and transverse tubules. This results in increased sodium influx and resulting myofiber necrosis. Some snake venoms, such as cobra and viperidae venom, contain peptides with phospholipase A2 activity, which can cause rapid mus-cle–fiber necrosis within a few hours.[31]

Treatment
Snakebite is usually a medical emergency requiring consultation with expert who can be contacted at a regional poison control center.[32]

AMPHIPHILLIC DRUG MYOPATHY (DRUG-INDUCED AUTOPHAGIC LYSOSOMAL MYOPATHY)

Amphiphilic drugs contain separate hydrophobic and hydrophilic domains, which allow the drugs to interact with the anionic phospholipids of cell membranes and organelles.

Chloroquine

Clinical features
Chloroquine, a quinolone derivative, is used for treatment and prevention of malaria due to its ability to disrupt the metabolism of heme. Chloroquine and

hydroxychloroquine are also used to treat dermatomyositis, sarcoidosis, systemic lupus erythematosus, and other connective tissue diseases due to their immunomodulatory effect. Some patients develop slowly progressive, painless, proximal weakness and atrophy, which are worse in the legs than in the arms.[33] A cardiomyopathy can also occur.[34] Sensation is often reduced as are muscle stretch reflexes, particularly at the ankle, secondary to a concomitant neuropathy.[33] This neuromyopathy usually occurs in patients who take 500 mg/d for a year or more but has been reported with doses as low as 200 mg/d. The neuromyopathy improves after chloroquine discontinuation. In a 3-year longitudinal study of patients with rheumatic diseases taking antimalarials, the prevalence of myopathy was 9.2% and the annual incidence of myopathy was 1.2%.[35]

Laboratory features and neurophysiology
Serum CK levels are usually elevated. Motor and sensory NCSs reveal mild to moderate reduction in the amplitudes with slightly reduced velocities in patients with superimposed neuropathy.[36] Individuals with only the myopathy usually have normal motor and sensory studies. Fibrillation potentials and myotonic discharges are seen primarily, but not exclusively, in the proximal limb muscles. Early recruitment of small-amplitude, short-duration polyphasic MUAPs are appreciated in weak proximal muscles. Neurogenic-appearing units and reduced recruitment may be seen in distal muscles that are more affected by toxic neuropathy.

Histopathology
Autophagic vacuoles are evident in as many as 50% of skeletal and cardiac muscle fibers.[33,36,37] Type 1 fibers seem preferentially affected. The vacuoles stain positive for acid phosphatase, suggesting lysosomal origin. On electron microscope (EM), the vacuoles are noted to contain typical concentric lamellar myeloid debris and curvilinear structures. Autophagic vacuoles are also evident in nerve biopsies.

Pathogenesis
Chloroquine is believed to interact with lipid membranes, forming drug-lipid complexes that are resistant to digestion by lysosomal enzymes. This results in the formation of the autophagic vacuoles filled with myeloid debris.

Hydroxychloroquine
Hydroxychloroquine is structurally similar to chloroquine and can cause a neuromyopathy.[33,38] The myopathy is usually not as severe as seen in chloroquine and vacuoles are less prominent on routine light microscopy, but EM still usually demonstrates abnormal accumulation of myeloid and curvilinear bodies.

Amiodarone

Clinical features
Amiodarone is an antiarrhythmic medication that may cause a tremor or ataxia and neuromyopathy.[39,40] The neuromyopathy is characterized by severe proximal and distal weakness along with distal sensory loss and reduced muscle stretch reflexes. The legs are more affected than the arms. The myotoxic effects may be exacerbated in patients who also develop amiodarone-induced hypothyroidism. Patients with renal insufficiency are predisposed to developing the toxic neuromyopathy. Concurrent use of amiodarone and statin increases the risk of statin myopathy.[41]

Laboratory features
Serum CK levels are elevated. Motor and sensory NCSs reveal reduced amplitudes and slowed conduction velocities, particularly in the lower extremities. EMG

demonstrates fibrillation potentials and positive sharp waves in proximal and distal muscles. In proximal muscles, MUAPs are typically polyphasic, short in duration, and small in amplitude and recruit early. Distal muscles are more likely to have large-amplitude, long-duration polyphasic MUAPs with decreased recruitment.

Histopathology
Muscle biopsies demonstrate scattered fibers with autophagic vacuoles. In addition, neurogenic atrophy can also be appreciated, particularly in distal muscles. EM reveals myofibrillar disorganization and autophagic vacuoles filled with myeloid debris. Myeloid inclusions are also apparent on nerve biopsies. These lipid membrane inclusions may be evident in muscle and nerve biopsies as long as 2 years after discontinuation of amiodarone.

Pathogenesis
The pathogenesis is presumably similar to other amphiphilic medications (eg, chloroquine).

Treatment
Muscle strength gradually improves after discontinuation of amiodarone and may take up to 6 months.

ANTIMICROTUBULAR DRUG MYOPATHIES
Colchicine

Clinical features
Colchicine is commonly prescribed for gout and also used for management of familial Mediterranean fever. Colchicine can cause a generalized toxic neuromyopathy.[42] It is weakly amphiphilic, but the toxic effect is believed to arise secondary to its binding with tubulin and prevention of tubulin's polymerization into microtubular structures. The neuromyopathy usually develops after chronic administration but it can also develop secondary to acute intoxication.[42–44] Chronic renal failure, concomitant statin use, and age over 50 years are risk factors for the development of neuromyopathy.[45] Patients usually manifest with progressive proximal muscle weakness over several months. Clinical myotonia has been described.[46,47] A superimposed toxic neuropathy leads to distal sensory loss as well as diminished reflexes.

Laboratory features
Serum CK level is elevated up to 50-fold in symptomatic patients. Serum CK may also be mildly elevated in asymptomatic patients taking colchicine.

Electrophysiologic findings
NCSs reveal reduced amplitudes, slightly prolonged latencies, and mildly slow conduction velocities of motor and sensory nerves in the arms and legs.[42,43] Needle EMG demonstrates positive sharp waves, fibrillation potentials, and complex repetitive discharges, which are detected with ease in all muscle regions. Myotonic discharges may also be seen.[47] The myopathic MUAP abnormalities can be masked in the distal limb muscles secondary to the superimposed peripheral neuropathy.

Histopathology
Muscle biopsies revealed vacuolar changes characterized by acid phosphatase-positive vacuoles and myofibrillar disarray foci. Ultrastructural study demonstrates autophagic vacuoles. Most of the vacuoles express dystrophin but not merosin. One study by Fernandez and colleagues[48] showed several fibers reacted with anti-MHC class I antibody, and granular deposits of membrane attack complex were

observed on the surface of numerous myofibers. Anti–alpha B crystallin antibody strongly reacted with vacuolar content. In addition, nerve biopsies can reveal evidence suggestive of a mild axonal neuropathy.

Pathogenesis
The abnormal assembly of microtubules most likely disrupts intracellular movement of localization of lysosomes, leading to accumulation of autophagic vacuoles. The selective type I involvement is probably due to the higher tubulin amount in type I fibers. Alpha B crystallin overexpression is related to its microtubule protection properties. Fernandez and colleagues[48] suggested that vacuoles randomly floating in sarcoplasm might occasionally meet the plasma membrane and open in the extracellular space, leading to complement activation.

Treatment
Weakness typically resolves within 3 to 4 weeks after discontinuing colchicine.

Vincristine

Clinical features
Vincristine is a chemotherapeutic agent that disrupts gene transcription and promotes the polymerization of tubulin into microtubules. A more common side effect of vincristine is a toxic axonal sensorimotor polyneuropathy that is associated with distal muscle weakness and sensory loss. Proximal muscle weakness and myalgias are less common.[49]

Laboratory features
Serum CK levels have not been reported in patients suspected of having a superimposed myopathy. NCSs demonstrate markedly reduced amplitudes of SNAPs and CMAPs, whereas the distal latencies are slightly prolonged and conduction velocities are mildly slow.[49] Needle EMG demonstrates positive sharp waves, fibrillation potentials, and neurogenic-appearing MUAPS in the distally located muscles of the upper and lower extremities.

Histopathology
Biopsies of distal muscles demonstrate evidence of neurogenic atrophy and, occasionally, the accumulation of lipofuscin granules. Proximal muscle biopsies reveal scattered necrotic fibers.[49] On EM, there is prominent myofibrillar disarray and subsarcolemmal accumulation of osmiophilic material. In addition, some myonuclei contain membrane-bound inclusions. Autophagic vacuoles with spheromembranous debris have been noted in research animals but have not been appreciated in humans.

Pathogenesis
The pathogenic basis of the neuromyopathy is presumably similar to that of colchicine.

DRUG-INDUCED MITOCHONDRIAL MYOPATHIES
Zidovudine (Azidothymidine)

Clinical features
Azidothymidine (AZT), an analog of thymidine, is the nucleoside reverse transcriptase inhibitor (NRTI) that is commonly associated with myopathy.[50] Patients usually present with an insidious onset of progressive proximal muscle weakness and myalgias.[51] These clinical features do not help to distinguish AZT myopathy from other HIV-related myopathies, however, such as polymyositis and inclusion body myositis. Such myopathies related to HIV infection are heterogenous and include inflammatory myopathy, microvasculitis, noninflammatory necrotizing myopathy, type 2 muscle

fiber atrophy secondary to disuse, and wasting due to chronic debility and a toxic myopathy secondary to AZT.[51,52] Regardless of the cause of the myopathy, patients manifest with progressive proximal muscle weakness and myalgias. In addition, muscle weakness may be multifactorial. Given the advent of modern antiretroviral therapies, AZT myopathy is rarely seen.

Laboratory features
Serum CK levels are normal or only mildly elevated in AZT myopathy. Similar elevations are evident, however, in other forms of HIV-related myopathy. A markedly elevated serum CK (eg, greater than 5 times the upper limit of normal) is more suggestive or an HIV-associated polymyositis. Motor and sensory NCSs are normal unless there is a concomitant peripheral neuropathy. Needle EMG may demonstrate positive sharp waves and fibrillation potentials and early recruitment of short-duration, small-amplitude polyphasic MUAPs.[53–55]

Histopathology
An HIV-positive individual patient may have 1 or more of the following: HIV-associated myositis, nemaline rod myopathy, AZT-induced mitochondrial myopathy, and type 2 muscle fiber atrophy. Thus, muscle biopsy may be helpful to differentiate these. Muscle biopsies are remarkable for the presence of ragged red fibers, suggesting mitochondrial abnormalities in AZT myopathy. The number of ragged red fibers correlates with the cumulative dose of AZT.[56] Necrotic fibers, cytoplasmic bodies, nemaline rods, and fibers with microvacuolization may be seen in addition to ragged red fibers.[51,57] In contrast to HIV-associated inflammatory myopathy, significant endomysial inflammation with or without invasion of non-necrotic fibers should not be present in cases of pure AZT myopathy.[58] EM reveals abnormalities of the mitochondria and myofilaments.

Pathogenesis
AZT acts as a false substitute for the viral reverse transcriptase, thereby limiting its enzymatic activity and replication of the HIV virus. AZT also inhibits, however, the activity of mitochondrial DNA polymerase, which probably accounts for the mitochondrial abnormalities. When treated with AZT, patients with HIV have a decrease in quantity of mitochondrial DNA and decline in respiratory chain enzymatic activity compared with untreated infected patients.[59,60] Although AZT is responsible for at least some of the mitochondrial abnormalities evident on muscle biopsy, the contribution of these mitochondrial abnormalities to the muscle weakness remains controversial.

Treatment
Patients with AZT myopathy usually improve after discontinuation of the medication.[51,55] The histologic and molecular abnormalities on repeat muscle biopsies resolve coinciding with clinical improvement after discontinuation of AZT.[61] The major drawback of discontinuing AZT is the possible increase in HIV replication. In patients with normal or only mildly elevated serum CK and normal or only slightly increased spontaneous activity on EMG, it is impossible to distinguish AZT myopathy from other HIV-associated myopathies. One approach is starting a nonsteroidal anti-inflammatory drug with or without decreasing the dose of AZT.[51] If there is still no objective improvement in strength, discontinuation of AZT should be considered. If there is still no objective improvement, patients should undergo a muscle biopsy and be considered for immunomodulating therapy (eg, intravenous immunoglobulin or corticosteroid treatment), if there is histologic evidence of an inflammatory myopathy. Patients can be rechallenged with AZT, particularly if there are no ragged red

fibers on biopsy. Newer therapies have reduced significantly reliance on AZT in HIV treatment.

Other Antiviral Agents

The risk of mitochondrial myopathy with other NRTIs (eg, lamivudine, zalcitabine, and didanosine) is probably less than that of AZT.[62,63] These agents are clearly associated, however, with mitochondrial toxicity, and patients may develop associated hyperlactemia and hepatic steatosis on these medications.[64] In patients with HIV infection, it is unclear if the myopathy was thought due to mitochondrial toxicity, myositis, or wasting syndrome.

DRUG-INDUCED INFLAMMATORY MYOPATHIES
Cholesterol-Lowering Agents

Cholesterol-lowering agents are discussed later.

L-tryptophan/Eosinophilia Myalgia Syndrome

Clinical features
Eosinophilia-myalgia syndrome was described in the late 1980s and 1990s and found caused by a contaminant used in the production of L-tryptophan.[65–69] The clinical, laboratory, electrophysiologic, and histopathologic features were similar to those seen in diffuse fasciitis with eosinophilia (Shulman syndrome[70]). Patients developed a subacute onset of generalized muscle pain and tenderness with variable degrees of weakness. Onset could have been within a few weeks or several years after starting tryptophan. Numbness, paresthesias, arthralgias, lymphadenopathy, dyspnea, abdominal pain, mucocutaneous ulcers, and an erythematous rash were also common. Some patients developed a severe generalized sensorimotor polyneuropathy mimicking Guillain-Barré syndrome[71,72] or multiple mononeuropathies suggestive of a vasculitis.[73]

Laboratory features
The serum CK levels were normal or elevated. Autoantibodies were absent and ESR was usually normal. The absolute eosinophil count was elevated. Decreased amplitudes of compound muscle action potentials (CMAPs) and sensory nerve action potentials (SNAPs) with normal or mildly reduced conduction velocities were evident in patients with a polyneuropathy.[72,73] A few patients with severe Guillain-Barré syndrome had electrophysiologic studies showing multifocal conduction block and slowing of conduction velocities.[74] Needle EMG revealed fibrillation potentials, complex repetitive discharges,[72–74] and small and large polyphasic MUAPs.[72] The electrophysiologic abnormalities improve with discontinuation of tryptophan.

Histopathology
Muscle biopsies demonstrated diffuse or perivascular inflammatory infiltrate in the fascia, perimysium, and to a lesser extent, in the endomysium.[72] A majority of inflammatory cells were CD8+ T cells and macrophages, whereas eosinophils and B cells comprised less than 3% of the infiltrating cells. There was no deposition of membrane attack complex on small blood vessels. Nerve biopsies showed predominantly perivascular inflammatory infiltrate, mainly mononuclear, with occasional eosinophils in the epineurium, endoneurium, and/or perineurium with axonal degeneration.[72,73]

Pathogenesis
The disorder was caused by a contaminant(s) in the manufacture of tryptophan. Two trace adulterants have been identified as the possible toxins: 3-(phenylamino)alanine

and 1,1'-ethylidenebis(tryptophan). The mechanism by which the contaminant resulted in the disorder is unknown, but the eosinophilia and eosinophilic infiltrate in tissues suggest some form of allergic reaction.

Treatment

Discontinuation of L-tryptophan and treatment with high-dose corticosteroids were usually effective in resolution of most of the symptoms.[71]

Toxic oil syndrome

The toxic oil syndrome was similar to the eosinophilia-myalgia syndrome associated with tryptophan.[75] This condition was restricted to a single epidemic in Spain and has not recurred since 1981–1982. The disorder was found significantly associated with consumption of contaminated rapeseed oil produced by a particular refinery. Two compounds, 1,2-di-oleyl ester and oleic anilide, are considered biologically relevant contaminants that may contribute to disease development.

D-Penicillamine

D-Penicillamine is rarely used nowadays to treat Wilson disease, rheumatoid arthritis, and other connective tissue disorders. Besides autoimmune myasthenia gravis, approximately 0.2% to 1.4% of patients treated with D-penicillamine developed an inflammatory myopathy reminiscent of polymyositis or dermatomyositis.[76,77] Discontinuation of the drug results in resolution of the symptoms. The medication may be restarted at a lower dosage without recurrence of the inflammatory myopathy.

Cimetidine

Rare cases of inflammatory myopathy have been reported with cimetidine, a histamine H_2 receptor antagonist. Patients develop generalized weakness and myalgias associated with CK elevations up to 40,000 U/L and interstitial nephritis.[78,79] Muscle biopsy shows perivascular inflammation, predominantly consisting of CD8[+] lymphocytes. There is no deposition of immunoglobulin or complement on small blood vessels nor did patients have a cutaneous rash to suggest dermatomyositis. Cases of cutaneous vasculitis have been described, however, with cimetidine use.[80]

Procainamide

Proximal muscle weakness and myalgias rarely occur with procainamide usage.[81] Serum CK levels are elevated, and EMGs are reported as consistent with a patchy myopathy. Muscle biopsies demonstrate nonspecific perivascular inflammation and rare necrotic muscle fibers. The pathogenesis may be related to lupus-like vasculitis, which can occur in patients treated with procainamide. In one study, Antirapsyn antibodies were reported in chronic procainamide-associated myopathy.[82] The myopathy resolves after withdrawal of procainamide.

Phenytoin

Myalgias and weakness may develop in patients treated with phenytoin due to hypersensitivity reactions.[83] Serum CK levels can be significantly elevated, and muscle biopsies show scattered necrotic, regenerating muscle fibers without evidence of inflammation.[84] EMG can reveal increased spontaneous activity with fibrillation potentials and positive sharp waves. Small-amplitude, short-duration, polyphasic MUAPs, which recruit early, may be observed. The myopathy improves with discontinuation of the phenytoin and a short course of corticosteroids.

Lamotrigine

A case of severe myoglobinuria and renal failure associated with a generalized rash, anemia, leukopenia, and thrombocytopenia shortly after the patient was started on antiepileptic medication, lamotrigine, was reported.[4] Clinical and laboratory features resemble thrombocytic thrombocytopenic purpura. The patient was treated with plasmapheresis and discontinuation of lamotrigine.

Interferon Alfa

Interferon alfa is used in the treatment of viral hepatitis and certain malignancies (eg, chronic myelogenous leukemia [CML] and melanoma). A rare side effect of alpha-interferon is the occurrence of autoimmune disorders, including myasthenia gravis and myositis.[85,86] Overproduction of type 1 interferons, such as interferon alfa, have been implicated in the pathogenesis of dermatomyositis in some studies.[87,88]

Imatinib Mesylate (Gleevic)

Imatinib mesylate (Gleevic) is a tyrosine kinase inhibitor use to treat patients with CML and other solid tumors. Myaglias occur in 21% to 52% of patients[89] and CK elevations in 45%. One patient with CML developed polymyositis while taking imatinib.[90] CML28 antibodies were detected in the patient's serum. CML28 is identical to hRrp46p, a component of the human exosome, a multiprotein complex involved in processing of RNA. Antibodies directed against hRrp46p and other components of the human exome (eg, PM/Scl 100 and PM/Scl 75) have been noted in patients with polymyositis. The patient's strength and serum CK normalized with discontinuation of the imatinib and a course of corticosteroids.

MYOPATHIES DUE TO IMPAIRED PROTEIN SYNTHESIS OR INCREASED CATABOLISM
Steroid Myopathy

Clinical features

Chronic exposure to high-dose oral steroids causes greatest risk of developing steroid myopathy. Prednisone at doses of 30 mg/d or more (or equivalent doses of other corticosteroids) is associated with an increased risk of myopathy.[91] Steroid myopathy may occur, however, after just a few weeks of treatment. Steroid myopathy manifests as proximal muscle weakness and atrophy affecting the legs more than the arms.[91–93] The distal extremities, oculobulbar, facial muscles, sensation, and muscle stretch reflexes are normal. Most patients exhibit a cushingoid appearance with facial edema and increased truncal adipose tissue.[94] Any synthetic glucocorticoid can cause the myopathy, but those that are fluorinated are more likely to result in muscle weakness than the nonflourinated compounds.[95] Women seem more at risk than men (approximately 2:1) of developing a steroid myopathy. Alternate-day dosing may reduce the risk of corticosteroid-induced weakness. Acute onset of severe generalized weakness can occur in patients receiving high dosages of intravenous corticosteroids with or without concomitant administration of neuromuscular blocking agents or sepsis.

Laboratory and electrophysiologic features

Serum CK is normal. Serum potassium can be low as a result of glucocorticoid excess and cause some degree of weakness. Motor and sensory nerve conductions are normal in steroid myopathy.[96,97] Repetitive stimulation studies should not demonstrate a significant decrement or increment. Needle EMG is normal as well as or with subtle myopathic changes without any fibrillation potentials. The paucity of abnormalities is understandable, because corticosteroids preferentially affect type 2 muscle fibers. The first recruited motor units are composed of type 1 muscle fibers. Because these are not affected as severely as type 2 fibers, there is little in the way of electrophysiologic pathology to observe.

Histopathology
Muscle biopsies reveal atrophy of type 2 fibers, especially the fast-twitch, glycolytic-type 2B fibers.[94] There may also be a lesser degree of atrophy of type 1 muscle fibers. Lipid droplets are commonly noted in type 1 fibers, and rare mitochondrial abnormalities have been seen on EM.

Pathogenesis
Corticosteroids bind to receptors on target cells and are subsequently internalized into the nuclei, where these regulate the transcription of specific genes. Exact pathogenesis of corticosteroid myopathy is not known but could be the result of decreased protein synthesis, increased protein degradation, alterations in carbohydrate metabolism, mitochondrial alterations, or reduced sarcolemmal excitability.[94]

Treatment
Reduction in the dose, tapering to an alternate-day regimen, or switching to a non-flourinated steroid along with a low-carbohydrate diet and exercise to prevent concomitant disuse atrophy are major modes of therapy.[94,95]

It is important to distinguish steroid myopathy from an exacerbation of underlying immune-mediated neuromuscular disorder (eg inflammatory myopathy, myasthenia gravis, and chronic inflammatory demyelinating polyneuropathy) in patients treated with corticosteroids.[98] If the weakness developed while a patient was on chronic high doses of steroids, a steroid myopathy should be considered. In cases of inflammatory myopathy, an increasing serum CK and an EMG with prominent increase in insertional and spontaneous activity point to an exacerbation of the myositis.

Finasteride

Clincal features
Finasteride is a used to treat benign prostatic hypertrophy. It is a 4-azasteroid that inhibits 5α-reductase and thus blocks dihydrotestosterone production and androgen action in the prostate and skin. One patient developed severe proximal greater than distal weakness and atrophy while treated with finasteride (5 mg/d)[99]; another patient treated for baldness reported severe myalgias and had elevated CK. Sensation and muscle stretch reflexes were normal.

Laboratory features
Serum CK levels were normal or elevated.

Electrophysiologic findings
NCSs were normal, whereas the EMG demonstrated showed small polyphasic MUAPs.

Histopathology
Muscle biopsy revealed only mild variability in fiber size, type 2 muscle fiber atrophy, and increased central nuclei.

Pathogenesis
The pathophysiologic mechanism for the myopathy is not known. Finasteride is one of the 4-azosteroids and has structural similarity to corticosteroids. Thus, the pathogenic mechanism may be similar to that seen of steroid myopathy.

Treatment
Discontinuation of finasteride was associated with normalization of strength and improvement in CK level and EMG abnormalities.

Emetine

Clinical features
Emetine hydrochloride (ipecac) is an emetic agent that has been abused, particularly in patients with anorexia nervosa and bulimia. A severe proximal myopathy and cardiomyopathy can occur with overuse of emetine (500–600 mg/d for more than 10 days).[100–102] Patients also complain of muscle pain, tenderness, and stiffness. Muscle stretch reflexes are usually diminished, but the sensory examination is completely normal.

Laboratory features
The serum CK levels may be mildly to moderately elevated. Needle EMG examination can be normal, although positive sharp waves and fibrillation potentials are usually apparent. There is early recruitment of small-amplitude, short-duration MUAPs.

Histopathology
Muscle biopsies reveal scattered necrotic fibers, small atrophic and regenerating fibers, and many fibers containing cytoplasmic bodies. Oxidative enzyme stains demonstrate targetoid or moth-eaten structures. On EM, there is evidence of myofibrillar degeneration in addition to compacted myofibrillar debris (cytoplasmic bodies). The histologic appearance of light and electron microscopy is similar to myofibrillar myopathy.[103]

Pathogenesis
The exact pathogenic basis for the disorder is not known, but it is postulated that emetine might inhibit the synthesis of important muscle proteins.

Treatment
The myopathy resolves after discontinued use of emetine.

TOXIC MYOPATHIES WITH UNKNOWN PATHOGENIC MECHANISM
Acute Quadriplegic Myopathy/Critical Illness Myopathy

Clinical features
High-dose corticosteroids may trigger critical illness myopathy, in particular among patients with prolonged ICU stay, mechanical ventilation, or persistent systemic inflammation,[104,105] especially in those who also received nondepolarizing, neuromuscular blocking agents.[106] The first patient reported with this acute form of steroid myopathy was a 24-year-old woman placed on large doses of intravenous hydrocortisone (up to 3 g/d) for status asthmaticus.[107] After 8 days, her airway obstruction resolved, but she was unable to resist gravity in both proximal and distal muscles. She gradually improved and could walk unassisted after 3 weeks but continued to have distal leg weakness after 2 months. Since this initial description, many additional patients have been reported in the literature.[106,108,109] Most prospective studies could not identify corticosteroids, however, as an independent risk factor for critical illness myopathy, summarized in a recent Cochrane review.[110] Similarly, ICU-acquired neuromyopathy was common (34%) among 128 survivors of persistent acute respiratory distress syndrome but was not significantly associated with methylprednisolone treatment.[111] Diffuse weakness develops as early as 4 to 7 days after initiation of corticosteroids.[111,112] Complete flaccid quadriplegia develops in some patients, especially those receiving more than 80 mg total of vecuronium.[109] In a series, distal limb and facial weakness were present in most patients.[109] Extraocular muscles were involved in 1 of 14 patients.

Laboratory features and electrophysiologic findings
In most patients, CK is normal or mildly elevated. EMG findings in this myopathy are variable. Insertional activity may be normal or show fibrillation potentials.[113] Myopathic motor units may be recorded on voluntary contraction,[93] but in severe cases, patients may not be able to recruit any motor units.

Histopathology
Muscle biopsy reveals type II atrophy, necrotic muscle fibers, and/or loss of myosin thick filaments as visualized on the ATPase stain.

Pathogenesis
The mechanism of muscle injury is poorly understood.

Treatment
Supportive care and treating underlying systemic abnormalities. Mortality is high due to the sepsis and organ failure. Corticosteroids and neuromuscular blockers should be discontinued if possible. Physical therapy and occupational therapy to prevent contractures and help regain muscle strength and functional abilities.

Omeprazole

Omeprazole inhibits H^+/K^+ ATPase enzyme system (proton pump) and is used for treatment of gastric and duodenal ulcers and reflux. Rare cases of neuromyopathy have been reported with this. Patients develop proximal weakness and myalgias along with paresthesias and stocking distribution of sensory loss. Muscle reflexes are diminished or absent. Serum CK levels are usually normal or mildly elevated. NCSs may be normal or reveal an axonal sensorimotor polyneuropathy. EMG can be normal or show small polyphasic MUAPs. Muscle biopsies showed type 2 muscle fiber atrophy. Symptoms improve with discontinuation of omeprazole.[114–116]

Isoretinion

Isoretinion (Accutane) is used for treatment of severe acne. Exercise-induced myalgias are common and rarely can develop proximal weakness. Serum CK can be normal or elevated. Rhabdomyolysis has also been reported in few cases. Decreased serum carnitine levels may be seen. EMG shows myopathic MUAPs. Muscle biopsy shows atrophy of muscle fibers. Pathogenic mechanism is not clear. Symptoms improve with discontinuation of medication.[117,118]

MYOPATHIES ASSOCIATED WITH ANESTHETIC AGENTS AND CENTRALLY ACTING MEDICATIONS
Malignant Hyperthermia

Clinical features
Malignant hyperthermia is a rare, genetically heterogenous group of disorders and is characterized by severe muscle rigidity, myoglobinuria, fever, tachycardia, cyanosis, and cardiac arrhythmias precipitated by depolarizing muscle relaxants (eg, succinylcholine) and inhalational anesthetic agents (eg, halothane).[119] The incidence of malignant hyperthermia ranges from 0.5% to 0.0005%. At least 50% of patients had previous anesthesia without any problems. The signs of malignant hyperthermia usually appear during surgery but can develop in the postoperative period and time for first signs could differ among anesthetic drugs.[120] Rarely, attacks of malignant hyperthermia have been triggered by exercise, ingestion of caffeine, and stress. The halothane contracture test or caffeine contracture test can be used to screen for susceptibility to malignant hyperthermia,[121] besides the genetic testing. These tests

are usually available at specialized centers only, however. Minimally invasive, intramuscular halothane, and caffeine test also has been described recently.[122]

Laboratory features and electrophysiologic studies

Serum CK can be normal or high between the attacks. During the attacks, serum CK levels are markedly elevated and myoglobinuria can be seen. Hyperkalemia, hypoxia, and hypercarbia can also be seen during an attack.[123] NCSs and EMG are usually normal in the interictal periods. EMG performed immediately after an attack of malignant hyperthermia may, however, demonstrate increased spontaneous activity and, perhaps, small polyphasic MUAPs recruiting early.

Histopathology

Muscle biopsies demonstrate nonspecific myopathic features and necrotic fibers after an attack.

Pathogenesis and molecular genetics

Numerous susceptibility loci have been identified (**Table 3**) and are associated with mutations of the ryanodine receptor malignant hyperthermia susceptibility (MHS) 1, sodium channels (MHS2), calcium channels (MHS3 and MHS5), and other proteins (including MHS4 and MHS5) and CPT2.

Treatment

Depolarizing muscle relaxants and inhalational anesthetic agents should be avoided in subjects with known susceptibility factors. In those who develop malignant hyperthermia, the anesthetic agent must be stopped and aggressive cooling measures muscle be instituted. In addition to supportive measures, dantrolene (2 mg/kg to 3 mg/kg rapid IV every 5 minutes for a total cumulative dose of 10 mg/kg) should be given.

MYOPATHIES SECONDARY TO DRUGS OF ABUSE
Alcoholic Myopathy

Chronic alcohol abuse more commonly than myopathy causes neuropathy. Several forms of toxic myopathy due to alcohol, however, have been described: acute necrotizing myopathy, acute hypokalemic myopathy, chronic alcoholic myopathy, asymptomatic alcoholic myopathy, and alcoholic cardiomyopathy.[124,125] Acute necrotizing

Table 3
Malignant hyperthermia

Susceptibility Genes	Inheritance Patterns
Ryanodine receptor	Autosomal dominant
SCN4A sodium channel	Autosomal dominant
CACNL2A calcium channel	Autosomal dominant
CACNA1S calcium channel	Autosomal dominant
Carnitine palmitoyltransferase II	Autosomal dominant
Dystrophin	X linked recessive
Myotonin protein kinase	Autosomal dominant
Myotonin protein kinase	Autosomal dominant
CLCN1 chloride channel	Autosomal dominant
Perclan	Autosomal recessive

Data from Mammen AL. Toxic myopathies. Continuum (Minneap Minn) 2013;19(6 Muscle Disease):1634–49.

myopathy patients present with myalgias, muscle cramping, swelling, and weakness after an intense binge drinking. Symptoms are usually associated with elevated CK levels and irritable myopathy on EMG, and, in severe cases, acute renal failure. Muscle biopsies reveal widespread muscle fiber necrosis. CK levels and muscle symptoms may resolve over several weeks; however, they may recur with repeated exposure to alcohol in those who are susceptible to this form of toxic myopathy. Some patients develop acute hypokalemia with weakness evolving over period of 1 to 2 days, low potassium (<2 meq/L), and elevated CK levels. Muscle biopsy may reveal vacuoles. This myopathy resolves with potassium supplementation.

Some alcoholics develop primarily proximal limb-girdle weakness, especially in lower limbs attributed to chonic alcoholic myopathy. Asymptomatic alcoholic myopathy has been suggested in patients with elevated serum CK levels without any weakness. The pathogenic basis for the various forms of alcoholic myopathies is not known and may involve direct toxic effects or malnutrition. The metabolism of alcohol may lead to accumulation of toxic metabolites or free radicals that may be damaging to lipid membranes.

Other Drugs

Illicit drugs and controlled narcotics (heroin, mepeidine, cocaine, pentazocine, pritramide, amphetamine, and so forth) may be myotoxic. Inhalation of volatile agent (eg, toluene) can also cause generalized weakness.

SUMMARY

Many drugs have potential to cause muscle damage, including commonly prescribed medications, such as statins. A good medical history, including current and previous medication history, should be obtained, because stopping the offending agent usually leads to improvement of myopathy because muscle cells have the capacity to regenerate. Continued use, however, and immune-mediated myopathies can be associated with significant morbidity and mortality. SANAM required chronic immunosuppression.

REFERENCES

1. Dalakas MC. Toxic and drug-induced myopathies. J Neurol Neurosurg Psychiatry 2009;80(8):832–8.
2. Kuncl RW. Agents and mechanisms of toxic myopathy. Curr Opin Neurol 2009; 22(5):506–15.
3. Mammen AL. Toxic myopathies. Continuum (Minneap Minn) 2013;19(6 Muscle Disease):1634–49.
4. Amato AA, Rusell JA. Neuromuscular disorders. In: Amato AA, Russell JA, editors. Toxic myopathies. Chapter 32. New York: McGraw Hill Companies Inc; 2008. p. 737–61.
5. Argov Z, Mastaglia FL. Drug-induced neuromuscular disorders in man. Disorders of voluntary muscle. 6th edition. Edinburgh (United Kingdom): Churchill-Livingstone; 1994. p. 989–1029.
6. Needham M, Mastaglia FL. Statin myotoxicity: a review of genetic susceptibility factors. Neuromuscul Disord 2014;24(1):4–15.
7. El-Salem K, Ababneh B, Rudnicki S, et al. Prevalence and risk factors of muscle complications secondary to statins. Muscle Nerve 2011;44(6):877–81.
8. Greenberg SA, Amato AA. Statin myopathies. Continuum 2006;12(3):169–84.

9. Mohassel P, Mammen AL. The spectrum of statin myopathy. Curr Opin Rheumatol 2013;25(6):747–52.

10. Walsh RJ, Amato AA. Toxic myopathies. Neurol Clin 2005;23(2):397–428.

11. Franc S, Dejager S, Bruckert E, et al. A comprehensive description of muscle symptoms associated with lipid-lowering drugs. Cardiovasc Drugs Ther 2003; 17(5–6):459–65.

12. Sakaeda T, Kadoyama K, Okuno Y. Statin-associated muscular and renal adverse events: data mining of the public version of the FDA adverse event reporting system. PLoS One 2011;6(12):e28124. http://dx.doi.org/10.1371/journal.pone.0028124.

13. Muzyka I, Barohn RJ, Dimachkie M, et al. Necrotizing autoimmune statin-associated myopathy. J Clin Neuromuscul Dis 2011;12(3):17.

14. Phillips PS, Haas RH, Bannykh S, et al, Scripps Mercy Clinical Research Center. Statin-associated myopathy with normal creatine kinase levels. Ann Intern Med 2002;137(7):581–5.

15. Needham M, Fabian V, Knezevic W, et al. Progressive myopathy with up-regulation of MHC-I associated with statin therapy. Neuromuscul Disord 2007; 17(2):194–200.

16. Mammen AL, Pak K, Williams EK, et al. Rarity of anti-3-hydroxy-3-methylglutaryl-coenzyme A reductase antibodies in statin users, including those with self-limited musculoskeletal side effects. Arthritis Care Res (Hoboken) 2012;64(2): 269–72.

17. Grable-Esposito P, Katzberg HD, Greenberg SA, et al. Immune-mediated necrotizing myopathy associated with statins. Muscle Nerve 2010;41(2):185–90. http://dx.doi.org/10.1002/mus.21486.

18. Mammen AL, Chung T, Christopher-Stine L, et al. Autoantibodies against 3-hydroxy-3-methylglutaryl-coenzyme A reductase in patients with statin-associated autoimmune myopathy. Arthritis Rheum 2011;63(3):713–21. http://dx.doi.org/10.1002/art.30156.

19. Werner JL, Christopher-Stine L, Ghazarian SR, et al. Antibody levels correlate with creatine kinase levels and strength in anti-3-hydroxy-3-methylglutaryl-coenzyme A reductase-associated autoimmune myopathy. Arthritis Rheum 2012;64(12):4087–93.

20. Slim H, Thompson PD. Ezetimibe-related myopathy: a systematic review. J Clin Lipidol 2008;2(5):328–34.

21. Alsheikh-Ali AA, Kuvin JT, Karas RH. Risk of adverse events with fibrates. Am J Cardiol 2004;94(7):935–8.

22. Noppen M, Velkeniers B, Dierckx R, et al. Cyclosporine and myopathy. Ann Intern Med 1987;107:945–6.

23. Atkison P, Joubert G, Barron A, et al. Hypertrophic cardiomyopathy associated with tacrolimus in paediatric transplant patients. Lancet 1995;345(8954):894–6.

24. Breil M, Chariot P. Muscle disorders associated with cyclosporine treatment. Muscle Nerve 1999;22(12):1631–6.

25. Teicher A, Rosenthal T, Kissin E, et al. Labetalol-induced toxic myopathy. Br Med J (Clin Res Ed) 1981;282(6279):1824–5.

26. Willis JK, Tilton AH, Harkin JC, et al. Reversible myopathy due to labetalol. Pediatr Neurol 1990;6(4):275–6.

27. Short TG, Young Y. Toxicity of intravenous anaesthetics. Best Pract Res Clin Anaesthesiol 2003;17(1):77–89.

28. Hanson P, Dive A, Brucher JM, et al. Acute corticosteroid myopathy in intensive care patients. Muscle Nerve 1997;20(11):1371–80.

29. Francis L, Bonilla E, Soforo E, et al. Fatal toxic myopathy attributed to propofol, methylprednisolone, and cyclosporine after prior exposure to colchicine and simvastatin. Clin Rheumatol 2008;27(1):129–31.

30. Strickland RA, Murray MJ. Fatal metabolic acidosis in a pediatric patient receiving an infusion of propofol in the intensive care unit: is there a relationship? Crit Care Med 1995;23(2):405–9.

31. Harris JB, Scott-Davey T. Secreted phospholipases A2 of snake venoms: effects on the peripheral neuromuscular system with comments on the role of phospholipases A2 in disorders of the CNS and their uses in industry. Toxins (Basel) 2013;5(12):2533–71. http://dx.doi.org/10.3390/toxins5122533.

32. Gold BS, Dart RC, Barish RA. Bites of venomous snakes [review]. N Engl J Med 2002;347(5):347–56.

33. Estes ML, Ewing-Wilson D, Chou SM, et al. Chloroquine neuromyotoxicity. Clinical and pathologic perspective. Am J Med 1987;82(3):447–55.

34. Azimian M, Gultekin SH, Hata JL, et al. Fatal antimalarial-induced cardiomyopathy: report of 2 cases. J Clin Rheumatol 2012;18(7):363–6.

35. Casado E, Gratacós J, Tolosa C, et al. Antimalarial myopathy: an underdiagnosed complication? Prospective longitudinal study of 119 patients. Ann Rheum Dis 2006;65(3):385–90.

36. Mastaglia FL, Papadimitriou JM, Dawkins RL, et al. Vacuolar myopathy associated with chloroquine, lupus erythematosus and thymoma. Report of a case with unusual mitochondrial changes and lipid accumulation in muscle. J Neurol Sci 1977;34(3):315–28.

37. Le Quintrec JS, Le Quintrec JL. Drug-induced myopathies. Baillieres Clin Rheumatol 1991;5(1):21–38.

38. Abdel-Hamid H, Oddis CV, Lacomis D. Severe hydroxychloroquine myopathy. Muscle Nerve 2008;38(3):1206–10.

39. Pulipaka U, Lacomis D, Omalu B. Amiodarone-induced neuromyopathy: three cases and a review of the literature. J Clin Neuromuscul Dis 2002;3(3):97–105.

40. Fernando Roth R, Itabashi H, Louie J, et al. Amiodarone toxicity: myopathy and neuropathy. Am Heart J 1990;119(5):1223–5.

41. Alsheikh-Ali AA, Karas RH. Adverse events with concomitant amiodarone and statin therapy. Prev Cardiol 2005;8(2):95–7.

42. Kuncl RW, Duncan G, Watson D, et al. Colchicine myopathy and neuropathy. N Engl J Med 1987;316(25):1562–8.

43. Kuncl RW, Cornblath DR, Avila O, et al. Electrodiagnosis of human colchicine myoneuropathy. Muscle Nerve 1989;12(5):360–4.

44. Teener JW. Inflammatory and toxic myopathy. Semin Neurol 2012;32(5):491–9.

45. Baker SK, Goodwin S, Sur M, et al. Cytoskeletal myotoxicity from simvastatin and colchicine. Muscle Nerve 2004;30(6):799–802.

46. Caglar K, Odabasi Z, Safali M, et al. Colchicine-induced myopathy with myotonia in a patient with chronic renal failure. Clin Neurol Neurosurg 2003;105(4):274–6.

47. Rutkove SB, De Girolami U, Preston DC, et al. Myotonia in colchicine myoneuropathy. Muscle Nerve 1996;19(7):870–5.

48. Fernandez C, Figarella-Branger D, Alla P, et al. Colchicine myopathy: a vacuolar myopathy with selective type I muscle fiber involvement. An immunohistochemical and electron microscopic study of two cases. Acta Neuropathol 2002;103(2):100–6.

49. Bradley WG, Lassman LP, Pearce GW, et al. The neuromyopathy of vincristine in man. Clinical, electrophysiological and pathological studies. J Neurol Sci 1970; 10(2):107–31.

50. Scruggs ER, Dirks Naylor AJ. Mechanisms of zidovudine-induced mitochondrial toxicity and myopathy. Pharmacology 2008;82(2):83–8. http://dx.doi.org/10. 1159/000134943.

51. Dalakas MC, Illa I, Pezeshkpour GH, et al. Mitochondrial myopathy caused by long-term zidovudine therapy. N Engl J Med 1990;322(16):1098–105.

52. Robinson-Papp J, Simpson DM. Neuromuscular diseases associated with HIV-1 infection. Muscle Nerve 2009;40(6):1043–53.

53. Simpson DM, Bender AN. Human immunodeficiency virus-associated myopathy: analysis of 11 patients. Ann Neurol 1988;24(1):79–84.

54. Simpson DM, Slasor P, Dafni U, et al. Analysis of myopathy in a placebo-controlled zidovudine trial. Muscle Nerve 1997;20(3):382–5.

55. Chalmers AC, Greco CM, Miller RG. Prognosis in AZT myopathy. Neurology 1991;41(8):1181–4.

56. Cupler EJ, Danon MJ, Jay C, et al. Early features of zidovudine-associated myopathy: histopathological findings and clinical correlations. Acta Neuropathol 1995;90(1):1–6.

57. Feinberg DM, Spiro AJ, Weidenheim KM. Distinct light microscopic changes in human immunodeficiency virus-associated nemaline myopathy. Neurology 1998;50(2):529–31.

58. Johnson RW, Williams FM, Kazi S, et al. Human immunodeficiency virus-associated polymyositis: a longitudinal study of outcome. Arthritis Rheum 2003;49(2):172–8.

59. Arnaudo E, Dalakas M, Shanske S, et al. Depletion of muscle mitochondrial DNA in AIDS patients with zidovudine-induced myopathy. Lancet 1991;337(8740): 508–10.

60. Mhiri C, Baudrimont M, Bonne G, et al. Zidovudine myopathy: a distinctive disorder associated with mitochondrial dysfunction. Ann Neurol 1991;29(6):606–14.

61. Masanés F, Barrientos A, Cebrián M, et al. Clinical, histological and molecular reversibility of zidovudine myopathy. J Neurol Sci 1998;159(2):226–8.

62. Benbrik E, Chariot P, Bonavaud S, et al. Cellular and mitochondrial toxicity of zidovudine (AZT), didanosine (ddI) and zalcitabine (ddC) on cultured human muscle cells. J Neurol Sci 1997;149(1):19–25.

63. Pedrol E, Masanés F, Fernández-Solá J, et al. Lack of muscle toxicity with didanosine (ddI). Clinical and experimental studies. J Neurol Sci 1996;138(1–2):42–8.

64. Simpson DM, Katzenstein DA, Hughes MD, et al. Neuromuscular function in HIV infection: analysis of a placebo-controlled combination antiretroviral trial. AIDS Clinical Group 175/801 Study Team. AIDS 1998;12(18):2425–32.

65. Fernstrom JD. Effects and side effects associated with the non-nutritional use of tryptophan by humans. J Nutr 2012;142(12):2236S–44S.

66. Hertzman PA, Blevins WL, Mayer J, et al. Association of the eosinophilia-myalgia syndrome with the ingestion of tryptophan. N Engl J Med 1990;322:869–73.

67. Kamb ML, Murphy JJ, Jones JL, et al. Eosinophilia-myalgia syndrome in L-tryptophan-exposed patients. JAMA 1992;267:77–82.

68. Kaufman LD, Philen RM. Tryptophan: current status and future trends for oral administration. Drug Saf 1993;8:89–98.

69. Kaufman LD, Gruber BL, Gregersen PK. Clinical follow-up and immunogenetic studies of 32 patients with eosinophilia-myalgia syndrome. Lancet 1991;337: 1071–4.

70. Owens WE 4th, Bertorini TE, Holt HT Jr, et al. Diffuse fasciitis with eosinophilia (shulman syndrome). J Clin Neuromuscul Dis 2004;6(2):99–101.

71. Hertzman PA, Clauw DJ, Kaufman LD, et al. The eosinophilia-myalgia syndrome: status of 205 patients and results of treatment 2 years after onset. Ann Intern Med 1995;122(11):851–5.

72. Smith BE, Dyck PJ. Peripheral neuropathy in the eosinophilia-myalgia syndrome associated with L-tryptophan ingestion. Neurology 1990;40(7):1035–40.

73. Burns SM, Lange DJ, Jaffe I, et al. Axonal neuropathy in eosinophilia-myalgia syndrome. Muscle Nerve 1994;17(3):293–8.

74. Donofrio PD, Stanton C, Miller VS, et al. Demyelinating polyneuropathy in eosinophilia-myalgia syndrome. Muscle Nerve 1992;15(7):796–805.

75. Patterson R, Germolec D. Review article toxic oil syndrome: review of immune aspects of the disease. J Immunotoxicol 2005;2(1):51–8.

76. Chappel R, Willems J. D-penicillamine-induced myositis in rheumatoid arthritis. Clin Rheumatol 1996;15(1):86–7.

77. Halla JT, Fallahi S, Koopman WJ. Penicillamine-induced myositis. Observations and unique features in two patients and review of the literature. Am J Med 1984; 77(4):719–22.

78. Watson AJ, Dalbow MH, Stachura I, et al. Immunologic studies in cimetidine-induced nephropathy and polymyositis. N Engl J Med 1983;308(3):142–5.

79. Hawkins RA, Eckhoff PJ Jr, MacCarter DK, et al. Cimetidine and polymyositis. N Engl J Med 1983;309(3):187–8.

80. Mitchell GG, Magnusson AR, Weiler JM. Cimetidine-induced cutaneous vasculitis. Am J Med 1983;75(5):875–6.

81. Lewis CA, Boheimer N, Rose P, et al. Myopathy after short term administration of procainamide. Br Med J (Clin Res Ed) 1986;292(6520):593–4.

82. Agius MA, Zhu S, Fairclough RH. Antirapsyn antibodies in chronic procainamide-associated myopathy (CPAM). Ann N Y Acad Sci 1998;841:527–9.

83. Engel JN, Mellul VG, Goodman DB. Phenytoin hypersensitivity: a case of severe acute rhabdomyolysis. Am J Med 1986;81(5):928–30.

84. Dimachkie MM, Vriesendorp FJ, Heck KA. Phenytoin-induced dermatomyositis: case report and literature review. Child Neurol 1998;13(11):577–80.

85. Cirigliano G, Della Rossa A, Tavoni A, et al. Polymyositis occurring during alpha-interferon treatment for malignant melanoma: a case report and review of the literature. Rheumatol Int 1999;19(1–2):65–7.

86. Hengstman GJ, Vogels OJ, ter Laak HJ, et al. Myositis during long-term interferon-alpha treatment. Neurology 2000;54(11):2186.

87. Greenberg SA. Type 1 interferons and myositis. Arthritis Res Ther 2010; 12(Suppl 1):S4. http://dx.doi.org/10.1186/ar2885.

88. Walsh RJ, Kong SW, Yao Y, et al. Type I interferon-inducible gene expression in blood is present and reflects disease activity in dermatomyositis and polymyositis. Arthritis Rheum 2007;56(11):3784–92.

89. Adenis A, Bouché O, Bertucci F, et al. Serum creatine kinase increase in patients treated with tyrosine kinase inhibitors for solid tumors. JMed Oncol 2012;29(4):3003–8. http://dx.doi.org/10.1007/s12032-012-0204-1.

90. Srinivasan J, Wu CJ, Amato AA. Inflammatory myopathy associated with imatinib mesylate therapy. Clin Neuromuscul Dis 2004;5(3):119–21.

91. Bowyer SL, LaMothe MP, Hollister JR. Steroid myopathy: incidence and detection in a population with asthma. J Allergy Clin Immunol 1985;76:234–42.

92. Hollister JR. The untoward effects of steroid treatment on the musculoskeletal system and what to do about them. J Asthma 1992;29:363–8.

93. Khaleeli AA, Edwards RH, Gohil K, et al. Corticosteroid myopathy: a clinical and pathological study. Clin Endocrinol 1983;18:155–66.
94. Kissel JT, Mendell JR. The endocrine myopathies. In: Rowland LP, Dimauro S, editors. Handbook of clinical neurology vol. 18, no. 62 myopathies. Amsterdam: Elsevier Science Publishers BV; 1992. p. 527–51.
95. Faludi G, Gotlieb J, Meyers J. Factors influencing the development of steroid-induced myopathies. Ann N Y Acad Sci 1966;138(1):62–72.
96. Buchthal F. Electrophysiological abnormalities in metabolic myopathies and neuropathies. Acta Neurol Scand 1970;46(Suppl 43):129–76.
97. Srinivasan J, Amato AA. Myopathies. Phys Med Rehabil Clin N Am 2003;14(2):403–34.
98. Dimachkie MM, Barohn RJ. Idiopathic inflammatory myopathies. Semin Neurol 2012;32(3):227–36. http://dx.doi.org/10.1055/s-0032-1329201.
99. Haan J, Hollander JM, van Duinen SG, et al. Reversible severe myopathy during treatment with finasteride. Muscle Nerve 1997;20(4):502–4.
100. Thyagarajan D, Day BJ, Wodak J, et al. Emetine myopathy in a patient with an eating disorder. Med J Aust 1993;159(11–12):757–60.
101. Dresser LP, Massey EW, Johnson EE, et al. Ipecac myopathy and cardiomyopathy. Neurol Neurosurg Psychiatry 1993;56(5):560–2.
102. Lacomis D. Case of the month. June 1996–anorexia nervosa. Brain Pathol 1996;6(4):535–6.
103. Kuntzer T, Bogousslavsky J, Deruaz JP, et al. Reversible emetine-induced myopathy with ECG abnormalities: a toxic myopathy. J Neurol 1989;236(4):246–8.
104. Latronico N, Tomelleri G, Filosto M. Critical illness myopathy. Curr Opin Rheumatol 2012;24(6):616–22.
105. Dimachkie MM. Critical illness myopathy and polyneuropathy. Medlink, 2013.
106. Hirano M, Ott BR, Raps EC, et al. Acute quadriplegic myopathy: a complication of treatment with steroids, nondepolarizing blocking agents, or both. Neurology 1992;42:2082–7.
107. MacFarlane I, Rosenthal F. Severe myopathy after status asthmaticus. Lancet 1977;2:615.
108. Lacomis D, Chad DA, Aronin N, et al. The myopathy of Cushing's syndrome. Muscle Nerve 1993;16:880–1.
109. Lacomis D, Giuliani MJ, Van Cott A, et al. Acute myopathy of intensive care: clinical, electromyographic, and pathological aspects. Ann Neurol 1996;40:645–54.
110. Hermans G, De Jonghe B, Bruyninckx F, et al. Interventions for preventing critical illness polyneuropathy and critical illness myopathy. Cochrane Database Syst Rev 2009;(1):CD006832.
111. Hough CL, Steinberg KP, Taylor Thompson B, et al. Intensive care unit-acquired neuromyopathy and corticosteroids in survivors of persistent ARDS. Intensive Care Med 2009;35(1):63–8.
112. Barohn RJ, Jackson CE, Rogers SJ, et al. Prolonged paralysis due to nondepolarizing neuromuscular blocking agents and corticosteroids. Muscle Nerve 1994;17:647–54.
113. Kaminski HJ, Ruff RL. Endocrine myopathies (hyper- and hypofunction of adrenal, thyroid, pituitary, and parathyroid glands and iatrogenic corticosteroid myopathy). In: Engel AG, Franzini-Armstrong C, editors. Myology. 2nd edition. New York: McGraw-Hill; 1994. p. 1726–53.
114. Clark DW, Strandell J. Myopathy including polymyositis: a likely class adverse effect of proton pump inhibitors? Eur J Clin Pharmacol 2006;62(6):473–9.

115. Garrote FJ, Lacambra C, del Ser T, et al. Subacute myopathy during omeprazole therapy. Lancet 1992;340(8820):672.
116. Faucheux JM, Tournebize P, Viguier A, et al. Neuromyopathy secondary to omeprazole treatment. Muscle Nerve 1998;21(2):261–2.
117. Chroni E, Monastirli A, Tsambaos D. Neuromuscular adverse effects associated with systemic retinoid dermatotherapy: monitoring and treatment algorithm for clinicians. Drug Saf 2010;33(1):25–34.
118. Sarifakioglu E, Onur O, Kart H, et al. Acute myopathy and acne fulminans triggered by isotretinoin therapy. Eur J Dermatol 2011;21(5):794–5.
119. Klingler W, Heiderich S, Girard T, et al. Functional and genetic characterization of clinical malignant hyperthermia crises: a multi-centre study. Orphanet J Rare Dis 2014;9(1):8. http://dx.doi.org/10.1186/1750-1172-9-8.
120. Visoiu M, Young MC, Wieland K, et al. Anesthetic drugs and onset of malignant hyperthermia. Anesth Analg 2014;118(2):388–96.
121. Schuster F, Johannsen S, Roewer N. A minimal-invasive metabolic test detects malignant hyperthermia susceptibility in a patient after sevoflurane-induced metabolic crisis. Case Rep Anesthesiol 2013;2013:953859.
122. Schuster F, Johannsen S, Schneiderbanger D, et al. Evaluation of suspected malignant hyperthermia events during anesthesia. BMC Anesthesiol 2013; 13(1):24. http://dx.doi.org/10.1186/1471-2253-13-24.
123. Nelson P, Litman RS. Malignant hyperthermia in children: an analysis of the north american malignant hyperthermia registry. Anesth Analg 2014;118(2):369–74.
124. Lang CH, Frost RA, Summer AD, et al. Molecular mechanisms responsible for alcohol-induced myopathy in skeletal muscle and heart. Int J Biochem Cell Biol 2005;37(10):2180–95.
125. Preedy VR, Ohlendieck K, Adachi J, et al. The importance of alcohol-induced muscle disease. J Muscle Res Cell Motil 2003;24(1):55–63.

Duchenne and Becker Muscular Dystrophies

Kevin M. Flanigan, MD

KEYWORDS

- Duchenne muscular dystrophy • Becker muscular dystrophy • Dystrophin
- Exon skipping

KEY POINTS

- Duchenne and Becker muscular dystrophies are due to mutations in the *DMD* gene.
- Mutational analysis of blood samples can lead to the diagnosis of a dystrophinopathy in around 95% of cases.
- Muscle biopsy may still be required in selected cases.
- The corticosteroids prednisone and deflazacort are the mainstays of therapy, which should be initiated by the age of 5 years.
- Management of the side effects of corticosteroids is a significant challenge.
- Optimal management of DMD requires multidisciplinary care including neurology, cardiology, pulmonary, physical medicine and rehabilitation, nutrition, physical therapy, and occupational therapy.
- A variety of novel and promising therapies are on the horizon or have entered clinical trials.

INTRODUCTION

The X-linked Duchenne and Becker muscular dystrophies (DMD and BMD) are allelic disorders occurring due to mutations in the *DMD* gene, which consists of 79 exons encoding the dystrophin protein. DMD has a commonly cited incidence of 1 in 3500 live male births,[1] but a recent survey of published data from a variety of newborn screening studies shows the reported incidence to range from 1:3802 to 1:6291.[2] BMD is about one-third as frequent as DMD.[1,3]

   The molecular difference between the more severe DMD and the milder BMD is due to differences in dystrophin expression and is explained in most cases by the "reading frame rule."[4] Originally defined in the case of exonic deletion mutations, this rule stated that *DMD* deletions that preserve an open reading frame allow translation of an internally truncated protein with a functional C-terminus, whereas out-of-frame deletions result in a truncated reading frame. Thus, DMD is nearly always associated

Center for Gene Therapy, Room 3014, The Research Institute of Nationwide Children's Hospital, 700 Children's Drive, Columbus, OH 43209, USA
E-mail address: kevin.flanigan@nationwidechildrens.org

Neurol Clin 32 (2014) 671–688
http://dx.doi.org/10.1016/j.ncl.2014.05.002
0733-8619/14/$ – see front matter © 2014 Elsevier Inc. All rights reserved.
neurologic.theclinics.com

with a complete absence of dystrophin, whereas the milder BMD is associated with the presence of variable amounts of partially functional dystrophin.

One of the primary roles of dystrophin is to link the cytoskeleton to the extracellular matrix, via the transmembrane dystroglycan protein and its associated protein complex including the sarcoglycans. Dystrophin binds to cytoskeletal actin via its N-terminal actin-binding domain 1 (ABD1) and to β-dystroglycan via its C-terminal domain, with the central rod domain, consisting of 24 spectrin-like repeats, in between. In the absence of dystrophin, the muscle membrane is susceptible to damage and muscle fiber deterioration occurs, resulting in cycles of regeneration and degeneration that result in fibrosis and fatty replacement of muscle. The partially functional nature of internally truncated dystrophin provides a route for novel therapies, as discussed later.

CLINICAL FINDINGS
Duchenne Muscular Dystrophy

Boys with DMD are typically brought to the attention of a clinician between the ages of 2 and 5 years. Delayed gait is sometimes described, but alteration of gait is the most common presenting symptom, and toe walking often leads to referral to physical therapists or orthopedic physicians before recognition of DMD. However, recent studies show that motor function is impaired in the infantile phase of DMD,[5] and assessment of serum creatine kinase (CK) is recommended as part of the routine screening of all infants with motor delay.[6] Cognition is also affected, and language development is delayed.[7] Intelligence quotient (IQ) is diminished by one standard deviation, although verbal IQ improves with age.[8,9] There is an increased risk of autism, attention deficit hyperactivity disorder, and obsessive-compulsive disorder in DMD boys.[10]

Proximal weakness is typically evident to the examiner at the time of presentation, seen as difficulty in climbing stairs, hopping, or arising from the floor (nearly always with use of the Gower maneuver). Muscle enlargement, particularly of the calves, is common; although classically called "pseudohypertrophy"[11] and attributed to fibrosis and fatty replacement, true hypertrophy of contractile mass is also present.[12] Tight heel cords and mild lordosis are frequently seen at diagnosis and along with gait disturbance often result in boys being the first sent to orthopedic physicians or physical therapists. A search for orthopedic causes may contribute to a delay in clinical diagnosis, which is common, with a mean age at first evaluation of 3.6 years and at diagnosis of 4.9 years.[13]

DMD follows a predictable clinical course.[14–17] Although lagging behind peers, strength may improve into the 6th or 7th year, followed by a plateau in function of 1 to 2 years before weakness begins a clear decline to wheelchair dependence. In the absence of steroids, the loss of independent ambulation occurs by the age of 12 years. Thereafter, arm function declines, but the major determinant of morbidity is progressive respiratory insufficiency. Forced vital capacity declines after loss of ambulation,[16,18] and scoliosis is frequent. Cardiomyopathy occurs increasing in frequency with age, and without ventilatory intervention, death in the absence of steroid therapy typically occurs by the age of 20 years.

Becker Muscular Dystrophy

BMD is in general significantly less severe than DMD, as demonstrated by its first description as a "benign variant" of muscle disease.[19,20] Patients may present as "mild DMD", appearing with limb-girdle weakness and calf hypertrophy similar to that seen in DMD but presenting in childhood, and half of BMD patients demonstrate symptoms of weakness by age 10 years.[21] BMD with childhood onset are distinct from DMD in that they remain ambulant until older than age 12 years. However, because there is clearly an overlap with DMD in this range, many clinicians find the concept of "intermediate muscular dystrophy" (IMD) useful to describe boys who walk past age 12 years but stop walking by age 15 years, reserving the classification of BMD for patients who lose ambulation after the age of 15 years. The IMD group thus encompasses patients who are more severe than most BMD but less severe than typical DMD.[17,22]

BMD nevertheless represents a quite widely variable phenotype, and patients may present with much milder weakness, with onset into mid- or late adulthood[23,24] or limited to the quadriceps muscles.[25] Other variants include cramp-myalgia syndrome,[21,26] exercise-induced myoglobinuria,[27] and asymptomatic hyperCKemia.[28] With some alleles, variation within families is seen, as is the case with a North American founder allele; some who carry it have minimal weakness or cramp-myalgia, whereas others are entirely asymptomatic into their 8th decade.[29] In BMD, cognition is generally spared,[30] although isolated cognitive impairment has been reported.[31]

Rating Scales

No specific rating scales have been established for BMD. For DMD, a variety of outcome measures have been used in the clinical trial setting or natural history settings, including modified Medical Research Council grading of up to 34 muscles,[14,32] quantitative muscle testing,[33] and the 6-minute walk test, which has become a de facto standard in trials over the past several years.[34,35] Subparts of the Motor Function Measure assessment have been shown to be sensitive to change in DMD.[36] Recently, the DMD-specific North Star Ambulatory Assessment has demonstrated robustness and sensitivity for change in boys with DMD.[37,38] Among tests commonly performed in the clinic, the 10-m walk test (time to walk 10 m) is the only one that has been shown to have prognostic value: a time of greater than 12 seconds predicts wheelchair use within 1 year in 100% of patients.[16]

DIAGNOSIS
Serum Chemistries

Serum CK is universally elevated in both DMD and BMD, presumably due to increased permeability of the sarcolemmal membrane, and this is nearly always the initial diagnostic test performed. In DMD it is often 50 to 100 times normal values; in BMD, it is lower, reaching a maximum value around 10 to 15 years of age.[39] BMD may occasionally present with episodes of extremely elevated CK associated with myoglobinuria leading to a clinical diagnosis of rhabdomyolysis, generally in patients with mild weakness that presumably allows more strenuous activity that precipitates these episodes.[27,29,40–42] Serum CK is elevated at birth, providing the opportunity for newborn screening.[43–48] A two-tiered system making use of CK level screening followed by mutational analysis of DNA extracted from the same blood spot provides a route to definitive newborn screening, without requiring families to return for a subsequent DNA sample.[2]

Although not a specific finding, the transaminases aspartate aminotransferase and alanine aminotransferase are also elevated[49–53] due to muscle damage, not liver injury, yet unnecessary liver biopsies are sometimes reported as part of a family's diagnostic odyssey. Gamma-glutamyl transferase level is instead a useful marker of liver injury.[54] In this population, assessment of renal function should make use of cystatin C rather than serum creatinine or creatinine clearance, both of which are diminished in DMD.[55]

Muscle Biopsy

Although the advances in molecular diagnostics discussed later have diminished the role of muscle biopsy in the diagnosis of DMD and BMD, muscle biopsy is still in relatively common use. Absent or altered dystrophin expression in a muscle biopsy specimen remains a gold standard of diagnosis, and it is important to remember that current methods of genomic analysis detect only around 93% to 96% of mutations.[56,57] The remainder consists of mRNA rearrangements, including pseudoexon insertions[58,59] that require analysis of muscle-derived mRNA to detect.

Histopathology

The histopathologic changes seen in DMD muscle result from deficiency of dystrophin. The resulting loss of muscle fiber integrity leads to myofiber necrosis, muscle fibrosis, and failure of regenerative capacity. The chronic and severe myopathic changes that lead to the description of dystrophic findings include fibrosis and fatty replacement, which increase with time, leading to end-stage myopathic change. In BMD, histopathology varies. In more severely affected muscles, all of the features of DMD muscle may be seen, whereas in less-affected cases the pathology may be limited to variation in fiber size and mild fibrosis, with varying degrees of degeneration or necrosis.

Assessment of Dystrophin Expression

Because these histopathologic changes are not specific — similar changes may be seen in many muscular dystrophies and in particular, the limb-girdle muscular dystrophies due to sarcoglycan mutations — diagnosis from muscle biopsy depends on analysis of dystrophin expression. This diagnosis may be achieved by immunohistochemical (IHC) or immunofluorescent (IF) analysis of muscle sections or by immunoblot (IB) of muscle homogenates. In the clinical laboratory, IHC or IF is performed using antibodies directed toward the N-terminal, the central rod, and the C-terminal domains. The use of rod domain antibodies alone may result in a mistaken interpretation of dystrophin absence, if an internally truncated BMD-associated protein lacks the epitope toward which the antibody is directed.

If appropriate antibodies are used, a complete absence of dystrophin reliably predicts a DMD phenotype, whereas in BMD dystrophin staining is typically patchy and incompletely surrounds muscle fibers. However, under conditions of increased sensitivity, IF of DMD muscle can show fibers with "traces" of dystrophin staining.[60] More clinically relevant, under standard staining DMD muscle biopsies frequently show small foci or clusters of fibers that show significant dystrophin expression. These are revertant fibers, due to secondary alterations in the gene such as altered pre-mRNA splicing that allow expression of some dystrophin, and can be found in up to 50% of patient biopsies[61–65] without a clear association with disease severity.

In contrast to IF or IHC staining, IB provides information on both the size and the amount of dystrophin. In regards to quantification, values of less than 3% as consistent with DMD and levels greater than 20% consistent with mild BMD were described[66] and are still used by some diagnostic laboratories. Although significant differences in methodology among laboratories make an absolute threshold difficult to establish, the presence of significant dystrophin expression by IB is generally useful. Dystrophin proteins of altered size most commonly demonstrate the effects of in-frame deletions in BMD patients, although exceptions to the rule — such as patients with abundant dystrophin of small size, which is evidently nonfunctional dystrophin based on clinical phenotype[67] — highlight the need for caution in interpretation and correlation with clinical phenotype.

Mutational Analysis

Complete mutational analysis of the DMD gene from lymphocyte-derived DNA is now a readily available clinical test. In the appropriate clinical setting, it is typically ordered after serum CK results are returned. Detailed characterization of the mutation now is considered the standard of care, because it allows the confirmation of the diagnosis of dystrophinopathy and provides information essential to counseling the family. Furthermore, mutation class–specific molecular therapies are in or are nearing clinical trials, and it is imperative to consider the suitability of the patient for these.

The size of the gene has historically presented a challenge for complete molecular diagnosis. The DMD gene is the largest gene known, consisting of 79 exons spread across 2.4 million nucleotides on the X chromosome. Deletions of one or more exons account for approximately 65% of DMD and BMD mutations.[22,68] Early efforts at mutation detection were directed toward the detection of deletions contained or ending within 2 deletion "hot-spots" near the N-terminus and within the central rod region. For many years, the standard clinical test was the economical multiplex polymerase chain reaction test, which checked for the presence of around 25 exons by use of multiple primer sets.[69,70] Useful in males who are hemizygous at the DMD locus, this test was not useful for detection of carriers or patients with duplications or point mutations. This test has been superseded by methods that test the copy number of every exon, including multiplex ligation-dependent probe amplification[71,72] and comparative genomic hybridization using either custom or commercial microarrays.[73–75] These tests readily identify exon duplication mutations (6% of all mutations), define the extent of contiguous exon deletions that extend out of the "hot-spot" exons, and diagnose female carriers.

The remainder of mutations require sequence analysis for detection, including nonsense, small subexonic insertions or deletions, missense, or splice site mutations. A variety of methods are in clinical use, including traditional Sanger sequencing of exons as well as next-generation sequencing approaches. What is important is that sequencing must be performed over the entire DMD coding region (ie, all exons), because nearly all point mutations are "private" and do not occur in hotspots. The distribution of DMD mutation classes varies slightly depending on the sample tested. In an unselected clinic cohort of 68 index cases, exonic deletions accounted for 65% of mutations and exonic duplications for 6%; nonsense mutations for 13%; missense mutations for 4%; and small insertions/deletions for 3%.[56] These numbers differ somewhat for reports from referral laboratory settings. For example, in a large cohort enriched for nondeletion patients, the distribution of mutation classes for all DMD and BMD patients was as follows: exon deletions 42.9%, nonsense mutations 26.5%, small frameshifts 11.4%, duplications 11.0%, splice site mutations 5.8%, and missense mutations 1.4%.[22]

Patients with no mutation detectable by modern genomic methods but who have either an X-linked family history or biopsy evidence for a dystrophinopathy frequently have pseudoexon mutations in which a deep intronic mutation creates a cryptic splice donor or acceptor site, resulting in the inclusion of intronic sequencing into the mature mRNA.[58,59] Sequencing of the DMD cDNA derived from muscle mRNA is required for this diagnosis; the same test will identify unusual mutations such as exon inversions, which may go undetected by standard analyses.[76–79]

Consistent with the Haldane rule for an X-linked lethal disorder, one-third of DMD cases are de novo. Carrier testing should always be considered for mothers of DMD boys, although it is not required in the setting of a clear X-linked history consistent with an obligate carrier status. Genetic counseling should be provided and address the risk of germline mosaicism in mothers with negative DNA tests, because it may occur in up to 10%.[80,81]

IMAGING

Imaging has historically been of little use in the diagnosis of DMD, but very recent work has highlighted the sensitivity of muscle magnetic resonance imaging (MRI) and in particular T2 signal and lipid fraction to longitudinal progression of disease, raising the possibility that MRI may become a robust outcome measure for clinical trials.[82-85]

DIAGNOSTIC DILEMMAS

The diagnosis of DMD can be made on clinical grounds with essentially complete certainty in the presence of an X-linked family history, but even in its absence the classic presentation and the prevalence of the disorder allows diagnosis with very high reliability. The classic mimic of DMD includes the severe forms of the sarcoglycanopathies, those autosomal recessive limb-girdle muscular dystrophies (LGMD2s) that occur due to mutations in the α-sarcoglycan (SGCA; LGMD2D), β-sarcoglycan (SGCB; LGMD2E), γ-sarcoglycan (SGCG; LGMD2C), and δ-sarcoglycan (SGCD; LGMD2F) genes. In their severe form, historically called severe childhood autosomal recessive muscular dystrophy,[86,87] they can be indistinguishable from DMD except for the pattern of inheritance (which allows girls to be affected). LGMD2I, because of mutations in the FKRP gene, can also result in either a Duchenne or a Beckerlike phenotype, including cardiomyopathy.[88,89] In the setting of negative DMD mutational analysis, these syndromes can be diagnosed by muscle biopsy characterization of sarcoglycan expression and α-dystroglycan glycosylation or by mutational analysis of all of these genes (now available in various diagnostic sequencing panels).

Exceptions to the Reading Frame Rule

One diagnostic challenge is that the reading frame rule is accurate 90% of the time, making it necessary for clinicians to recognize that exceptions to it exist. Examples include large in-frame deletions that affect the N-terminal dystrophin actin-binding domain 1 and extend into the central rod domain, which often result in DMD. Conversely, 14% of nonsense mutations (as predicted by genomic analysis) are associated with BMD, rather than the predicted DMD[90]; typically, this occurs due to altered pre-mRNA splicing within the flanking in-frame context of exons 23–42, resulting in an open reading frame and continued protein translation.[90-92] Other classic examples include the relatively common out-of-frame deletion of exons 3–7, which results in both DMD and BMD phenotypes due to downstream translational initiation.[93,94] Examples such as these highlight that prognostication, or phenotypic classification, cannot rely solely on the predicted reading frame; the entire clinical picture must be taken into account, including age at presentation, consistency of examination findings with predicted phenotype, and results of dystrophin expression studies.

GENETIC MODIFIERS

Although the largest predictor of phenotype is whether the causative DMD mutation follows the reading-frame rule, other genes that modify the severity of DMD have recently been defined. The first is SPP1, which encodes osteopontin, a cytokine active in the transforming growth factor β (TGFβ) pathway.[95] A polymorphism in the SPP1 5' untranslated regions has been found to associate with prolonged ambulation in DMD patients.[96,97] The second is LTBP4, which encodes the latent TGFβ binding protein 4. Variations in this gene were identified as modifiers in a sarcoglycanopathy mouse model of sarcoglycanopathy[98] and confirmed to have an effect on ambulation in a large cohort of dystrophinopathy patients, with patients homozygous for the protective allele walking a mean of 1.8 years longer.[99] The identification of these and future genetic modifiers offer potential pathways for future therapeutic approaches.

MANAGEMENT

Management of DMD must take into account the multiple systems affected in patients; the significant psychosocial and familial stressors induced by the disease; the burdens of proposed interventions; and the complications induced by the sole therapy to date, corticosteroids. Management may ideally be provided within a multidisciplinary care setting, which can be organized to provide the components of universal care standards, to which the clinician is referred.[100,101] At a minimum, patients should be seen yearly by a neurologist or rehabilitation physician, cardiologist, pulmonologist, physical and occupational therapists, and nutritionist. Other specialists and consultants often play critical roles in the management of the DMD patient, including endocrinologists, orthopedic surgeons, and social workers, among others.

The management goals of both DMD and BMD are similar, except that a large part of the management of DMD is directed toward managing complications of corticosteroid therapy, which is not used in BMD. An exhaustive review of management targets for DMD is found in a recent pair of reviews.[100,101] A briefer list of key points follows:

Management Goals in DMD

- Preservation of strength and ambulation
- Minimization of steroid complications
  - Obesity
  - Delayed puberty
  - Osteoporosis
  - Cataracts
- Prevention of complications including contractures
- Minimization of injury risk from falls
- Preservation of ventilatory function
- Prophylaxis or treatment of cardiomyopathy
- Avoidance or treatment of scoliosis
- Appropriate school environment
- Treatment of family stressors

PHARMACOLOGIC THERAPY
Corticosteroids

In DMD, the only medications that have been conclusively demonstrated to affect muscle function are glucocorticoid corticosteroids, prednisone and deflazacort. Their mechanism of action in DMD is unclear, but multiple studies have confirmed a beneficial effect. The original seminal trial established a prednisone dose of 0.75 mg per kilogram per day as the standard dose, resulting in improved muscle strength at 6 months of therapy.[32] Comparable efficacy results are found with deflazacort, 0.9 mg per kilogram per day, with potentially fewer complications and in particular less pronounced weight gain.[102] Multiple trials have confirmed positive effects, leading to a consensus that treatment may result in prolongation of ambulation by 1 to 3 years compared with no treatment.[32,103–109]

The side effects of corticosteroid therapy included small stature, weight gain (due to both fat accumulation and increased appetite), increased osteoporosis, an increased risk of cataracts, delayed puberty, and a tendency toward behavioral disturbance. These side effects frequently require careful monitoring, discussed in detail elsewhere.[100] Nutritional input is critical, and bone health screening is essential, with vitamin D supplementation where appropriate and DEXA scans yearly while on steroids.

Alternative regimens designed to minimize these side effects include prednisone, 0.75 mg/kg, on the first 10 days of each month or the same dose taken alternating 10 days on and off. Determination of the efficacy of this intermittent dosing in comparison to daily prednisone and daily deflazacort is the goal of the ongoing double-blinded National Institutes of Health–sponsored FOR-DMD trial. Another alternate regimen is weekend dosing, in which prednisone, 10 mg/kg per week, is divided between a Saturday and Sunday dose (ie, 5 mg/kg each weekend day); in a brief trial, this showed nearly equal efficacy to daily prednisone along with similar side effects.[110]

Knowing when to initiate and when to stop corticosteroids is a challenge. Current recommendations for initiation suggest starting corticosteroids therapy between the age of 2 and 5 years if a boy has either plateaued in strength (in which case it is recommended) or is declining (in which case it is "highly recommended").[100] There is a general consensus that it should be initiated during the phase of functional motor plateau, whenever that occurs,[100] although treatment by age 5 years is common. Earlier treatment may be associated with a more significant long-term benefit, although this is anecdotal.[111,112] No consensus exists as to whether corticosteroid therapy should be stopped at loss of ambulation,[100] and although this practice is common, some retrospective data suggest that use of low-dose steroids in nonambulant boys results in less scoliosis and improved ventilation.[109]

Cardiac Care

Cardiomyopathy is a nearly universal feature of DMD, with an estimated incidence as high as 25% by age 6 years and 59% by age 10 years,[113,114] although other studies suggest the median age of onset is around 14 to 15 years.[115,116] Although cardiac fibrosis and diastolic dysfunction may precede systolic dysfunction,[117–119] the systolic dysfunction that is commonly detected on standard clinical echocardiograms may be the earliest feature noticed in most clinics. Screening echocardiograms are recommended at diagnosis or by age 6 years; every 2 years up to 8 years; and yearly after 10 years.[101] Treatment of cardiomyopathy typically begins with afterload reduction using angiotensin-converting enzyme inhibitors or angiotensin receptor blockers, which likely have similar efficacy.[120] The timing of initiation of these medications remains debatable, although limited studies suggest that they should be initiated before the identification of systolic dysfunction.[121,122] Cardiac conduction disturbance is frequent, requiring Holter monitoring for assessment[123–125]; these may precede systolic dysfunction[126] and necessitate treatment.

NONPHARMACOLOGIC THERAPIES
Pulmonary Care

Ventilatory insufficiency eventually supervenes in essentially all cases of DMD and is the major cause of mortality.[127] Forced vital capacity declines after loss of ambulation because the diaphragm weakens, thoracic capacity declines, and pulmonary morbidity increases. However, the use of a mechanical insufflator/exsufflator may decrease the frequency of respiratory infections, and early acquisition of and training with this device should be considered after loss of ambulation. The second critical intervention is the recognition and treatment of nocturnal ventilatory insufficiency; early and appropriate nocturnal ventilation resulted in increasing the percentage of patients surviving to age 25 years to 53% of patients a retrospective study of 197 patients.[128] Snoring, morning headaches, or excessive daytime sleepiness should lead to a polysomnogram, which may be repeated yearly in nonambulant patients, because they are at increasing risk each year for nocturnal hypoventilation. Patients with either obstructive apnea or hypercapnia are typically treated with bilevel continuous positive airway pressure ventilation.[127]

Scoliosis

Once a boy is in a wheelchair full time, the risk of scoliosis increases; it ultimately affects up to 77% of boys,[129] although it may be delayed by proper wheelchair fitting and by use of steroids.[129,130] Data on the effect of scoliosis surgery are largely retrospective[131] or anecdotal, but evidence for a significant impact on survival was found in one clinic cohort, where with noninvasive ventilatory support it increased survival by nearly 8 years.[132] Once scoliosis is clinically evident on examination of the nonambulant boy, yearly spinal radiographs are warranted to assess progression and the need for orthopedic intervention. Orthopedic consultation should be considered for curves past 20 degrees.[101]

NOVEL THERAPIES

Novel therapies are directed toward a variety of gene corrective, gene replacement, and surrogate gene approaches.

Nonsense Suppression

Nonsense suppression therapies induce "readthrough" of nonsense mutations, such that instead of translational termination, an amino acid is inserted into the nascent peptide chain and translation continues. The nonsense suppression agent ataluren has shown promise in preclinical studies in the standard DMD mouse model, *mdx*, which carries a nonsense mutation in exon 23,[133] as well as in an early phase human trial.[134] Other agents directed toward the same mechanism are undergoing preclinical studies.[135,136]

Exon Skipping

Exon skipping therapy makes use of the clinical observations inherent in the reading frame rule. Antisense oligonucleotides (AONs) complementary to exon definition elements within a target exon induce the ribosome to ignore an exon during pre-mRNA splicing, which results in an mRNA with a larger but in-frame deletion that can be translated through the C-terminus. Targeting of one exon would theoretically be able to correct multiple DMD mutations. Skipping of exon 45 would correct both deletions of exons 46–47 and exons 46–48, among others. Because of this, targeting a limited number of exons (44, 45, 51, and 53) would be expected to be beneficial to around 35% of all DMD patients and skipping of 2 exons could theoretically be beneficial to 83%.[137]

Two different AON chemistries directed toward exon 51 skipping have been used in DMD patient trials: 2'O-methyl phosphorothioate AONs and phosphorodiamidate morpholino oligomers. Initial results for each were promising.[138–141] However, the recent small trial (n = 12) of the morpholino shows a significant difference in distance walked between patients treated with the compound immediately versus those initially treated with placebo, as measured at 48 weeks of treatment,[142] with essentially no side effects, which is a very promising result. If confirmed, this approach may be extended to other exons, and to other mutation classes such as single exon duplications, where skipping would restore a wild-type rather than a BMD-like mRNA.

Gene Transfer

Gene transfer approaches now in clinical development use adeno-associated viruses (AAVs) to deliver a transgene of interest to muscle. A challenge to the use of AAV is that these viruses can only carry a transgene of around 5 kb, smaller than the DMD cDNA of nearly 14 kb. As a result, current strategies make use of micro- or mini-dystrophin transgenes containing only 4 spectrinlike repeats in the central rod domain and missing the C-terminus. Expression in an initial trial was poor,[143] but a trial of an improved vector is planned, and other vectors are in preclinical development.[144]

SUMMARY

- Duchenne and Becker muscular dystrophies are due to mutations in the *DMD* gene.
- Mutational analysis of blood samples can lead to the diagnosis of a dystrophinopathy in around 95% of cases.
- Muscle biopsy may still be required in selected cases.
- The corticosteroids prednisone and deflazacort are the mainstays of therapy, which should be initiated by the age of 5 years.
- Management of the side effects of corticosteroids is a significant challenge.
- Optimal management of DMD requires multidisciplinary care including neurology, cardiology, pulmonary, physical medicine and rehabilitation, nutrition, physical therapy, and occupational therapy.
- A variety of novel and promising therapies are on the horizon or have entered clinical trials.

REFERENCES

1. Emery AE. Population frequencies of neuromuscular diseases–II. Amyotrophic lateral sclerosis (motor neurone disease). Neuromuscul Disord 1991;1(5): 323–5.
2. Mendell JR, Shilling C, Leslie ND, et al. Evidence-based path to newborn screening for Duchenne muscular dystrophy. Ann Neurol 2012;71(3):304–13.
3. Bushby KM, Thambyayah M, Gardner-Medwin D. Prevalence and incidence of Becker muscular dystrophy. Lancet 1991;337(8748):1022–4.
4. Monaco AP, Bertelson CJ, Liechti-Gallati S, et al. An explanation for the phenotypic differences between patients bearing partial deletions of the DMD locus. Genomics 1988;2(1):90–5.
5. Connolly AM, Florence JM, Cradock MM, et al. Motor and cognitive assessment of infants and young boys with duchenne muscular dystrophy: results from the Muscular Dystrophy Association DMD Clinical Research Network. Neuromuscul Disord 2013;23(7):529–39.
6. Noritz GH, Murphy NA, Neuromotor Screening Expert Panel. Motor delays: early identification and evaluation. Pediatrics 2013;131(6):e2016–27.
7. Cyrulnik SE, Fee RJ, De Vivo DC, et al. Delayed developmental language milestones in children with Duchenne's muscular dystrophy. J Pediatr 2007;150(5): 474–8.
8. Cotton SM, Voudouris NJ, Greenwood KM. Association between intellectual functioning and age in children and young adults with Duchenne muscular

dystrophy: further results from a meta-analysis. Dev Med Child Neurol 2005; 47(4):257–65.

9. Cotton S, Voudouris NJ, Greenwood KM. Intelligence and duchenne muscular dystrophy: full-scale, verbal, and performance intelligence quotients. Dev Med Child Neurol 2001;43(7):497–501.

10. Hendriksen JG, Vles JS. Neuropsychiatric disorders in males with duchenne muscular dystrophy: frequency rate of attention-deficit hyperactivity disorder (ADHD), autism spectrum disorder, and obsessive–compulsive disorder. J Child Neurol 2008;23(5):477–81.

11. Duchenne GB. Récherches sur la paralysie musculaire pseudohypertrophique, ou paralysie myosclérosique. Arch Gén Méd 1868;11(5).

12. Kornegay JN, Childers MK, Bogan DJ, et al. The paradox of muscle hypertrophy in muscular dystrophy. Phys Med Rehabil Clin N Am 2012;23(1):149–72, xii.

13. Ciafaloni E, Fox DJ, Pandya S, et al. Delayed diagnosis in duchenne muscular dystrophy: data from the muscular dystrophy surveillance, tracking, and research network (MD STARnet). J Pediatr 2009;155(3):380–5.

14. Brooke MH, Fenichel GM, Griggs RC, et al. Clinical investigation in Duchenne dystrophy: 2. Determination of the "power" of therapeutic trials based on the natural history. Muscle Nerve 1983;6(2):91–103.

15. Brooke MH, Griggs RC, Mendell JR, et al. The natural history of Duchenne muscular dystrophy: a caveat for therapeutic trials. Trans Am Neurol Assoc 1981;106:195–9.

16. McDonald CM, Abresch RT, Carter GT, et al. Profiles of neuromuscular diseases. Duchenne muscular dystrophy. Am J Phys Med Rehabil 1995;74(Suppl 5): S70–92.

17. Nicholson LV, Johnson MA, Bushby KM, et al. Integrated study of 100 patients with Xp21 linked muscular dystrophy using clinical, genetic, immunochemical, and histopathological data. Part 1. Trends across the clinical groups. J Med Genet 1993;30(9):728–36.

18. Tangsrud S, Petersen IL, Lodrup Carlsen KC, et al. Lung function in children with Duchenne's muscular dystrophy. Respir Med 2001;95(11):898–903.

19. Becker PE. Dystrophia Musculorum Progressiva. Eine genetische und klinische Untersuchung der Muskeldystrophien. Stuttgart (Germany): Thieme; 1953.

20. Becker PE. Two families of benign sex-linked recessive muscular dystrophy. Rev Can Biol 1962;21:551–66.

21. Bushby KM, Gardner-Medwin D. The clinical, genetic and dystrophin characteristics of Becker muscular dystrophy. I. Natural history. J Neurol 1993;240(2): 98–104.

22. Flanigan KM, Dunn DM, von Niederhausern A, et al. Mutational spectrum of DMD mutations in dystrophinopathy patients: application of modern diagnostic techniques to a large cohort. Hum Mutat 2009;30(12):1657–66.

23. Yazaki M, Yoshida K, Nakamura A, et al. Clinical characteristics of aged Becker muscular dystrophy patients with onset after 30 years. Eur Neurol 1999;42(3): 145–9.

24. Heald A, Anderson LV, Bushby KM, et al. Becker muscular dystrophy with onset after 60 years. Neurology 1994;44(12):2388–90.

25. Sunohara N, Arahata K, Hoffman EP, et al. Quadriceps myopathy: forme fruste of Becker muscular dystrophy. Ann Neurol 1990;28(5):634–9.

26. Bushby KM, Cleghorn NJ, Curtis A, et al. Identification of a mutation in the promoter region of the dystrophin gene in a patient with atypical Becker muscular dystrophy. Hum Genet 1991;88(2):195–9.

27. Minetti C, Tanji K, Chang HW, et al. Dystrophinopathy in two young boys with exercise-induced cramps and myoglobinuria. Eur J Pediatr 1993;152(10): 848–51.
28. Melis MA, Cau M, Muntoni F, et al. Elevation of serum creatine kinase as the only manifestation of an intragenic deletion of the dystrophin gene in three unrelated families. Eur J Paediatr Neurol 1998;2(5):255–61.
29. Flanigan KM, Dunn DM, von Niederhausern A, et al. DMD Trp3X nonsense mutation associated with a founder effect in North American families with mild Becker muscular dystrophy. Neuromuscul Disord 2009;19(11):743–8.
30. Young HK, Barton BA, Waisbren S, et al. Cognitive and psychological profile of males with Becker muscular dystrophy. J Child Neurol 2008;23(2):155–62.
31. North KN, Miller G, Iannaccone ST, et al. Cognitive dysfunction as the major presenting feature of Becker's muscular dystrophy. Neurology 1996;46(2):461–5.
32. Mendell JR, Moxley RT, Griggs RC, et al. Randomized, double-blind six-month trial of prednisone in Duchenne's muscular dystrophy. N Engl J Med 1989; 320(24):1592–7.
33. Lerario A, Bonfiglio S, Sormani M, et al. Quantitative muscle strength assessment in duchenne muscular dystrophy: longitudinal study and correlation with functional measures. BMC Neurol 2012;12:91.
34. McDonald CM, Henricson EK, Abresch RT, et al. The 6-minute walk test and other clinical endpoints in duchenne muscular dystrophy: reliability, concurrent validity, and minimal clinically important differences from a multicenter study. Muscle Nerve 2013;48(3):357–68.
35. McDonald CM, Henricson EK, Abresch RT, et al. The 6-minute walk test and other endpoints in Duchenne muscular dystrophy: longitudinal natural history observations over 48 weeks from a multicenter study. Muscle Nerve 2013; 48(3):343–56.
36. Vuillerot C, Girardot F, Payan C, et al. Monitoring changes and predicting loss of ambulation in Duchenne muscular dystrophy with the Motor Function Measure. Dev Med Child Neurol 2010;52(1):60–5.
37. Mazzone ES, Messina S, Vasco G, et al. Reliability of the north star ambulatory assessment in a multicentric setting. Neuromuscul Disord 2009;19(7):458–61.
38. Mazzone E, Vasco G, Sormani MP, et al. Functional changes in duchenne muscular dystrophy: a 12-month longitudinal cohort study. Neurology 2011; 77(3):250–6.
39. Zatz M, Rapaport D, Vainzof M, et al. Serum creatine-kinase (CK) and pyruvate-kinase (PK) activities in Duchenne (DMD) as compared with Becker (BMD) muscular dystrophy. J Neurol Sci 1991;102(2):190–6.
40. Thakker PB, Sharma A. Becker muscular dystrophy: an unusual presentation. Arch Dis Child 1993;69(1):158–9.
41. Doriguzzi C, Palmucci L, Mongini T, et al. Exercise intolerance and recurrent myoglobinuria as the only expression of Xp21 Becker type muscular dystrophy. J Neurol 1993;240(5):269–71.
42. Shoji T, Nishikawa Y, Saito N, et al. A case of Becker muscular dystrophy and massive myoglobinuria with minimal renal manifestations. Nephrol Dial Transplant 1998;13(3):759–60.
43. Drummond LM. Creatine phosphokinase levels in the newborn and their use in screening for Duchenne muscular dystrophy. Arch Dis Child 1979;54(5):362–6.
44. Pearce JM, Pennington RJ, Walton JN. Serum enzyme studies in muscle disease. III. Serum creatine kinase activity in relatives of patients with the duchenne type of muscular dystrophy. J Neurol Neurosurg Psychiatry 1964;27:181–5.

45. Drousiotou A, Ioannou P, Georgiou T, et al. Neonatal screening for duchenne muscular dystrophy: a novel semiquantitative application of the bioluminescence test for creatine kinase in a pilot national program in Cyprus. Genet Test 1998;2(1):55–60.

46. Bradley DM, Parsons EP, Clarke AJ. Experience with screening newborns for duchenne muscular dystrophy in Wales. BMJ 1993;306(6874):357–60.

47. Plauchu H, Dorche C, Cordier MP, et al. Duchenne muscular dystrophy: neonatal screening and prenatal diagnosis. Lancet 1989;1(8639):669.

48. Skinner R, Emery AE, Scheuerbrandt G, et al. Feasibility of neonatal screening for duchenne muscular dystrophy. J Med Genet 1982;19(1):1–3.

49. Morse RP, Rosman NP. Diagnosis of occult muscular dystrophy: importance of the "chance" finding of elevated serum aminotransferase activities. J Pediatr 1993;122(2):254–6.

50. Zamora S, Adams C, Butzner JD, et al. Elevated aminotransferase activity as an indication of muscular dystrophy: case reports and review of the literature. Can J Gastroenterol 1996;10(6):389–93.

51. Vajro P, Del Giudice E, Veropalumbo C. Muscular dystrophy revealed by incidentally discovered elevated aminotransferase levels. J Pediatr 2010;156(4):689.

52. Veropalumbo C, Del Giudice E, Esposito G, et al. Aminotransferases and muscular diseases: a disregarded lesson. Case reports and review of the literature. J Paediatr Child Health 2012;48(10):886–90.

53. McMillan HJ, Gregas M, Darras BT, et al. Serum transaminase levels in boys with Duchenne and Becker muscular dystrophy. Pediatrics 2011;127(1):e132–6.

54. Rosales XQ, Chu ML, Shilling C, et al. Fidelity of gamma-glutamyl transferase (GGT) in differentiating skeletal muscle from liver damage. J Child Neurol 2008;23(7):748–51.

55. Viollet L, Gailey S, Thornton DJ, et al. Utility of cystatin C to monitor renal function in Duchenne muscular dystrophy. Muscle Nerve 2009;40(3):438–42.

56. Dent KM, Dunn D, von Niederhausern AC, et al. Improved molecular diagnosis of dystrophinopathies in an unselected clinical cohort. Am J Med Genet A 2005; 134:295–8.

57. Yan J, Feng J, Buzin CH, et al. Three-tiered noninvasive diagnosis in 96% of patients with Duchenne muscular dystrophy (DMD). Hum Mutat 2004;23(2):203–4.

58. Gurvich OL, Tuohy TM, Howard MT, et al. DMD pseudoexon mutations: splicing efficiency, phenotype, and potential therapy. Ann Neurol 2008;63(1):81–9.

59. Tuffery-Giraud S, Saquet C, Chambert S, et al. Pseudoexon activation in the DMD gene as a novel mechanism for Becker muscular dystrophy. Hum Mutat 2003;21(6):608–14.

60. Arechavala-Gomeza V, Kinali M, Feng L, et al. Revertant fibres and dystrophin traces in Duchenne muscular dystrophy: implication for clinical trials. Neuromuscul Disord 2010;20(5):295–301.

61. Nicholson LV, Davison K, Johnson MA, et al. Dystrophin in skeletal muscle. II. Immunoreactivity in patients with Xp21 muscular dystrophy. J Neurol Sci 1989;94(1–3):137–46.

62. Nicholson LV, Johnson MA, Gardner Medwin D, et al. Heterogeneity of dystrophin expression in patients with Duchenne and Becker muscular dystrophy. Acta Neuropathol 1990;80(3):239–50.

63. Klein CJ, Coovert DD, Bulman DE, et al. Somatic reversion/suppression in Duchenne muscular dystrophy (DMD): evidence supporting a frame-restoring mechanism in rare dystrophin-positive fibers. Am J Hum Genet 1992;50(5): 950–9.

64. Fanin M, Danieli GA, Vitiello L, et al. Prevalence of dystrophin-positive fibers in 85 Duchenne muscular dystrophy patients. Neuromuscul Disord 1992;2(1):41–5.

65. Burrow KL, Coovert DD, Klein CJ, et al. Dystrophin expression and somatic reversion in prednisone-treated and untreated Duchenne dystrophy. CIDD Study Group. Neurology 1991;41(5):661–6.

66. Hoffman EP, Kunkel LM, Angelini C, et al. Improved diagnosis of Becker muscular dystrophy by dystrophin testing. Neurology 1989;39(8):1011–7.

67. Taylor LE, Kaminoh YJ, Rodesch CK, et al. Quantification of dystrophin immuno-fluorescence in dystrophinopathy muscle specimens. Neuropathol Appl Neuro-biol 2012;38(6):591–601.

68. Tuffery-Giraud S, Beroud C, Leturcq F, et al. Genotype-phenotype analysis in 2,405 patients with a dystrophinopathy using the UMD-DMD database: a model of nationwide knowledgebase. Hum Mutat 2009;30(6):934–45.

69. Beggs AH, Koenig M, Boyce FM, et al. Detection of 98% of DMD/BMD gene deletions by polymerase chain reaction. Hum Genet 1990;86(1):45–8.

70. Chamberlain JS, Gibbs RA, Ranier JE, et al. Multiplex PCR for the diagnosis of Duchenne muscular dystrophy. In: Innis MA, Gelfand DH, Sninsky JJ, et al, editors. PCR protocols: a guide to methods and applications. San Francisco (CA): Academic Press; 1990. p. 272–81.

71. Janssen B, Hartmann C, Scholz V, et al. MLPA analysis for the detection of deletions, duplications and complex rearrangements in the dystrophin gene: potential and pitfalls. Neurogenetics 2005;6:29–35.

72. Schwartz M, Duno M. Improved molecular diagnosis of dystrophin gene muta-tions using the multiplex ligation-dependent probe amplification method. Genet Test 2004;8(4):361–7.

73. del Gaudio D, Yang Y, Boggs BA, et al. Molecular diagnosis of Duchenne/Becker muscular dystrophy: enhanced detection of dystrophin gene rearrange-ments by oligonucleotide array-comparative genomic hybridization. Hum Mutat 2008;29(9):1100–7.

74. Hegde MR, Chin EL, Mulle JG, et al. Microarray-based mutation detection in the dystrophin gene. Hum Mutat 2008;29(9):1091–9.

75. Saillour Y, Cossee M, Leturcq F, et al. Detection of exonic copy-number changes us-ing a highly efficient oligonucleotide-based comparative genomic hybridization-array method. Hum Mutat 2008;29(9):1083–90.

76. Madden HR, Fletcher S, Davis MR, et al. Characterization of a complex Duchenne muscular dystrophy-causing dystrophin gene inversion and restora-tion of the reading frame by induced exon skipping. Hum Mutat 2009;30(1): 22–8.

77. Flanigan KM, Dunn D, Larsen CA, et al. Becker muscular dystrophy due to an inversion of exons 23 and 24 of the DMD gene. Muscle Nerve 2011;44(5):822–5.

78. Cagliani R, Sironi M, Ciafaloni E, et al. An intragenic deletion/inversion event in the DMD gene determines a novel exon creation and results in a BMD pheno-type. Hum Genet 2004;115(1):13–8.

79. Bettecken T, Muller CR. Identification of a 220-kb insertion into the Duchenne gene in a family with an atypical course of muscular dystrophy. Genomics 1989;4(4):592–6.

80. Grimm T, Muller B, Muller CR, et al. Theoretical considerations on germline mosaicism in Duchenne muscular dystrophy. J Med Genet 1990;27(11):683–7.

81. Barbujani G, Russo A, Danieli GA, et al. Segregation analysis of 1885 DMD fam-ilies: significant departure from the expected proportion of sporadic cases. Hum Genet 1990;84(6):522–6.

82. Arpan I, Forbes SC, Lott DJ, et al. T(2) mapping provides multiple approaches for the characterization of muscle involvement in neuromuscular diseases: a cross-sectional study of lower leg muscles in 5-15-year-old boys with Duchenne muscular dystrophy. NMR Biomed 2013;26(3):320–8.

83. Forbes SC, Walter GA, Rooney WD, et al. Skeletal muscles of ambulant children with Duchenne muscular dystrophy: validation of multicenter study of evaluation with MR imaging and MR spectroscopy. Radiology 2013;269(1):198–207.

84. Willcocks RJ, Arpan IA, Forbes SC, et al. Longitudinal measurements of MRI-T2 in boys with Duchenne muscular dystrophy: effects of age and disease progression. Neuromuscul Disord 2014;24(5):393–401.

85. Hollingsworth KG, Garrood P, Eagle M, et al. Magnetic resonance imaging in Duchenne muscular dystrophy: longitudinal assessment of natural history over 18 months. Muscle Nerve 2013;48(4):586–8.

86. Matsumura K, Tome FM, Collin H, et al. Deficiency of the 50K dystrophin-associated glycoprotein in severe childhood autosomal recessive muscular dystrophy. Nature 1992;359(6393):320–2.

87. Matsumura K, Campbell KP. Deficiency of dystrophin-associated proteins: a common mechanism leading to muscle cell necrosis in severe childhood muscular dystrophies. Neuromuscul Disord 1993;3(2):109–18.

88. Brockington M, Blake DJ, Prandini P, et al. Mutations in the fukutin-related protein gene (FKRP) cause a form of congenital muscular dystrophy with secondary laminin alpha2 deficiency and abnormal glycosylation of alpha-dystroglycan. Am J Hum Genet 2001;69(6):1198–209.

89. Schwartz M, Hertz JM, Sveen ML, et al. LGMD2I presenting with a characteristic Duchenne or Becker muscular dystrophy phenotype. Neurology 2005;64(9):1635–7.

90. Flanigan KM, Dunn DM, von Niederhausern A, et al. Nonsense mutation-associated Becker muscular dystrophy: interplay between exon definition and splicing regulatory elements within the DMD gene. Hum Mutat 2011;32(3):299–308.

91. Ginjaar IB, Kneppers AL, v d Meulen JD, et al. Dystrophin nonsense mutation induces different levels of exon 29 skipping and leads to variable phenotypes within one BMD family. Eur J Hum Genet 2000;8(10):793–6.

92. Disset A, Bourgeois CF, Benmalek N, et al. An exon skipping-associated nonsense mutation in the dystrophin gene uncovers a complex interplay between multiple antagonistic splicing elements. Hum Mol Genet 2006;15(6):999–1013.

93. Gangopadhyay SB, Sherratt TG, Heckmatt JZ, et al. Dystrophin in frameshift deletion patients with Becker muscular dystrophy. Am J Hum Genet 1992;51(3):562–70.

94. Winnard AV, Mendell JR, Prior TW, et al. Frameshift deletions of exons 3-7 and revertant fibers in Duchenne muscular dystrophy: mechanisms of dystrophin production. Am J Hum Genet 1995;56(1):158–66.

95. Vetrone SA, Montecino-Rodriguez E, Kudryashova E, et al. Osteopontin promotes fibrosis in dystrophic mouse muscle by modulating immune cell subsets and intramuscular TGF-beta. J Clin Invest 2009;119(6):1583–94.

96. Bello L, Piva L, Barp A, et al. Importance of SPP1 genotype as a covariate in clinical trials in Duchenne muscular dystrophy. Neurology 2012;79(2):159–62.

97. Pegoraro E, Hoffman EP, Piva L, et al. SPP1 genotype is a determinant of disease severity in Duchenne muscular dystrophy. Neurology 2011;76(3):219–26.

98. Heydemann A, Ceco E, Lim JE, et al. Latent TGF-beta-binding protein 4 modifies muscular dystrophy in mice. J Clin Invest 2009;119(12):3703–12.

99. Flanigan KM, Ceco E, Lamar KM, et al. LTBP4 genotype predicts age of ambulatory loss in duchenne muscular dystrophy. Ann Neurol 2013;73(4):481–8.

100. Bushby K, Finkel R, Birnkrant DJ, et al. Diagnosis and management of Duchenne muscular dystrophy, part 1: diagnosis, and pharmacological and psychosocial management. Lancet Neurol 2010;9(1):77–93.

101. Bushby K, Finkel R, Birnkrant DJ, et al. Diagnosis and management of Duchenne muscular dystrophy, part 2: implementation of multidisciplinary care. Lancet Neurol 2010;9(2):177–89.

102. Bonifati MD, Ruzza G, Bonometto P, et al. A multicenter, double-blind, randomized trial of deflazacort versus prednisone in Duchenne muscular dystrophy. Muscle Nerve 2000;23(9):1344–7.

103. Fenichel GM, Florence JM, Pestronk A, et al. Long-term benefit from prednisone therapy in Duchenne muscular dystrophy. Neurology 1991;41(12):1874–7.

104. Fenichel GM, Mendell JR, Moxley RT 3rd, et al. A comparison of daily and alternate-day prednisone therapy in the treatment of Duchenne muscular dystrophy. Arch Neurol 1991;48(6):575–9.

105. Griggs RC, Moxley RT 3rd, Mendell JR, et al. Prednisone in Duchenne dystrophy. A randomized, controlled trial defining the time course and dose response. Clinical Investigation of Duchenne Dystrophy Group. Arch Neurol 1991;48(4):383–8.

106. Griggs RC, Moxley RT 3rd, Mendell JR, et al. Duchenne dystrophy: randomized, controlled trial of prednisone (18 months) and azathioprine (12 months). Neurology 1993;43(3 Pt 1):520–7.

107. Manzur AY, Kuntzer T, Pike M, et al. Glucocorticoid corticosteroids for Duchenne muscular dystrophy. Cochrane Database Syst Rev 2008;(1):CD003725.

108. Wong BL, Christopher C. Corticosteroids in Duchenne muscular dystrophy: a reappraisal. J Child Neurol 2002;17(3):183–90.

109. Moxley RT 3rd, Pandya S, Ciafaloni E, et al. Change in natural history of Duchenne muscular dystrophy with long-term corticosteroid treatment: implications for management. J Child Neurol 2010;25(9):1116–29.

110. Escolar DM, Hache LP, Clemens PR, et al. Randomized, blinded trial of weekend vs daily prednisone in Duchenne muscular dystrophy. Neurology 2011; 77(5):444–52.

111. Merlini L, Cicognani A, Malaspina E, et al. Early prednisone treatment in Duchenne muscular dystrophy. Muscle Nerve 2003;27(2):222–7.

112. Merlini L, Gennari M, Malaspina E, et al. Early corticosteroid treatment in 4 Duchenne muscular dystrophy patients: 14-year follow-up. Muscle Nerve 2012;45(6):796–802.

113. Nigro G, Comi LI, Politano L, et al. The incidence and evolution of cardiomyopathy in Duchenne muscular dystrophy. Int J Cardiol 1990;26(3):271–7.

114. Cox GF, Kunkel LM. Dystrophies and heart disease. Curr Opin Cardiol 1997; 12(3):329–43.

115. Connuck DM, Sleeper LA, Colan SD, et al. Characteristics and outcomes of cardiomyopathy in children with Duchenne or Becker muscular dystrophy: a comparative study from the Pediatric Cardiomyopathy Registry. Am Heart J 2008;155(6):998–1005.

116. Viollet L, Thrush PT, Flanigan KM, et al. Effects of angiotensin-converting enzyme inhibitors and/or beta blockers on the cardiomyopathy in Duchenne muscular dystrophy. Am J Cardiol 2012;110(1):98–102.

117. Takenaka A, Yokota M, Iwase M, et al. Discrepancy between systolic and diastolic dysfunction of the left ventricle in patients with Duchenne muscular dystrophy. Eur Heart J 1993;14(5):669–76.

118. Giglio V, Pasceri V, Messano L, et al. Ultrasound tissue characterization detects preclinical myocardial structural changes in children affected by Duchenne muscular dystrophy. J Am Coll Cardiol 2003;42(2):309–16.
119. American Academy of Pediatrics Section on Cardiology and Cardiac Surgery. Cardiovascular health supervision for individuals affected by Duchenne or Becker muscular dystrophy. Pediatrics 2005;116(6):1569–73.
120. Allen HD, Flanigan KM, Thrush PT, et al. A randomized, double-blind trial of lisinopril and losartan for the treatment of cardiomyopathy in duchenne muscular dystrophy. PLoS Curr 2013;5. pii: ecurrents.md.2cc69a1dae4be7dfe2bcb420024ea865.
121. Duboc D, Meune C, Lerebours G, et al. Effect of perindopril on the onset and progression of left ventricular dysfunction in Duchenne muscular dystrophy. J Am Coll Cardiol 2005;45(6):855–7.
122. Stollberger C, Finsterer J. Can perindopril delay the onset of heart failure in duchenne muscular dystrophy? J Am Coll Cardiol 2005;46(9):1781 [author reply: 1782].
123. Corrado G, Lissoni A, Beretta S, et al. Prognostic value of electrocardiograms, ventricular late potentials, ventricular arrhythmias, and left ventricular systolic dysfunction in patients with Duchenne muscular dystrophy. Am J Cardiol 2002;89(7):838–41.
124. Thrush PT, Allen HD, Viollet L, et al. Re-examination of the electrocardiogram in boys with Duchenne muscular dystrophy and correlation with its dilated cardiomyopathy. Am J Cardiol 2009;103(2):262–5.
125. Chenard AA, Becane HM, Tertrain F, et al. Ventricular arrhythmia in Duchenne muscular dystrophy: prevalence, significance and prognosis. Neuromuscul Disord 1993;3(3):201–6.
126. James J, Kinnett K, Wang Y, et al. Electrocardiographic abnormalities in very young Duchenne muscular dystrophy patients precede the onset of cardiac dysfunction. Neuromuscul Disord 2011;21(7):462–7.
127. Birnkrant DJ, Bushby KM, Amin RS, et al. The respiratory management of patients with duchenne muscular dystrophy: a DMD care considerations working group specialty article. Pediatr Pulmonol 2010;45(8):739–48.
128. Eagle M, Baudouin SV, Chandler C, et al. Survival in Duchenne muscular dystrophy: improvements in life expectancy since 1967 and the impact of home nocturnal ventilation. Neuromuscul Disord 2002;12(10):926–9.
129. Kinali M, Main M, Eliahoo J, et al. Predictive factors for the development of scoliosis in Duchenne muscular dystrophy. Eur J Paediatr Neurol 2007;11(3):160–6.
130. King WM, Ruttencutter R, Nagaraja HN, et al. Orthopedic outcomes of long-term daily corticosteroid treatment in Duchenne muscular dystrophy. Neurology 2007;68(19):1607–13.
131. Cheuk DK, Wong V, Wraige E, et al. Surgery for scoliosis in Duchenne muscular dystrophy. Cochrane Database Syst Rev 2013;(2):CD005375.
132. Eagle M, Bourke J, Bullock R, et al. Managing Duchenne muscular dystrophy–the additive effect of spinal surgery and home nocturnal ventilation in improving survival. Neuromuscul Disord 2007;17(6):470–5.
133. Welch EM, Barton ER, Zhuo J, et al. PTC124 targets genetic disorders caused by nonsense mutations. Nature 2007;447(7140):87–91.
134. Finkel RS, Flanigan KM, Wong B, et al. Phase 2a study of ataluren-mediated dystrophin production in patients with nonsense mutation Duchenne muscular dystrophy. PLoS One 2013;8(12):e81302.
135. Du L, Damoiseaux R, Nahas S, et al. Nonaminoglycoside compounds induce readthrough of nonsense mutations. J Exp Med 2009;206(10):2285–97.

136. Kayali R, Ku JM, Khitrov G, et al. Read-through compound 13 restores dystrophin expression and improves muscle function in the mdx mouse model for Duchenne muscular dystrophy. Hum Mol Genet 2012;21(18):4007–20.
137. Aartsma-Rus A, Fokkema I, Verschuuren J, et al. Theoretic applicability of antisense-mediated exon skipping for Duchenne muscular dystrophy mutations. Hum Mutat 2009;30(3):293–9.
138. Cirak S, Arechavala-Gomeza V, Guglieri M, et al. Exon skipping and dystrophin restoration in patients with Duchenne muscular dystrophy after systemic phosphorodiamidate morpholino oligomer treatment: an open-label, phase 2, dose-escalation study. Lancet 2011;378(9791):595–605.
139. Goemans NM, Tulinius M, van den Akker JT, et al. Systemic administration of PRO051 in Duchenne's muscular dystrophy. N Engl J Med 2011;364(16):1513–22.
140. Kinali M, Arechavala-Gomeza V, Feng L, et al. Local restoration of dystrophin expression with the morpholino oligomer AVI-4658 in Duchenne muscular dystrophy: a single-blind, placebo-controlled, dose-escalation, proof-of-concept study. Lancet Neurol 2009;8(10):918–28.
141. van Deutekom JC, Janson AA, Ginjaar IB, et al. Local dystrophin restoration with antisense oligonucleotide PRO051. N Engl J Med 2007;357(26):2677–86.
142. Mendell JR, Rodino-Klapac LR, Sahenk Z, et al. Eteplirsen for the treatment of Duchenne muscular dystrophy. Ann Neurol 2013;74(5):637–47.
143. Mendell JR, Campbell K, Rodino-Klapac L, et al. Dystrophin immunity in Duchenne's muscular dystrophy. N Engl J Med 2010;363(15):1429–37.
144. Wang Z, Storb R, Halbert CL, et al. Successful regional delivery and long-term expression of a dystrophin gene in canine muscular dystrophy: a preclinical model for human therapies. Mol Ther 2012;20(8):1501–7.

Congenital Myopathies and Muscular Dystrophies

Heather R. Gilbreath, PA-C[a], Diana Castro, MD[b], Susan T. Iannaccone, MD[b],*

KEYWORDS

- Congenital muscular dystrophy • Congenital myopathy
- Ullrich congenital muscular dystrophy • Nemaline myopathy
- Central core myopathy • Centronuclear myopathy
- Merosin deficiency congenital muscular dystrophy

KEY POINTS

- Diagnosis most often depends on muscle biopsy and mutation analysis, but the physician in charge must be aware of the expertise of both the biopsy laboratory and that of the DNA diagnostic laboratory.
- There are many pitfalls that can result in misinterpretation of both the biopsy and the DNA; these are best avoided by working with laboratories that have the highest expertise.
- It is important that patients and families receive complete information regarding the diagnostic process and the results, including hard copies for their child's own records.
- There are now published guidelines for the management of children with congenital muscular dystrophies (CMD) and congenital myopathies (CM).
- Patient groups are lobbying for support of clinical trials for patients with CMD and CM, and some studies may well be seen coming online in the next few years.

INTRODUCTION

The congenital muscular dystrophies (CMD) and myopathies (CM) are a diverse group of diseases that share features such as early onset of symptoms (in the first year of life), genetic causes, and high risks for restrictive lung disease and orthopedic deformities. The classification of these disorders is historically based and first depended on muscle biopsy findings. CMDs were identified with dystrophic biopsies and CMs with peculiar structural changes seen with histochemistry or electron microscopy. Thus,

Funding Sources: NIH (NS077323), ISIS, GSK, PTC Therapeutics, MDA (259206), Santhera, Sarepta Therapeutics (S.T. Iannaccone, D. Castro).
Conflict of Interest: S.T. Iannaccone serves as advisor to Sarepta and ISIS; D. Castro: None.
[a] Department of Advanced Practice, Children's Medical Center of Dallas, 2350 Stemmons Freeway, Dallas, TX 75207, USA; [b] Departments of Pediatrics and Neurology and Neurotherapeutics, University of Texas Southwestern Medical Center, 5323 Harry Hines Boulevard, Dallas, TX 75390-9063, USA
* Corresponding author.
E-mail address: susan.iannaccone@utsouthwestern.edu

the CMDs were first described early in the twentieth century,[1] whereas CMs were not recognized until cryostat sections and histochemistry came into use in the late 1960s.[2] At that time, it was apparent that most patients with CMs had nonprogressive weakness, whereas the CMDs were thought to be similar to other dystrophies with progressive limb girdle weakness. As each of the entities was associated with unique gene mutations, some understanding for disease mechanism became available and a fairly well-structured genotype-phenotype correlation for all the CMDs and CMs is now available.

Diagnosis should begin with a suspicion, the consideration of whether creatine kinase (CK) is elevated, and a look at involvement outside the skeletal muscles. Abnormal brain imaging, cognitive involvement, early orthopedic deformities, epilepsy, and structural changes in the eye should suggest a CMD. Nondystrophic biopsy, facial and bulbar weakness, and no eye involvement other than gaze palsy would suggest a CM. Once brain imaging or muscle histology support a specific disease, then diagnosis should be confirmed by mutation analysis. This confirmation will allow for accurate prognostication, educated anticipatory guidance, and informed family planning.

To illustrate best the clinical spectrum and diagnostic algorithm for these diseases, this article presents 5 cases with discussion immediately following. The cases represent the most common forms of CMD and CM and provide an opportunity to review important clues to diagnosis and guidelines for management.

CASE 1

A 4-year-old boy was referred to the Neuromuscular Disease Clinic for joint laxity. Birth history was reported to be significant for hypotonia, respiratory difficulties requiring oxygen via nasal cannula, poor feeding, and congenital hip dislocation. The patient had motor delay. Specifically, he began sitting for brief periods of time at 7 months of age, and combat crawling after 1 year of age. He eventually walked without assistance but was noted to suffer from significant weakness. At presentation, he was unable to stand independently from a seated position. Social and language function was normal.

Physical examination demonstrated a well-developed child with long myopathic facies, a high palate, and mild ptosis bilaterally. Lung and heart examinations were normal. Musculoskeletal examination was significant for mild flexion contractures of both elbows and knees with hyperlaxity of both wrists. On neurologic examination, the patient was found to be hypotonic with decreased muscle bulk, proximal greater than distal muscle weakness, and decreased reflexes.

CK level was 280 iU/L. Electrodiagnostic studies were normal. Cardiac evaluation was negative. Muscle biopsy (**Fig. 1**) revealed dystrophic changes, including marked variability in fiber size with regenerating fibers and central nuclei. Immunohistochemistry demonstrated reduced reaction to 300 kDa merosin and sarcoglycan antibodies. Magnetic resonance imaging (MRI) of brain was normal. Skin fibroblast testing confirmed a splicing mutation in exon 16 of the COL6A gene.

The patient lost his ability to ambulate at 5 years of age. By late childhood, he had severe restrictive lung disease with a forced vital capacity of 0.4 L or 16% predicted and required noninvasive ventilation intermittently during the day and all night.

This young boy had symptoms from birth with hyptonia, weakness, and joint contractures. The differential diagnosis included CMD and CM, but the progressive nature of his contractures and restrictive lung disease are much more consistent with CMD. Furthermore, the distal laxity and normal CK level are typical of collagen mutations or

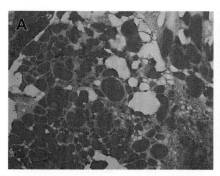
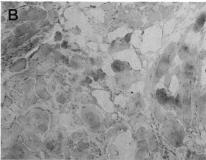

Fig. 1. (*A*) Hematoxylin and eosin (H&E) stain for light microscopy of muscle biopsy from Case 1 obtained when patient was 3 years old. There are many features of a dystrophic process including marked variation in fiber diameter, increased fibrosis and fat infiltration, and ring fibers (original magnification ×20). (*B*) Modified Gomori trichrome (GT) stain of the same biopsy. There is an increase in internal nuclei with hypertrophied and severely atrophied fibers (original magnification ×20).

Ullrich congenital muscular dystrophy (UCMD). Other characteristics of UCMD, the skin manifestations of keloid formation and follicular hyperkeratosis (hyperkeratosis pilaris), were not seen on presentation. However, skin changes may not be present in early childhood and often progress dramatically after puberty.[3] Biopsy in this case was dystrophic but the immunohistology was misleading, suggesting a merosin deficiency, whereas the normal brain imaging was against that diagnosis. Staining for collagen 6 may be normal or abnormal in UCMD, so diagnosis depends on mutation analysis that is now available on blood.[4]

Bethlem myopathy is allelic with UCMD and usually associated with dominant mutations. However, there is a spectrum of disease with many patients showing overlap, such as severe Bethlem caused by recessive mutations and mild UCMD caused by heterozygous mutations. Cardiomyopathy has never been reported associated with either recessive or dominant mutations in these patients, setting them apart from other CMD as well as the CM (**Table 1**).

Other forms of CMD are caused by mutations in laminin α2, α7 β1 integrin, and several genes responsible for glycosylation of dystroglycan (**Box 1**). The most common of these are mutations in laminin α2 (*LAMA*) that cause merosin deficiency CMD (see Case 3). Among people of Japanese origin, mutations of the fukutin gene (*FKN*) are the most common cause of CMD.[5] Abnormalities of merosin and glycosylation are usually associated with structural changes in the brain and brain stem. Patients may have epilepsy or mental retardation. Exceptions are patients who have a

Table 1 Characteristics of UCMD	
Onset of weakness	Neonatal or infancy
Congenital hip dislocation	Common
Joint contractures	Begin in infancy or early childhood
CK	Normal or slightly elevated
Restrictive lung disease	Severe and progressive
Cardiomyopathy	Never seen
Brain MRI	Normal

Box 1
Classification: CMD and linked genes

Ullrich	COL6A
MDC1A (Merosin deficiency)	LAMA2
Congenital muscular dystrophy with integrin α7 defect	ITGA7
Walker Warburg syndrome	POMT1,2; LARGE
Fukuyama CMD	FKTM
Muscle eye brain-like CMD	FKTM, FKRP
MDC1C (fukutin-related protein deficiency)	FKRP
MDC1D (LARGE deficiency)	LARGE
Muscle eye brain disease	POMGNT1, FKTM, FKRP
SEPN1-related myopathy	SEPN1
L-CMD (LMNA-related CMD)	LMNA

---

limb girdle dystrophy phenotype caused by mutations in glycosylation. They lie at the mild end of the spectrum and generally do not have any involvement of brain or eye.[6,7] Management is symptomatic and must include anticipatory guidance.

The patient presented here benefited from noninvasive ventilation and aggressive pulmonary toilet (airway clearance). Although he suffered from relentless contractures, reconstructive surgery was of limited help. Dynamic bracing may slow progression of contractures but there are no controlled studies to determine this. Most patients cannot maintain daily use of orthotics because of discomfort and many find recurrence of contractures after surgery. Unfortunately, for the typical child with UCMD, life expectancy is shortened and death from respiratory failure or infection is common in the second and third decades.

CASE 2

A 6-month-old boy presented to the Neuromuscular Disease Clinic with hypotonia and dysphagia. Pregnancy, labor, and delivery were reported to be uncomplicated. However, the patient had significant sucking and swallowing difficulties at birth, necessitating gavage feedings and then gastrostomy by age 1 month. Family members denied respiratory difficulties.

On physical examination, the patient was a well-developed, well-nourished boy in no acute distress. General examination was significant for a long myopathic face (**Fig. 2**) with a high, narrow palate as well as pectus excavatum deformity of the chest wall. Eye movements were normal as were lung and heart examinations. On neurologic examination, the patient was profoundly hypotonic with decreased muscle mass throughout and proximal muscle weakness. Deep tendon reflexes were absent.

CK was normal. A muscle biopsy (**Fig. 3**) demonstrated poor fiber-type differentiation and the presence of nemaline rods. Sequencing of the nebulin (NEB) gene was significant for heterozygous mutations: one at the junction of intron 11 and exon 12 predicted to disrupt the intron 11 splice acceptor site and another in exon 18 predicted to result in frame-shift and premature protein termination. These mutations confirmed a diagnosis of recessive nemaline myopathy.

The patient continued to gain developmental milestones slowly, ultimately walking independently near 30 months of age. However, he suffered from nonprogressive proximal muscle weakness and moderate restrictive lung disease. At 10 years of age, a polysomnogram revealed alveolar hypoventilation with bradypnea and hypercapnia. He was treated with noninvasive nocturnal ventilation (BiPAP).

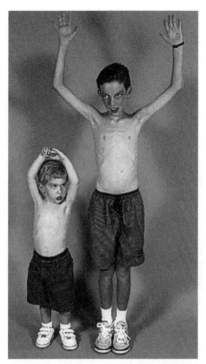

Fig. 2. Case 2, toddler with his older brother. Note the long, myopathic facies and asthenic body habitus in both, which are typical of patients with CM.

This baby had severe hypotonia with swallowing and breathing problems from birth. The differential diagnosis was spinal muscular atrophy (SMA) versus CM, although CMD could not be ruled out on physical examination. He had no tongue fasciculations, a finding against SMA. Although an electromyogram might have helped differentiate, it would most likely require anesthesia. More commonly, SMA can be ruled out by mutation analysis and the recommendation made for muscle biopsy.

The CM are best diagnosed by muscle biopsy using sophisticated histochemistry and electron microscopy (**Tables 2** and **3**). When the characteristic structural changes in the muscle fiber are found, mutation analysis is directed for genes at risk. In many patients, the characteristic rods are not seen, even after as many as 4 muscle biopsies. The absence of rods could be due to a sampling error with variation among muscles or related to stage of disease. When rods are not seen, there will be fiber size disproportion or lack of fiber type differentiation, both important clues to the diagnosis of CM.[8]

Nemaline and central core disease are the most common disorders of the CMs (see Case 5). In this case, there was an affected older brother that informed the workup. Nemaline myopathy, however, is not always a recessive disorder; there are several mutations that are heterozygous or dominant in nature. Central core disease is typically dominant in inheritance but can be seen with de novo or sporadic mutations and negative family history.

The management for nemaline myopathy is similar to that for the CMDs and SMA; see published guidelines (**Box 2**).[9,10] It is important to note that, although rare, cardiomyopathy occurs with some regularity and, thus, monitoring with echocardiography is

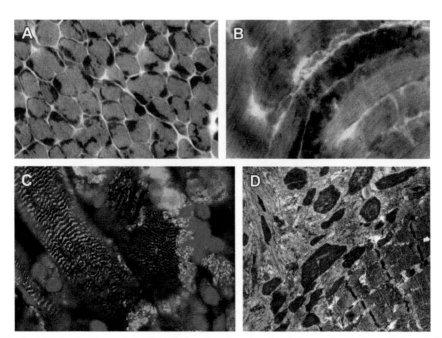

Fig. 3. (*A*) Muscle biopsy from Case 2 showing clusters of rods in nearly all fibers. This stain is GT and rods stain as dark blue. (*B*) High power view of the same muscle sample with GT stain shows the elongated shape of the rods. (*C*) Use of green fluorescent tag for ∂-actinin labels the rods in a high power view. Nuclei are labeled red. (*D*) Electron microscopy of a muscle biopsy from another nemaline patient shows several small rods disrupting the normal sarcomeric pattern. (*Courtesy of* M. Vainzof, University of Sao Paolo, Brazil.)

important.[11,12] More common are respiratory complications often with bulbar weakness. Patients are at high risk for sleep hypoventilation as well as airway obstruction regardless of the severity of their limb girdle weakness. There is a peculiar association between diaphragm paralysis and nemaline myopathy (with little genotype/phenotype correlation).[13] Thus, annual pulmonary function tests sitting and supine and sleep studies are crucial for preventing serious complications.

Table 2 Some phenotypic clues for CM	
Nemaline myopathy	Diaphragm weakness Distal weakness in lower extremities (LEs) Severe facial and bulbar weakness
Central core disease (including minicore)	Muscle pain/cramps MH Dominant inheritance
Fiber type disproportion	Low tone without other distinguishing characteristics
Centronuclear myopathy (including myotubular myopathy)	Progressive ophthalmoparesis Early respiratory failure in boys Progressive craniofacial deformities

Table 3
Congenital myopathies and their genes

Name	Genes Mutated	Inheritance
Nemaline myopathy	TPM3 (1q21.3)	AD or AR
	NEB (2q22.3)	AR
	ACTA 1 (1q42.13)	AD or sporadic, AR
	TPM2 (9p13.3)	AD
	TNNT1 (19q13.42)	AR (Amish private mutation)
	KBTBD 13 (15q22.31)	AD
	CFL2 (14q13.1)	AR
Core myopathy (including minicore)	RYR1 (19q13.1)	AR
	SEPN1 (1p36.11)	AR or sporadic
	TTN (2q31.2)	AR
	MYH7 (14q12)	AD
Fiber type disproportion	ACTA1 (1q42.1)	AD
	Locus 2 (Xq13.1-q22.1)	AR
	SEPN1 (1p36.11)	AR
	TPM3 (1q21.2)	AD
	TPM2 (9p13)	AD
	MYL2 (12q24.11)	AR
Centronuclear myopathy (including myotubular myopathy)	MTM1 (Xq28)	X-linked
	DNM2 (19q13.1)	AD
	MYF6 (12q21.31)	AD
	CCDC78 (16p13.3)	AD
	BIN1 (2q14.3)	AR

Abbreviations: AD, autosomal dominant; AR, autosomal recessive.

   Orthopedic complications are common as well but not so predictable. They typically affect the distal lower extremities and scoliosis is common. Many patients exhibit poor weight gain and experience significant fatigue. There are no guidelines for exercise beyond stretching, although some patients seem to benefit from aquatherapy (**Box 3**). As a CM, progressive weakness is not expected but occurs often by the fourth and fifth decades.

CASE 3

A 6-week-old baby boy presented to the Neuromuscular Disease Clinic for severe hypotonia. He was reported to have required an extended neonatal intensive care unit admission following birth due to respiratory and feeding difficulties.
   Physical examination demonstrated an alert infant with moderate facial weakness and pectus excavatum deformity. Lung and heart examinations were normal.

Box 2
Management pearls: annual monitoring for CM

Pulmonary function tests (PFTs), sitting and supine

Electrocardiogram, echocardiogram according to risk

Nutrition and growth parameters

Swallowing and bulbar weakness

Polysomnogram if PFTs less than 65% predicted or symptoms of sleep disturbance

Orthopedic: range of motion, scoliosis screen

Neurologic examination demonstrated markedly decreased tone throughout with severe head lag. Extraocular movements were full except for decreased upgaze bilaterally. In the supine position, there was no spontaneous movement of any muscle groups except fingers and toes. There were no tongue fasciculations. Deep tendon reflexes were absent throughout.

CK was elevated at 16,000. Electrodiagnostic studies demonstrated a mild axonal neuropathy. Brain MRI revealed abnormal white matter and pontine hypoplasia (**Fig. 4**).

Muscle biopsy was significant for active myopathic changes, including rare degenerating and regenerating myofibers (**Fig. 5**). Immunohistochemistry revealed absent α-2 laminin consistent with merosin-deficient congenital muscular dystrophy. DNA mutation analysis showed him to be compound heterozygous for mutations in LAMA2. He was heterozygous at the intron-exon 4 junction of the LAMA2 gene for a mutation defined as c.396+1G>T and he was also heterozygous in exon 4 of LAMA2 for a mutation defined as c.498G>A. At 8 years of age, the patient had significant dysphagia as well as restrictive lung disease and sleep-disordered breathing.

Merosin deficiency (MDC1A) represents the most common form of CMD after Ullrich among people of western European origin.[14] Mutations are recessive and affected

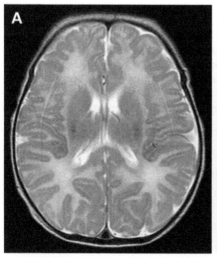
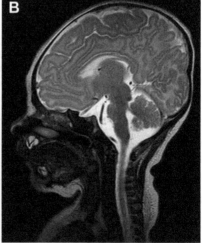

Fig. 4. (*A, B*) MRI images of the brain in Case 3. The white matter of both hemispheres is abnormal and the brain stem is flattened.

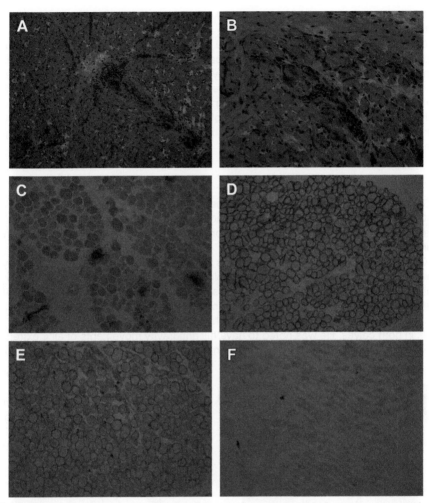

Fig. 5. (*A*) H&E section from the biopsy of Case 3 shows myopathic features and secondary inflammation by macrophages. (*B*) High power view of the same region emphasizes the predominance of macrophages, a characteristic of this disease early in its course. (*C*) Alkaline phosphatase labels regenerating fibers of which there are many, evidence that this is an active process such as muscular dystrophy. (*D*) Immunohistology using peroxidase tag shows that dystrophin labeling is normal. (*E*) Immunohistology using antibody for ∂-dystroglycan demonstrates normal labeling. (*F*) Immunohistology using 300-kDa antibody for merosin demonstrates nearly complete absence of that protein, diagnostic for merosin deficiency or MDC 1A. (*Courtesy of* D. Burns, UT Southwestern Medical Center, Dallas, TX.)

siblings and cousins are often encountered. Patients clinically look very similar to SMA type 1 or severe type 2 cases but do not have tongue fasciculations. Brain imaging and nerve conduction studies are usually abnormal after the age of 6 months and can aid in early diagnosis.[15] However, diagnosis should be confirmed by mutation analysis in all cases providing for accurate prognosis and family planning.

There is a spectrum of disease from the severe infantile form with symptoms at birth to mild weakness seen with partial merosin deficiency. Partial merosin deficiency is defined by immunohistochemistry on muscle biopsy. It requires the use of 2 antibodies for this protein against the 80-kDa and 300-kDa moieties. Most patients with complete deficiency never walk.

One clue in this case was the abnormal vertical gaze that has been described in many patients. The association with gaze palsies is seen in only a few CM and sometimes raises the possibility of congenital myasthenic syndrome. Cardiomyopathy has been described but is rare, although all patients, whether they have partial or complete deficiency, are at risk for epilepsy, of all types and at all ages.[16]

Management is as described above for other patients with CMs or CMDs. Patients should be monitored for seizures but their cognitive function remains normal through life (**Fig. 6**).

CASE 4

A 3-year-old boy presented to the Neuromuscular Disease Clinic with a history of intermittent toe walking and frequent falls. In addition, the patient had difficulty climbing stairs. He did not complain of muscle pain or muscle cramping and there were no concerns for bulbar or respiratory weakness.

On physical examination, the patient was a well-developed and well-nourished boy. General examination was significant for a slightly high and narrow palate. Respiratory and cardiac examinations were normal. Musculoskeletal examination did not show evidence of scoliosis but was concerning for scapular winging bilaterally. On neurologic examination, the patient was found to be hypotonic with a slight increase in muscle bulk in both calves. He was noted to have full antigravity movements of all 4 extremities. His gait demonstrated hyperextension of both knees, but he could heel and toe

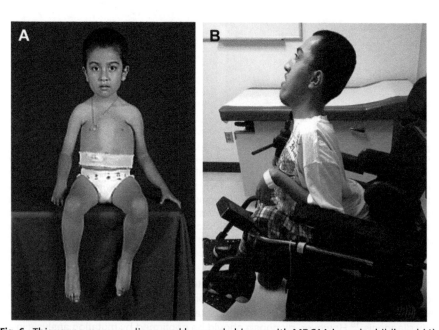

Fig. 6. This young man was diagnosed by muscle biopsy with MDC1A in early childhood (A), confirmed by mutation analysis later. He had dysphagia, gastrointestinal dysmotility, severe progressive restrictive lung disease, and relentless orthopedic deformities but no seizures. He uses BiPAP when asleep and enteral feedings. At the age of 21 years (B), he attended clinic appointments alone via public transportation.

walk appropriately. The Gowers sign was positive and deep tendon reflexes were absent except for ankle jerks that were 2+.

CK was elevated at 1300 iU/L. Electrodiagnosis did not demonstrate electrophysiologic evidence for a neuropathy or irritative myopathy, although voluntary motor units could not be assessed. A muscle biopsy was significant for disproportionately small type 1 myofibers that contained centrally located nuclei (**Figs. 7** and **8**). DNA testing for the *DMPK* (myotonic dystrophy) and *MTM1* (myotubular myopathy) genes was negative as was mutation analysis for *ACTA1* and *COL6* genes. Ultimately, the patient was confirmed to be a compound heterozygote for Gln23354Stop and c.100185delA mutations in the titin (*TTN*) gene, confirming his diagnosis of centronuclear myopathy.

This case is a good example of the "diagnostic odyssey" that many people with CM experience. If the biopsy shows only nonspecific changes or the mutation analysis for the most commonly associated genes (*DMPK* and *MTM1* in this case) are negative, it can be extremely difficult to counsel the patient and family regarding prognosis and inheritance. This patient's mutation was identified through collaboration with Dr Alan Beggs at Boston Childrens' Hospital.[17] There is high hope that next-generation sequencing will end such odysseys, but prohibitive costs, denied access, and variations in technique may prevent such hopes from being attained. The results of all gene sequencing must be interpreted in the clinical context. When results are unclear, consultation with a genetic counselor may be indicated. Therefore, for the CM, the muscle biopsy remains the best means of narrowing the search for gene mutations.

As with many patients with recessive centronuclear myopathy or central core disease (see discussion below), the limb girdle weakness is mild. Many patients have progressive ophthalmoparesis, an important clinical finding that can indicate diagnosis. This boy could still develop ophthalmoparesis in the second decade of life. There is not much propensity for cardiomyopathy, although the risk remains as does that for restrictive lung disease and orthopedic complications. Thus, the management is the same as described above.

CASE 5

A 10-year-old girl presented to the Neuromuscular Disease Clinic for hypotonia. Birth and developmental history were reported to be normal. However, family members

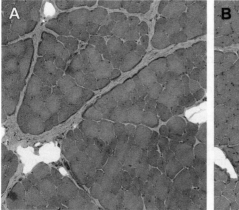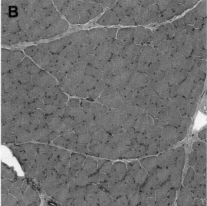

Fig. 7. (*A*) GT stain of biopsy from Case 4 shows some chronic but mild myopathic changes. (*B*) H&E section shows variation in fiber diameter and internal nuclei in nearly half of all fibers. (*Courtesy of* D. Burns, UT Southwestern Medical Center, Dallas, TX.)

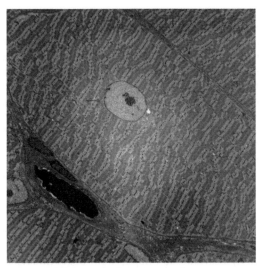

Fig. 8. Electron microscopy of the muscle from Case 4 shows a very small fiber with single internal nucleus (*arrow*) in cross-section, typical of centronuclear myopathy. (*Courtesy of* D. Burns, UT Southwestern Medical Center, Dallas, TX.)

recalled that the patient had been previously evaluated by an orthopedist as a toddler due to an abnormal gait. She was diagnosed as being "pigeon-toed" and no interventions were deemed necessary. At 8 years of age, the patient was noted to have difficulty arising from the floor. She was referred for physical therapy services and improved. Nevertheless, the patient continued to have difficulty climbing stairs as well as running and jumping. Family members denied a history of muscle fatigue or frequent falls.

On physical examination, the patient was a well-developed, well-nourished girl in no acute distress. Lung and heart examinations were normal. Musculoskeletal examination was significant for slight scapular winging. On neurologic examination, the patient was noted to have decreased muscle tone and decreased muscle bulk throughout. Minimal ptosis was evident in the right eye with facial weakness including difficulty burying eyelashes. Manual muscle testing demonstrated mild limb girdle weakness. Shoulder abduction was 4−, elbow flexion 4−, hip flexion 3, and knee extension 3+; all were symmetric. Her gait was significant for decreased heel strike bilaterally. The Gowers sign was positive. Deep tendon reflexes were absent in the upper extremities and 1+ in the lower extremities and symmetric.

Pulmonary function testing showed mild restrictive lung disease with forced vital capacity of 1.26 L or 63% predicted. CK was normal. The electromyogram was consistent with a myopathic process. A muscle biopsy showed marked type 1 fiber predominance and type 2 fiber atrophy. DNA testing of the *ACTA1* gene was normal.

The patient's weakness was nonprogressive. She had a repeat muscle biopsy performed approximately 3 years after the first that again demonstrated type 1 myofiber predominance (**Figs. 9** and **10**). There were rare fibers with core/targetoid-like change and a mild loss of randomness of fiber-type distribution. Mutation analysis of the *RYR1* gene was positive for a heterozygous mutation in exon 91, an undocumented variant of uncertain clinical significance defined as c.12727G>A, which was predicted to result in the amino acid substitution p.Glu4243Lys. Parental testing was negative, supporting the conclusion that the patient carried a de novo, clinically significant mutation.

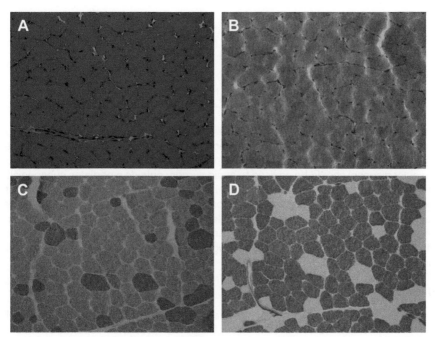

Fig. 9. (A) H&E stain of muscle biopsy from Case 5 shows minimal myopathic changes. (B) GT section. (C) ATPase stain at pH 9.4. (D) ATPase stain at pH 4.3. (Courtesy of D. Burns, UT Southwestern Medical Center, Dallas, TX.)

This patient had no history for malignant hyperthermia (MH) but RYRY1 (as well as SEPN1) mutations are commonly associated with a significant risk of MH.[18,19] Therefore, identification of the mutation in individual patients as well as their family members is crucial to avoid life-threatening events (**Box 4**). Although most pediatric-trained anesthesiologists avoid pharmacologic triggers when working with children with any neuromuscular disorder, it is cost-effective to know the exact risk for a given case.

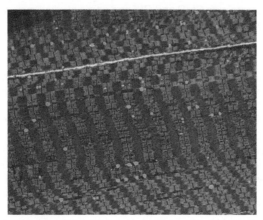

Fig. 10. Electron microscopy of muscle from Case 5 shows disruption of sarcomeric structure suggestive of minicore formation. (Courtesy of D. Burns, UT Southwestern Medical Center, Dallas, TX.)

> **Box 4**
> **Some triggers for MH/rhabdomyolysis**
>
> Succinylcholine (depolarizing muscle blockade)
>
> Halothane (inhalational agents)
>
> Excessive exercise, especially in heat with poor hydration

The general recommendation is that children with *RYR1* or *SEPN1* mutations or histologic evidence of core myopathy wear a medical alert in the form of dog tag or bracelet stating MH as a risk. Moreover, parents (and those of all children affected by neuromuscular disease) should be advised to avoid surgery outside a pediatric subspecialty hospital, not only because of the risk of MH but also because of many possible postoperative complications including respiratory failure, cardiac arrhythmias, and bowel paralysis. Such children at risk are particularly susceptible to narcotic effects. There are published guidelines for preoperative and postoperative management of children with Duchenne muscular dystrophy, although 2 consensus statements address CMD and CM specifically.[10,20–24]

SUMMARY

The cases presented in this article provide a survey of the CMDs and CMs commonly seen in the pediatric neuromuscular clinic. Diagnosis most often depends on muscle biopsy and mutation analysis, but the physician in charge must be aware of the expertise of the biopsy laboratory and that of the DNA diagnostic laboratory. There are many pitfalls that can result in misinterpretation of both the biopsy and the DNA; these are best avoided by working with laboratories that have the highest expertise. Furthermore, it is important that patients and families receive complete information regarding the diagnostic process and the results, including hard copies for their child's own records.

There are now published guidelines for the management of children with CMD and CM. The guidelines have been publicized and distributed by several patient advocacy/support organizations including the Muscular Dystrophy Association of USA, CureCMD, and the Joshua Frase Foundation. Such groups are lobbying for support of clinical trials for patients with CMD and CM and some studies may well be seen online in the next few years.

REFERENCES

1. Batten FE. Three cases of myopathy, infantile type. Brain 1903;26:147–8.
2. Magee KR, Shy GM. A new congenital non-progressive myopathy. Brain 1956;79: 610–21.
3. Nadeau A, Kinali M, Main M, et al. Natural history of Ullrich congenital muscular dystrophy. Neurology 2009;73(1):25–31.
4. Mercuri E, Yuva Y, Brown SC, et al. Collagen VI involvement in Ullrich syndrome: a clinical, genetic, and immunohistochemical study. Neurology 2002;58(9):1354–9.
5. Okada M, Kawahara G, Noguchi S, et al. Primary collagen VI deficiency is the second most common congenital muscular dystrophy in Japan. Neurology 2007;69(10):1035–42.
6. Riisager M, Duno M, Hansen FJ, et al. A new mutation of the fukutin gene causing late-onset limb girdle muscular dystrophy. Neuromuscul Disord 2013;23(7): 562–7.

7. Fiorillo C, Moro F, Astrea G, et al. Novel mutations in the fukutin gene in a boy with asymptomatic hyperCKemia. Neuromuscul Disord 2013;23(12):1010–5.

8. Ryan MM, Ilkovski B, Strickland CD, et al. Clinical course correlates poorly with muscle pathology in nemaline myopathy. Neurology 2003;60:665–73.

9. Vanasse M, Pare H, Zeller R. Medical and psychosocial considerations in rehabilitation care of childhood neuromuscular diseases. Handb Clin Neurol 2013;113: 1491–5.

10. Wang CH, Finkel RS, Bertini ES, et al, Participants of the International Conference on SMA Standard of Care. Consensus statement for standard of care in spinal muscular atrophy. J Child Neurol 2007;22:1027–49.

11. Gatayama R, Ueno K, Nakamura H, et al. Nemaline myopathy with dilated cardiomyopathy in childhood. Pediatrics 2013;131(6):e1986–90.

12. Mir A, Lemler M, Ramaciotti C, et al. Hypertrophic cardiomyopathy in a neonate associated with nemaline myopathy. Congenit Heart Dis 2012;7(4):E37–41.

13. Taglia A, D'Ambrosio P, Palladino A, et al. One case of respiratory failure due to diaphragmatic paralysis and dilated cardiomyopathy in a patient with nemaline myopathy. Acta Myol 2012;31(3):201–3.

14. Clement EM, Feng L, Mein R, et al. Relative frequency of congenital muscular dystrophy subtypes: analysis of the UK diagnostic service 2001-2008. Neuromuscul Disord 2012;22(6):522–7.

15. Quijano-Roy S, Renault F, Romero N, et al. EMG and nerve conduction studies in children with congenital muscular dystrophy. Muscle Nerve 2004;29(2):292–9.

16. Geranmayeh F, Clement E, Feng LH, et al. Genotype-phenotype correlation in a large population of muscular dystrophy patients with LAMA2 mutations. Neuromuscul Disord 2010;20(4):241–50.

17. Ceyhan-Birsoy O, Agrawal PB, Hidalgo C, et al. Recessive truncating titin gene, TTN, mutations presenting as centronuclear myopathy. Neurology 2013;81(14): 1205–14.

18. Taylor A, Lachlan K, Manners RM, et al. A study of a family with the skeletal muscle RYR1 mutation (c.7354C>T) associated with central core myopathy and malignant hyperthermia susceptibility. J Clin Neurosci 2012;19(1):65–70.

19. Malicdan MC, Nishino I. Central core disease. In: Pagon RA, Adam MP, Bird TD, et al, editors. GeneReviews™ [Internet]. Seattle (WA): University of Washington, Seattle; 2007. p. 1993–2013.

20. Birnkrant D, Panitch HB, Benditt JO, et al. American College of Chest Physicians Consensus statement on the respiratory and related management of patients with Duchenne muscular dystrophy undergoing anesthesia or sedation. Chest 2007; 132(6):1977–86.

21. Bushby K, Finkel R, Birnkrant DJ, et al, DMD Care Considerations Working Group. Diagnosis and management of Duchenne muscular dystrophy, part 1: diagnosis, and pharmacological and psychosocial management. Lancet Neurol 2010;9(1):77–93.

22. Wang CH, Bonnemann CG, Rutkowshi A, et al, International Standard of Care Committee for Congenital Muscular Dystrophy. Consensus statement on standard of care for congenital muscular dystrophies. J Child Neurol 2010;25(12): 1559–81.

23. Wang CH, Dowling JJ, North K, et al. Consensus statement on standard of care for congenital myopathies. J Child Neurol 2012;27(3):363–82.

24. Iannaccone ST, Castro D. Congenital muscular dystrophies and congenital myopathies. Continuum (Minneap Minn) 2013;19(6 Muscle Disease):1509–34.

Myotonic Dystrophy

Charles A. Thornton, MD

KEYWORDS

- Myotonic dystrophy • Electrophysiology • Myopathy • Expanded DNA repeat

KEY POINTS

- Myotonic dystrophy (dystrophia myotonica, DM) is one of the most common lethal monogenic disorders in populations of European descent.
- Myotonic dystrophy type 1 (DM1) was first described over a century ago.
- DM1 is caused by expansion of a CTG triplet repeat in the 3' noncoding region of *DMPK*, the gene encoding the DM protein kinase.
- More recently, a second form of the disease, myotonic dystrophy type 2, was recognized, which results from repeat expansion in a different gene.
- Both disorders have autosomal dominant inheritance and multisystem features, including myotonic myopathy, cataract, and cardiac conduction disease.

EPIDEMIOLOGY

A population-based screen to determine the genetic frequency of myotonic dystrophy (DM) is technically feasible but has not yet been performed on a large scale. The most ambitious screen to date showed a DM gene frequency of 1 in 1100 among Finnish blood donors, equally divided between myotonic dystrophy type 1 (DM1) and type 2 (DM2).[1] However, the 95% confidence intervals were broad (1 in 500 to 1 in 3700) because the sample size was small (*n* = 4520). It is also possible that DM1-affected individuals were underrepresented in the blood donor pool. A referral center in England found that DM1 was the most common genetic disease of skeletal muscle, accounting for 29% of the population in a muscle clinic.[2] The estimated point prevalence of 1 in 9400 was considered conservative because at-risk relatives were not systematically screened. Other DM1 prevalence estimates in Europe ranged from 1 in 8300 to 1 in 10,700.[3,4] Harper reviewed epidemiologic studies of DM1 in Europe and arrived at an estimated gene frequency of 1 in 7400.[5] Studies of non-European populations

Supported by National Institutes of Health U54NS48843 Paul Wellstone Muscular Dystrophy Cooperative Research Center.
Department of Neurology, Center for Neural Development and Disease, Center for RNA Biology, University of Rochester Medical Center, Box 645, 601 Elmwood Avenue, Rochester, NY 14642, USA
E-mail address: charles_thornton@urmc.rochester.edu

Neurol Clin 32 (2014) 705–719
http://dx.doi.org/10.1016/j.ncl.2014.04.011   **neurologic.theclinics.com**

indicated that DM1 was rare in Taiwan and sub-Saharan Africa, except among European descendants in South Africa.[6–8] DM1 is highly prevalent in certain founder populations. For example, the frequency was 1 in 550 among residents of Northeastern Quebec.[9] The epidemiology of DM1 in the United States has not been systematically studied.

There are fewer epidemiologic studies of DM2. The genetic diagnosis of DM1 and DM2 was made with similar frequency at a reference laboratory in Germany,[10] suggesting that the prevalence of the 2 disorders is similar in northern Europe. This observation agrees with the genetic screening studies in Finland cited earlier.[1] In Europeans the DM2 expansion is only found on a specific chromosomal haplotype, suggesting the occurrence of a predisposing mutation in a common ancestral founder.[11] In the United States, clinical experience suggests that DM2 is roughly 5-fold less common than DM1.

GENETICS

The discovery of the DM1 mutation in 1992 provided the third example (after Kennedy disease and fragile X syndrome) of a human genetic disease caused by expansion of a tandem repeat.[12] Nine years later, the expanded CCTG repeat was discovered in DM2.[13] Now the list of expanded repeat disorders has grown to more than 25.

The number of CTG repeats in the *DMPK* gene is variable in the general population, ranging from 5 to 37 repeats.[12] Individuals with DM1 have at least 50 and in some cases upwards of 3000 CTG repeats in *DMPK*. At the DM2 locus, the number of CCTG repeats in *ZNF9* is also polymorphic in the general population, ranging from 10 to 33 repeats.[13,14] Although DM2 has been reported with CCTG expansions as small as 75 repeats, more than 90% of patients have more than 1000 CCTG repeats, and the mean expansion size is around 5000 repeats.[15]

The clinical features of DM1 are shaped by 2 characteristics of the CTG expansion: (1) the expansion is highly unstable so that new alleles with different repeat sizes are frequently generated and (2) there is a bias for further expansion, rather than contraction, in the generation of new alleles. On average, the CTG expansion increases by more than 200 repeats when transmitted from one generation to the next.[16,17] This leads to anticipation, the genetic phenomenon whereby symptoms begin at an earlier age in successive generations. The CTG expansion is also unstable in somatic cells of a person throughout life. This process occurs at different rates in different cells, which leads to variability of repeat length in different tissues. Against expectations, the DM1 expansion is actually more unstable in nondividing cells of skeletal muscle, heart, and brain than in proliferating cells of the hematopoietic system.[18,19] In skeletal muscle, the DM1 expansion typically grows to more than 2000 repeats by 20 years of age,[20] and in patients older than 40 years the average repeat length in skeletal muscle was greater than 4000 repeats, which was 3- to 25-fold larger than in blood.[21] These dramatic changes in post-mitotic cells are believed to result from aberrant (incorrect) DNA repair, through a mechanism that is coupled to transcription across the repeat tract.[22] It is likely that the onset and progression of symptoms is fundamentally linked to the age-dependent growth of the CTG repeat in somatic cells.

Other aspects of DM1 genetics that are pertinent for clinical care include the following:

1. Caution should be exercised in using CTG repeat size to predict future symptoms. The most reliable correlation is that patients with small expansions generally have mild symptoms. For example, people with 50 to 70 repeats may have normal neurologic examinations even into the sixth decade.[23] Most commonly these individuals

come to light when their affected children develop symptoms. CTG expansions that are slightly larger, comprising 70 to 90 repeats, are usually associated with mild symptoms that began after 40 years of age. At the other end of the spectrum, congenital DM1 (CDM) is usually associated with expansions of more than 1000 repeats.[24] However, between these extremes, correlations between repeat size and disease severity are not highly robust.

2. Small expansions (50–80 repeats) may be transmitted for several generations with minor changes. These alleles display greater instability on passage through the male germline.[23,25] Accordingly, the jump from small expansion with minor symptoms to large expansion with classical DM1 is more likely to occur with paternal transmission.

3. In contrast, the massive intergenerational expansions to 1000 or more repeats are more likely to occur with maternal transmission.[17,24] This explains the near-exclusive maternal transmission of CDM.

4. Anticipation is not inevitable. Occasionally the expanded repeat undergoes an intergenerational contraction (<5% of transmissions).[26]

5. Around 5% of DM1 families have sequence interruptions within the CTG repeat.[27] Most commonly these are CCG or CGG triplets interspersed among CTG triplets. It appears that sequence interruptions tend to stabilize the repeat tract and reduce anticipation, and in some cases may lead to variant phenotypes. For example, one kindred with interrupted repeats had a variant phenotype of CMT-like polyneuropathy with paroxysmal encephalopathy.

In DM2, the CCTG expansions are also unstable in somatic cells and with intergenerational transmission. However, unlike DM1, DM2 does not have a strong bias for intergenerational expansion, and correlations between disease severity and expansion size are relatively weak.[15] Accordingly, there is less anticipation in DM2 than in DM1.[15,28]

CLINICAL PRESENTATION OF MYOTONIC DYSTROPHY

The spectrum of DM1 severity extends from lethal effects in infancy to mild, late-onset symptoms. Although DM1 commonly presents as an adult-onset multisystem degenerative disorder, it also may affect fetal development and post-natal growth in individuals who carry large expansions. The mix of developmental and degenerative features, and the patterns of multisystem involvement, are hugely variable between patients. Because the clinical heterogeneity is extreme, it is useful to subdivide DM1 into categories to provide a conceptual framework for pattern recognition and prognosis.

CONGENITAL DM1

Around 15% of DM1-affected individuals have fetal onset with involvement of muscle and the central nervous system (CNS).[29] CDM may occur with CTG expansions as small as 750 repeats, but more commonly it is caused by CTG expansions with more than 1000 repeats. As described earlier, expansions in this size range are generated more frequently during oogenesis than spermatogenesis. The prenatal manifestations of CDM may include reduced fetal movement, polyhydramnios, and ultrasound findings of talipes equinovarus or borderline ventriculomegaly.[30] At birth the cardinal features are neonatal hypotonia, poor feeding, and respiratory difficulty. A prospective study found that 79% of infants required nasogastric feeding and 53% required transient or prolonged ventilatory support.[31] The overall neonatal mortality was 18%. The possibility of CDM may be considered but incorrectly dismissed when there is no family history of DM1. However, it is important to note that more than half of the affected mothers do not carry a diagnosis of DM1 because their condition has gone unrecognized[31] or has not generated any symptoms.[32] Later in childhood, individuals with CDM exhibit delayed motor milestones and a range of learning disabilities, including autism spectrum disorder.[29,33] Oropharyngeal weakness is prominent, often producing a characteristic tented appearance of the upper lip, facial diplegia, marked dysarthria, and greater impairment of expressive than receptive communication. In the second or third decade, patients with CDM will develop the degenerative features of the disease, as described later under "classical DM1".

CHILDHOOD DM1

Children with onset of DM1 after the first year but before 10 years of age often present with predominant cognitive and behavioral features that are not accompanied by conspicuous muscle disease.[33-35] Around half of these children have intellectual impairment (full-scale IQ in the range of 50–70). A range of psychiatric symptoms may occur, including attention deficit disorder, anxiety, and mood disorder, but autism is uncommon.[34] Notably, the risk of childhood-onset DM1 appears similar with maternal or paternal transmission.

CLASSICAL DM1

Around 75% of patients develop symptoms in the second, third, or fourth decade. The most common initial symptom is myotonia. Similar to recessive generalized myotonia (RGM), the myotonia in DM is more pronounced after rest and improves with muscle activity, the "warm-up phenomenon". In contrast to RGM, the action myotonia in DM1 shows selective involvement of specific muscle groups of the forearm, hand, tongue, and jaw. The cardinal finding on examination is myotonic myopathy, consisting of action and percussion myotonia, weakness, and muscle wasting in a characteristic distribution, with preferential involvement of cranial, trunk, and distal limb muscles. All cranial muscles are potentially affected, producing a characteristic appearance of ptosis, wasting of temporalis and masseter, and facial weakness. The neck flexors are affected early. Diaphragmatic weakness may occur before there is any weakness of the limb-girdle muscles. Among limb muscles, the long finger flexors and ankle dorsiflexors are preferentially affected. As symptoms progress, some patients continue to exhibit a strong distal to proximal gradient, whereas others develop shoulder and hip-girdle weakness at a much earlier time. Severe weakness of the ankle dorsi- and plantar-flexors often produces a flail ankle with marked instability of stance. In contrast to most other dystrophies, including DM2, DM1 causes obvious tongue weakness and often there is modest limitation of ocular motility.

MINIMAL DM1

Small CTG expansions (in the range of 70–100 repeat) are usually associated with mild weakness, myotonia, and cataracts that begin after 40 years of age.

NEUROMUSCULAR FEATURES OF DM2

Symptoms of DM2 usually begin in the second to sixth decade (median age 48 years).[15] For many patients the first symptom is grip myotonia. However, in others the myotonia is not apparent and the presentation resembles an indolent form of limb-girdle dystrophy. Although progression is slow, in some patients it seems to accelerate after 50 years of age. DM2 selectively affects the limb-girdle, neck flexor, and elbow extensor muscles. The long finger flexors are often affected, but to a lesser extent than in DM1, and other distal limb muscles are usually spared until later in the course. Compared with DM1, there is no congenital disease in DM2, and there is much less cranial and respiratory muscle weakness. Muscle wasting is less pronounced, and some patients exhibit hypertrophy of calf and thigh muscles, which on histologic examination is true hypertrophy with conspicuous enlargement of muscle fibers. Pain is a common feature that seems to be muscular in origin but not necessarily connected to myotonia. A prior diagnosis of fibromyalgia is relatively common.

SYSTEMIC FEATURES
Cardiac Disease

The cardiac impact of DM1 falls mainly on the conduction system. Cardiac dysrhythmia, particularly heart block, is the second leading cause of death after respiratory failure.[36] In a prospective study, the risk of sudden death in a clinic population was 1.1% per year.[37] Sixty-five percent of patients show prolongation of the PR interval or QRS duration. The conduction defects are progressive and may lead to severe bradycardia or asystole due to atrioventricular block. Atrial tachycardias (flutter, fibrillation, or sinus tachycardia) are relatively common, and risk of ventricular tachycardia is also elevated. Although the cardiac contractility is relatively preserved, heart failure may occur at later ages. Ten percent of patients in a large study had clinical or echocardiographic evidence of left ventricular systolic dysfunction (LVSD).[38] LVSD was rare before 40 years of age, but after this age the frequency steadily increased, reaching a high of 30% by the age of 70 years.

Few studies have examined the cardiac effects of DM2, but it is clear that conduction disease and heart failure may both occur. One study found that the frequency of conduction disease was lower in DM2 than in DM1, but LVSD was more common.[39] DM2 is also associated with increased risk of sudden death.[40]

Ocular

Cataracts before the age of 55 years, or family history of premature cataracts, suggest the diagnosis of DM1 or DM2 in patients with muscle symptoms. By direct ophthalmoscopy the cataracts of DM are nonspecific and appear as punctate opacities. By slit lamp examination they have a multicolored iridescent appearance and are located in the posterior lens capsule, findings that are highly suggestive of DM1 or DM2. Premature cataracts may also occur in mitochondrial, centronuclear, or myofibrillar (αB-crystallin) myopathies.

CNS

The neuropsychiatric features of congenital and childhood-onset DM1 were discussed earlier. The CNS features of classical DM1 have been the subject of several recent reviews[41,42] and will be briefly summarized here. Although the CNS features are highly variable between patients, DM1 is commonly associated with sleep disturbance, behavioral effects, and changes of cognition. The most common CNS symptom, affecting around 80% of patients, is daytime hypersomnolence. In some individuals this is coupled with a global disorganization of sleep habits and diurnal rhythm. Studies have shown sleep-onset rapid eye movement in 26% to 54% of patients.[43–45] DM1 is also associated with a variable constellation of behavioral and cognitive changes, which may include anxiety, avoidant behavior, apathy, memory impairment, executive dysfunction, and problems with visuospatial processing (reviewed in Refs.[41,42]). Brain MRI scans may demonstrate extensive alterations of white matter signal intensity in both types of DM, especially in the frontal and temporal lobes.[46,47] The underlying cellular and neuropathologic basis for this finding has not been determined.

Other Systemic Features

1. Gastrointestinal symptoms are highly prevalent in DM1.[48] The frequency of chole-lithiasis is increased, which may reflect involvement of smooth muscle in the gall-bladder.[49] Intestinal dysmotility is common, producing symptoms of bowel urgency and diarrhea, often alternating with constipation. Whether these symptoms result from involvement of smooth muscle, enteric neurons, or both has not been determined.
2. Epidemiologic studies have confirmed the clinical impression that DM1 is associated with higher risk of cancer, most notably involving the thyroid gland, ovary, colon, endometrium, brain, and eye (choroidal melanoma).[50–52]
3. Primary hypogonadism is common in men with DM1, and to a lesser extent in DM2. This condition may produce testicular atrophy, reduced fertility, erectile dysfunction, and low testosterone.[53]
4. DM1 is associated with metabolic derangements including insulin resistance, increased cholesterol, and hypertriglyceridemia.[54,55]
5. Abnormal liver function tests are common in DM1 and DM2.[55,56] Modest elevations of alanine and aspartate aminotransferase levels, gamma-glutamyltransferase, and alkaline phosphatase may occur. Generally these abnormalities are nonprogressive and do not require liver biopsy unless there is corollary evidence of another disease process. It is unknown whether these changes represent a primary effect of DM on hepatocytes or a secondary consequence of metabolic derangements, biliary stasis, or fatty liver.
6. Balding can occur in men and women with DM1.

LABORATORY AND ELECTROPHYSIOLOGIC TESTING
Genetic Testing

Genetic testing for DM is definitive and cost-effective. Except for rare examples of laboratory error, a negative genetic test excludes the diagnosis. Therefore, when clinical signs point to DM, no diagnostic evaluation other than genetic testing is necessary. Repeat-primed polymerase chain reaction (PCR) is a low-cost method to determine whether an expanded repeat is present or absent, without measuring the size of the repeat tract. In most cases, a Southern blot is still required to determine the CTG or CCTG expansion size, but this may change as new PCR methods and sequencing technologies become available. Because DM1 and DM2 are distinguishable on clinical grounds, it is usually reasonable to test for one disorder or the other, as opposed to automatic testing for both.

Electrophysiology

The needle examination in DM1 is characterized by distal predominant myotonic discharges, myopathic motor units, and early recruitment. The short exercise test often shows a transient drop of compound muscle action potential amplitude in DM1,[57,58] a finding that is qualitatively similar to RGM and consistent with chloride channelopathy (see later discussion). The distribution of myotonic discharges is less consistent in DM2. In some DM2 patients, the electromyographic myotonia is altogether absent or confined to paraspinal or proximal muscles.[15,59] Compared to DM1, a predominance of waning myotonic discharges occurs in DM2. Notably, the finding of electromyographic myotonia that is not accompanied by action or percussion myotonia may prompt a fruitless search for DM1 or DM2. Myotonic or high-frequency discharges without clinical myotonia can be observed in late-onset Pompe disease, centronuclear myopathies, several myofibrillar myopathies, and myopathies with inclusion bodies.[60]

Muscle Pathology

Muscle biopsy was never a key diagnostic procedure for DM1, and now is entirely superseded by genetic testing. If, however, muscle tissue is examined, the pathologist is likely to provide the correct diagnosis. There is no pathognomonic feature on conventional stains, but the constellation of dramatically increased central nuclei, ring fibers, pyknotic nuclear clumps, and selective atrophy of type 1 fibers is strongly suggestive of DM1. Compared to other dystrophies, muscle fiber necrosis and collagen deposition is less conspicuous in DM1, but fiber atrophy is more profound. DM2 shares many of the same findings, except that there is selective atrophy of type 2 fibers and a population of fibers with marked hypertrophy.[61] As described below, both disorders exhibit nuclear inclusions of CUG/CCUG repeat RNA and muscleblind-like (MBNL) proteins.[62] These staining procedures are diagnostic of DM but have not been implemented in most laboratories, presumably because processing of DM samples is relatively uncommon.

PATHOGENESIS
RNA Toxicity

The DM1 and DM2 gene discoveries were perplexing because DMPK and ZNF9 have no functional connections yet the clinical features are similar. Also, the repeat expansions in both disorders are located in genomic regions that do not encode proteins. The evidence now supports a unifying theory of RNA-mediated pathogenesis in which both disorders result from toxicity of repetitive RNA.[63,64] DM1 has been examined in more detail but it appears that the disease process is broadly similar in DM2.

Sequestration of MBNL Proteins

The expanded repeat in DM1 is located in the terminal part of the DMPK gene, close to the signal for polyadenylation. Even when highly expanded, the repeat sequence does not block the synthesis or processing of DMPK RNA. This results in production of a mutant mRNA that contains several thousand CUG repeats. These unusual transcripts are not exported to the cytoplasm, but instead are retained in the nucleus in discrete clumps or "foci".[65,66] These collections of mutant RNA were not previously observed by conventional histochemical stains. They were first revealed by staining tissue with probes that hybridize to the repetitive RNA. As expected, the foci are most conspicuous in cells with large expansions and high levels of DMPK expression: muscle fibers, smooth muscle cells, cardiomyocytes, and neurons.[67–69]

Proteins in the MBNL family bind to CUG repeat RNA with high affinity.[70] These proteins normally act to regulate splicing of several hundred transcripts.[71] They also have a role in regulating RNA transport and decay.[72] However, these functions are lost when MBNL proteins are trapped in nuclear foci of CUG repeats.[70,73] This results in expression of many incorrect splice products and protein isoforms. For example, mis-splicing of the ClC-1 chloride channel leads to reduced chloride conductance in muscle fibers,[74,75] a physiological alteration that is known to produce myotonia. Splicing defects of other transcripts, including insulin receptor, BIN1, dystrophin, and L-type calcium channels, are suspected to cause insulin resistance and myopathy.[21,76–78] However, not all investigators agree that MBNL sequestration is an important determinant of DM disease.[79]

Signaling Changes and Aberrant Translation of Expanded Repeats

Studies suggest that RNA toxicity also involves the activation of signaling pathways by mutant *DMPK* RNA.[80] Although the mechanisms for this effect are not clearly defined, it is possible that components of the innate immune system, which normally detect the intrusion of viral RNAs, are mistakenly activated by the RNA with expanded CUG repeats.[81] One downstream consequence is to induce phosphorylation and stabilization of another splicing factor, CUGBP1.[80] When CUGBP1 accumulates to high levels, it further aggravates the problem with splicing regulation.[82] Recent studies also show that expanded repeat RNAs may have unusual interactions with the protein synthesis machinery, which leads to translation of the repeat sequence even though it is not located in a conventional protein-coding region.[83] If this occurs *in vivo*, the repetitive peptides would be expected to have cellular toxicity.

Other Effects

The transcripts from the mutant *DMPK* allele are retained in the nucleus and therefore are not efficiently translated,[66] which leads to a partial (around 50%) reduction of DMPK protein.[84] Some studies also suggest that CCTG expansions cause reduction of ZNF9 protein in DM2,[85–87] but there are conflicting data on this point.[88] Although these effects may contribute to pathogenesis at some level, they do not appear to be the major determinants of disease.

Pathophysiology of Congenital DM1

A major unresolved question regarding DM1 relates to the pathophysiology of congenital disease. There is little information on this topic from studies of affected infants or animal models. In flies, MBNL protein is required for normal muscle development.[89] In mice, combinatorial knockout of 2 MBNL proteins, MBNL1 and MBNL2, is lethal during prenatal development (note that both of these proteins are sequestered by CUG repeat RNA).[90] Cell culture experiments have shown that expression of expanded CUG repeat RNA can interfere with myogenic differentiation.[91] Taken together, these observations are consistent with the concept that RNA toxicity, and possibly MBNL sequestration, may contribute to developmental phenotypes of DM1. However, if that is the case, it is unclear why congenital disease does not also occur in DM2, considering that CCUG repeats are similarly effective for sequestering MBNL proteins.

Therapy and Management for DM1 and DM2

No treatments are currently available that fundamentally alter the course of DM1 or DM2. The management of DM is based on genetic counseling; preserving function and independence; preventing cardiopulmonary complications; and providing symptomatic treatment of myotonia, hypersomnolence, and pain.

In DM1, the combined effects of sleep-disordered breathing, increased abdominal adipose, and weakness of the diaphragm and oropharyngeal muscles often lead to respiratory impairment and nocturnal hypoventilation. It is useful to monitor forced vital capacity and forced expiratory volume in 1 second in the sitting and supine position.[92] The threshold for obtaining polysomnography in this population should be low. Many patients will progress to a point of requiring noninvasive nighttime ventilatory support.

Pacemakers and cardiac defibrillators can be lifesaving in DM1, but presently there is no consensus about the indications for cardiac referral or device implantation. The electrocardiogram should be monitored annually. Holter monitoring is a useful adjunct to detect nocturnal bradycardia or other intermittent arrhythmias. One expert recommended annual echocardiograms,[93] although the utility of this before age 40 is unclear. The risk of sudden death in DM1 increases if the PR interval is greater than 240 ms, the QRS duration greater than 120 ms, or with atrial tachyarrhythmia.[37] It is reasonable, therefore, to refer patients with these findings for further cardiac evaluation. The size of the CTG repeat expansion is not particularly useful for stratifying risk, as it does not predict sudden death or LVSD.[38] Patients and family members should be educated that symptoms of palpitations, syncope, or near-syncope require prompt evaluation.

Case series and observational studies have suggested that daytime hypersomnolence in DM1 can be successfully managed with stimulant medications, such as methylphenidate.[94] Small therapeutic trials of modafinil have shown mixed results.[95,96]

Anabolic agents were tested in DM1 in an effort to overcome the muscle wasting. However, despite some improvement of muscle mass with testosterone or recombinant insulinlike growth factor, consistent improvement of functional ability was not achieved.[97–99]

Improvement of myotonia has been reported in DM1 using various anticonvulsant or antiarrhythmic drugs.[100] A randomized placebo-controlled crossover study of mexiletine showed reduction of grip myotonia by up to 50% in DM1 patients after 7 weeks of treatment.[101] A study to assess safety and functional improvement with longer-term treatment is currently underway (RT Moxley, personal communication, 2014).

Experimental Treatments for DM1 and DM2

Elucidation of disease mechanisms in DM1 and DM2 has led to the identification of novel targets for therapeutic intervention. In preclinical studies, evidence for engagement of these targets and therapeutic benefit has been obtained using several different approaches. Antisense oligonucleotides (ASOs), gene therapy vectors, and small molecules have been used to reduce the levels of toxic RNA.[102–105] Small molecules and ASOs have also been used to inhibit MBNL binding to CUG/CCUG repeats or block the signaling pathways that lead to overexpression of CUGBP1.[106–109] Gene therapy vectors have been used to increase the expression of MBNL1 protein.[110] Taken together, these studies have suggested that DM-associated biochemical and physiologic defects are reversible in transgenic mouse models. Further chemical optimization and preclinical testing is necessary, but it seems possible that several of these therapeutic strategies may advance to clinical trials.

REFERENCES

1. Suominen T, Bachinski LL, Auvinen S, et al. Population frequency of myotonic dystrophy: higher than expected frequency of myotonic dystrophy type 2 (DM2) mutation in Finland. Eur J Hum Genet 2011;19:776–82.
2. Norwood FL, Harling C, Chinnery PF, et al. Prevalence of genetic muscle disease in Northern England: in-depth analysis of a muscle clinic population. Brain 2009;132:3175–86.
3. Siciliano G, Manca M, Gennarelli M, et al. Epidemiology of myotonic dystrophy in Italy: re-appraisal after genetic diagnosis. Clin Genet 2001;59:344–9.
4. Magee A, Nevin NC. The epidemiology of myotonic dystrophy in Northern Ireland. Community Genet 1999;2:179–83.
5. Harper PS. Myotonic dystrophy. London: W.B. Saunders Company; 2001.
6. Lotz BP, van der Meyden CH. Myotonic dystrophy. Part I. A genealogical study in the northern Transvaal. S Afr Med J 1985;67:812–4.

7. Ashizawa T, Epstein HF. Ethnic distribution of myotonic dystrophy gene. Lancet 1991;338:642–3.

8. Hsiao KM, Chen SS, Li SY, et al. Epidemiological and genetic studies of myotonic dystrophy type 1 in Taiwan. Neuroepidemiology 2003;22:283–9.

9. Yotova V, Labuda D, Zietkiewicz E, et al. Anatomy of a founder effect: myotonic dystrophy in Northeastern Quebec. Hum Genet 2005;117:177–87.

10. Udd B, Meola G, Krahe R, et al. 140th ENMC International Workshop: Myotonic Dystrophy DM2/PROMM and other myotonic dystrophies with guidelines on management. Neuromuscul Disord 2006;16:403–13.

11. Bachinski LL, Udd B, Meola G, et al. Confirmation of the type 2 myotonic dystrophy (CCTG)n expansion mutation in patients with proximal myotonic myopathy/proximal myotonic dystrophy of different European origins: a single shared haplotype indicates an ancestral founder effect. Am J Hum Genet 2003;73:835–48.

12. Brook JD, McCurrach ME, Harley HG, et al. Molecular basis of myotonic dystrophy: expansion of a trinucleotide (CTG) repeat at the 3' end of a transcript encoding a protein kinase family member. Cell 1992;68:799–808.

13. Liquori CL, Ricker K, Moseley ML, et al. Myotonic dystrophy type 2 caused by a CCTG expansion in intron 1 of ZNF9. Science 2001;293:864–7.

14. Bachinski LL, Czernuszewicz T, Ramagli LS, et al. Premutation allele pool in myotonic dystrophy type 2. Neurology 2009;72:490–7.

15. Day JW, Ricker K, Jacobsen JF, et al. Myotonic dystrophy type 2: molecular, diagnostic and clinical spectrum. Neurology 2003;60:657–64.

16. Redman JB, Fenwick RG Jr, Fu YH, et al. Relationship between parental trinucleotide GCT repeat length and severity of myotonic dystrophy in offspring. JAMA 1993;269:1960–5.

17. De Temmerman N, Sermon K, Seneca S, et al. Intergenerational instability of the expanded CTG repeat in the DMPK gene: studies in human gametes and pre-implantation embryos. Am J Hum Genet 2004;75:325–9.

18. Ashizawa T, Dubel JR, Harati Y. Somatic instability of CTG repeat in myotonic dystrophy. Neurology 1993;43:2674–8.

19. Thornton CA, Johnson K, Moxley RT. Myotonic dystrophy patients have larger CTG expansions in skeletal muscle than in leukocytes. Ann Neurol 1994;35:104–7.

20. Zatz M, Passos-Bueno MR, Cerqueira A, et al. Analysis of the CTG repeat in skeletal muscle of young and adult myotonic dystrophy patients: when does the expansion occur? Hum Mol Genet 1995;4:401–6.

21. Nakamori M, Sobczak K, Puwanant A, et al. Splicing biomarkers of disease severity in myotonic dystrophy. Ann Neurol 2013;74:862–72.

22. Pearson CE, Nichol EK, Cleary JD. Repeat instability: mechanisms of dynamic mutations. Nat Rev Genet 2005;6:729–42.

23. Barcelo JM, Mahadevan MS, Tsilfidis C, et al. Intergenerational stability of the myotonic dystrophy protomutation. Hum Mol Genet 1993;2:705–9.

24. Tsilfidis C, MacKenzie AE, Mettler G, et al. Correlation between CTG trinucleotide repeat length and frequency of severe congenital myotonic dystrophy. Nat Genet 1992;1:192–5.

25. Martorell L, Monckton DG, Sanchez A, et al. Frequency and stability of the myotonic dystrophy type 1 premutation. Neurology 2001;56:328–35.

26. Ashizawa T, Anvret M, Baiget M, et al. Characteristics of intergenerational contractions of the CTG repeat in myotonic dystrophy. Am J Hum Genet 1994;54:414–23.

27. Braida C, Stefanatos RK, Adam B, et al. Variant CCG and GGC repeats within the CTG expansion dramatically modify mutational dynamics and likely contribute toward unusual symptoms in some myotonic dystrophy type 1 patients. Hum Mol Genet 2010;19:1399–412.

28. Schneider C, Ziegler A, Ricker K, et al. Proximal myotonic myopathy: evidence for anticipation in families with linkage to chromosome 3q. Neurology 2000;55:383–8.

29. Harper PS. Congenital myotonic dystrophy in Britain. I. Clinical aspects. Arch Dis Child 1975;50:505–13.

30. Zaki M, Boyd PA, Impey L, et al. Congenital myotonic dystrophy: prenatal ultrasound findings and pregnancy outcome. Ultrasound Obstet Gynecol 2007;29:284–8.

31. Campbell C, Levin S, Siu VM, et al. Congenital myotonic dystrophy: Canadian population-based surveillance study. J Pediatr 2013;163:120–5.

32. Martorell L, Cobo AM, Baiget M, et al. Prenatal diagnosis in myotonic dystrophy type 1. Thirteen years of experience: implications for reproductive counselling in DM1 families. Prenat Diagn 2007;27:68–72.

33. Ekstrom AB, Hakenas-Plate L, Tulinius M, et al. Cognition and adaptive skills in myotonic dystrophy type 1: a study of 55 individuals with congenital and childhood forms. Dev Med Child Neurol 2009;51:982–90.

34. Douniol M, Jacquette A, Cohen D, et al. Psychiatric and cognitive phenotype of childhood myotonic dystrophy type 1. Dev Med Child Neurol 2012;54:905–11.

35. Angeard N, Jacquette A, Gargiulo M, et al. A new window on neurocognitive dysfunction in the childhood form of myotonic dystrophy type 1 (DM1). Neuromuscul Disord 2011;21:468–76.

36. de Die-Smulders CE, Howeler CJ, Thijs C, et al. Age and causes of death in adult-onset myotonic dystrophy. Brain 1998;121:1557–63.

37. Groh WJ, Groh MR, Saha C, et al. Electrocardiographic abnormalities and sudden death in myotonic dystrophy type 1. N Engl J Med 2008;358:2688–97.

38. Bhakta D, Groh MR, Shen C, et al. Increased mortality with left ventricular systolic dysfunction and heart failure in adults with myotonic dystrophy type 1. Am Heart J 2010;160:1137–41.

39. Wahbi K, Meune C, Becane HM, et al. Left ventricular dysfunction and cardiac arrhythmias are frequent in type 2 myotonic dystrophy: a case control study. Neuromuscul Disord 2009;19:468–72.

40. Schoser BG, Ricker K, Schneider-Gold C, et al. Sudden cardiac death in myotonic dystrophy type 2. Neurology 2004;63:2402–4.

41. Bugiardini E, Meola G, on behalf of the DMCNSG. Consensus on cerebral involvement in myotonic dystrophy Workshop report. Neuromuscul Disord 2014;24(5):445–52.

42. Meola G, Sansone V. Cerebral involvement in myotonic dystrophies. Muscle Nerve 2007;36:294–306.

43. Ciafaloni E, Mignot E, Sansone V, et al. The Hypocretin Neurotransmission System in Myotonic Dystrophy Type 1. Neurology 2007;70:226–30.

44. Laberge L, Begin P, Dauvilliers Y, et al. A polysomnographic study of daytime sleepiness in myotonic dystrophy type 1. J Neurol Neurosurg Psychiatry 2009;80:642–6.

45. Yu H, Laberge L, Jaussent I, et al. Daytime sleepiness and REM sleep characteristics in myotonic dystrophy: a case-control study. Sleep 2011;34:165–70.

46. Minnerop M, Weber B, Schoene-Bake JC, et al. The brain in myotonic dystrophy 1 and 2: evidence for a predominant white matter disease. Brain 2011;134: 3530–46.
47. Wozniak JR, Mueller BA, Bell CJ, et al. Diffusion tensor imaging reveals widespread white matter abnormalities in children and adolescents with myotonic dystrophy type 1. J Neurol 2013;260:1122–31.
48. Heatwole C, Bode R, Johnson N, et al. Patient-reported impact of symptoms in myotonic dystrophy type 1 (PRISM-1). Neurology 2012;79:348–57.
49. Cardani R, Mancinelli E, Saino G, et al. A putative role of ribonuclear inclusions and MBNL1 in the impairment of gallbladder smooth muscle contractility with cholelithiasis in myotonic dystrophy type 1. Neuromuscul Disord 2008;18: 641–5.
50. Gadalla SM, Pfeiffer RM, Kristinsson SY, et al. Quantifying cancer absolute risk and cancer mortality in the presence of competing events after a myotonic dystrophy diagnosis. PLoS One 2013;8:e79851.
51. Gadalla SM, Lund M, Pfeiffer RM, et al. Cancer risk among patients with myotonic muscular dystrophy. JAMA 2011;306:2480–6.
52. Win AK, Perattur PG, Pulido JS, et al. Increased cancer risks in myotonic dystrophy. Mayo Clin Proc 2012;87:130–5.
53. Peric S, Nisic T, Milicev M, et al. Hypogonadism and erectile dysfunction in myotonic dystrophy type 1. Acta Myol 2013;32:106–9.
54. Moxley RT III, Griggs RC, Goldblatt D, et al. Decreased insulin sensitivity of forearm muscle in myotonic dystrophy. J Clin Invest 1978;62:857–67.
55. Heatwole CR, Miller J, Martens B, et al. Laboratory abnormalities in ambulatory patients with myotonic dystrophy type 1. Arch Neurol 2006;63:1149–53.
56. Achiron A, Barak Y, Magal N, et al. Abnormal liver test results in myotonic dystrophy. J Clin Gastroenterol 1998;26:292–5.
57. Sander HW, Tavoulareas GP, Quinto CM, et al. The exercise test distinguishes proximal myotonic myopathy from myotonic dystrophy. Muscle Nerve 1997;20: 235–7.
58. Fournier E, Viala K, Gervais H, et al. Cold extends electromyography distinction between ion channel mutations causing myotonia. Ann Neurol 2006;60:356–65.
59. Logigian EL, Ciafaloni E, Quinn LC, et al. Severity, type, and distribution of myotonic discharges are different in type 1 and type 2 myotonic dystrophy. Muscle Nerve 2007;35:479–85.
60. Hanisch F, Kronenberger C, Zierz S, et al. The significance of pathological spontaneous activity in various myopathies. Clin Neurophysiol 2013. [Epub ahead of print].
61. Vihola A, Bassez G, Meola G, et al. Histopathological differences of myotonic dystrophy type 1 (DM1) and PROMM/DM2. Neurology 2003;60:1854–7.
62. Mankodi A, Teng-umnuay P, Krym M, et al. Ribonuclear inclusions in skeletal muscle in myotonic dystrophy types 1 and 2. Ann Neurol 2003;54:760–8.
63. Osborne RJ, Thornton CA. RNA-dominant diseases. Hum Mol Genet 2006;15: R162–9.
64. Todd PK, Paulson HL. RNA-mediated neurodegeneration in repeat expansion disorders. Ann Neurol 2010;67:291–300.
65. Taneja KL, McCurrach M, Schalling M, et al. Foci of trinucleotide repeat transcripts in nuclei of myotonic dystrophy cells and tissues. J Cell Biol 1995;128: 995–1002.
66. Davis BM, McCurrach ME, Taneja KL, et al. Expansion of a CUG trinucleotide repeat in the 3' untranslated region of myotonic dystrophy protein kinase

transcripts results in nuclear retention of transcripts. Proc Natl Acad Sci U S A 1997;94:7388–93.

67. Mankodi A, Lin X, Blaxall BC, et al. Nuclear RNA foci in the heart in myotonic dystrophy. Circ Res 2005;97:1152–5.

68. Jiang H, Mankodi A, Swanson MS, et al. Myotonic dystrophy type 1 associated with nuclear foci of mutant RNA, sequestration of muscleblind proteins, and deregulated alternative splicing in neurons. Hum Mol Genet 2004;13:3079–88.

69. Mankodi A, Urbinati CR, Yuan QP, et al. Muscleblind localizes to nuclear foci of aberrant RNA in myotonic dystrophy types 1 and 2. Hum Mol Genet 2001;10:2165–70.

70. Miller JW, Urbinati CR, Teng-umnuay P, et al. Recruitment of human muscleblind proteins to (CUG)(n) expansions associated with myotonic dystrophy. EMBO J 2000;19:4439–48.

71. Ho TH, Charlet B, Poulos MG, et al. Muscleblind proteins regulate alternative splicing. EMBO J 2004;23:3103–12.

72. Wang ET, Cody NA, Jog S, et al. Transcriptome-wide Regulation of Pre-mRNA Splicing and mRNA Localization by Muscleblind Proteins. Cell 2012;150:710–24.

73. Lin X, Miller JW, Mankodi A, et al. Failure of MBNL1-dependent postnatal splicing transitions in myotonic dystrophy. Hum Mol Genet 2006;15:2087–97.

74. Mankodi A, Takahashi MP, Jiang H, et al. Expanded CUG repeats trigger aberrant splicing of ClC-1 chloride channel pre-mRNA and hyperexcitability of skeletal muscle in myotonic dystrophy. Mol Cell 2002;10:35–44.

75. Lueck JD, Mankodi A, Swanson MS, et al. Muscle chloride channel dysfunction in two mouse models of myotonic dystrophy. J Gen Physiol 2007;129:79–94.

76. Savkur RS, Philips AV, Cooper TA. Aberrant regulation of insulin receptor alternative splicing is associated with insulin resistance in myotonic dystrophy. Nat Genet 2001;29:40–7.

77. Fugier C, Klein AF, Hammer C, et al. Misregulated alternative splicing of BIN1 is associated with T tubule alterations and muscle weakness in myotonic dystrophy. Nat Med 2011;17:720–5.

78. Tang ZZ, Yarotskyy V, Wei L, et al. Muscle weakness in myotonic dystrophy associated with misregulated splicing and altered gating of CaV1.1 calcium channel. Hum Mol Genet 2011;21:1312–24.

79. Bachinski LL, Baggerly KA, Neubauer VL, et al. Most expression and splicing changes in myotonic dystrophy type 1 and type 2 skeletal muscle are shared with other muscular dystrophies. Neuromuscul Disord 2014;24(3):227–40.

80. Kuyumcu-Martinez NM, Wang GS, Cooper TA. Increased steady-state levels of CUGBP1 in myotonic dystrophy 1 are due to PKC-mediated hyperphosphorylation. Mol Cell 2007;28:68–78.

81. Tian B, White RJ, Xia T, et al. Expanded CUG repeat RNAs form hairpins that activate the double-stranded RNA-dependent protein kinase PKR. RNA 2000;6:79–87.

82. Philips AV, Timchenko LT, Cooper TA. Disruption of splicing regulated by a CUG-binding protein in myotonic dystrophy. Science 1998;280:737–41.

83. Zu T, Gibbens B, Doty NS, et al. Non-ATG-initiated translation directed by microsatellite expansions. Proc Natl Acad Sci U S A 2011;108:260–5.

84. Maeda M, Taft CS, Bush EW, et al. Identification, tissue-specific expression, and subcellular localization of the 80- and 71-kDa forms of myotonic dystrophy kinase protein. J Biol Chem 1995;270:20246–9.

85. Pelletier R, Hamel F, Beaulieu D, et al. Absence of a differentiation defect in muscle satellite cells from DM2 patients. Neurobiol Dis 2009;36:181–90.

86. Raheem O, Olufemi SE, Bachinski LL, et al. Mutant (CCTG)n expansion causes abnormal expression of zinc finger protein 9 (ZNF9) in myotonic dystrophy type 2. Am J Pathol 2010;177:3025–36.

87. Huichalaf C, Schoser B, Schneider-Gold C, et al. Reduction of the rate of protein translation in patients with myotonic dystrophy 2. J Neurosci 2009;29:9042–9.

88. Margolis JM, Schoser BG, Moseley ML, et al. DM2 intronic expansions: evidence for CCUG accumulation without flanking sequence or effects on ZNF9 mRNA processing or protein expression. Hum Mol Genet 2006;15:1808–15.

89. Artero R, Prokop A, Paricio N, et al. The muscleblind gene participates in the organization of Z-bands and epidermal attachments of Drosophila muscles and is regulated by Dmef2. Dev Biol 1998;195:131–43.

90. Lee KY, Li M, Manchanda M, et al. Compound loss of muscleblind-like function in myotonic dystrophy. EMBO molecular medicine 2013;5:1887–900.

91. Amack JD, Paguio AP, Mahadevan MS. Cis and trans effects of the myotonic dystrophy (DM) mutation in a cell culture model. Hum Mol Genet 1999;8:1975–84.

92. Poussel M, Kaminsky P, Renaud P, et al. Supine changes in lung function correlate with chronic respiratory failure in myotonic dystrophy patients. Respir Physiol Neurobiol 2014;193:43–51.

93. McNally EM, Sparano D. Mechanisms and management of the heart in myotonic dystrophy. Heart 2011;97:1094–100.

94. van der Meche FG, Bogaard JM, van der Sluys JC, et al. Daytime sleep in myotonic dystrophy is not caused by sleep apnoea. J Neurol Neurosurg Psychiatry 1994;57:626–8.

95. MacDonald JR, Hill JD, Tarnopolsky MA. Modafinil reduces excessive somnolence and enhances mood in patients with myotonic dystrophy. Neurology 2002;59:1876–80.

96. Orlikowski D, Chevret S, Quera-Salva MA, et al. Modafinil for the treatment of hypersomnia associated with myotonic muscular dystrophy in adults: a multicenter, prospective, randomized, double-blind, placebo-controlled, 4-week trial. Clin Ther 2009;31:1765–73.

97. Griggs RC, Pandya S, Florence JM, et al. Randomized controlled trial of testosterone in myotonic dystrophy. Neurology 1989;39:219–22.

98. Vlachopapadopoulou E, Zachwieja JJ, Gertner JM, et al. Metabolic and clinical response to recombinant human insulin-like growth factor I in myotonic dystrophy–a clinical research center study. J Clin Endocrinol Metab 1995;80:3715–23.

99. Heatwole CR, Eichinger KJ, Friedman DI, et al. Open-label trial of recombinant human insulin-like growth factor 1/recombinant human insulin-like growth factor binding protein 3 in myotonic dystrophy type 1. Arch Neurol 2011;68:37–44.

100. Trip J, Drost G, van Engelen BG, et al. Drug treatment for myotonia. Cochrane Database Syst Rev 2006;(25):CD004762.

101. Logigian EL, Martens WB, Moxley RT, et al. Mexiletine is an effective antimyotonia treatment in myotonic dystrophy type 1. Neurology 2010;74:1441–8.

102. Furling D, Doucet G, Langlois MA, et al. Viral vector producing antisense RNA restores myotonic dystrophy myoblast functions. Gene Ther 2003;10:795–802.

103. Mulders SA, van den Broek WJ, Wheeler TM, et al. Triplet-repeat oligonucleotide-mediated reversal of RNA toxicity in myotonic dystrophy. Proc Natl Acad Sci U S A 2009;106:13915–20.

104. Wheeler TM, Leger AJ, Pandey SK, et al. Targeting nuclear RNA for in vivo correction of myotonic dystrophy. Nature 2012;488:111–5.
105. Coonrod LA, Nakamori M, Wang W, et al. Reducing levels of toxic RNA with small molecules. ACS Chem Biol 2013;8:2528–37.
106. Childs-Disney JL, Hoskins J, Rzuczek SG, et al. Rationally designed small molecules targeting the RNA that causes myotonic dystrophy type 1 are potently bioactive. ACS Chem Biol 2012;7:856–62.
107. Arambula JF, Ramisetty SR, Baranger AM, et al. A simple ligand that selectively targets CUG trinucleotide repeats and inhibits MBNL protein binding. Proc Natl Acad Sci U S A 2009;106:16068–73.
108. Ofori LO, Hoskins J, Nakamori M, et al. From dynamic combinatorial 'hit' to lead: in vitro and in vivo activity of compounds targeting the pathogenic RNAs that cause myotonic dystrophy. Nucleic Acids Res 2012;40:6380–90.
109. Wang GS, Kuyumcu-Martinez MN, Sarma S, et al. PKC inhibition ameliorates the cardiac phenotype in a mouse model of myotonic dystrophy type 1. J Clin Invest 2009;119:3797–806.
110. Kanadia RN, Shin J, Yuan Y, et al. Reversal of RNA mis-splicing and myotonia following muscleblind overexpression in a mouse poly(CUG) model for myotonic dystrophy. Proc Natl Acad Sci U S A 2006;103:11748–53.

Facioscapulohumeral Muscular Dystrophy

 CrossMark

Jeffrey Statland, MD*, Rabi Tawil, MD

KEYWORDS

- Muscular dystrophy • Facioscapulohumeral muscular dystrophy • D4Z4 deletion
- DUX4 • SMCHD1 mutation

KEY POINTS

- Clinically, Facioscapulohumeral muscular dystrophy types 1 and 2 are similar: often asymmetric and descending weakness affecting the face, shoulder, and arms followed by the distal lower extremities and pelvic girdle.
- Facioscapulohumeral muscular dystrophy patients with the largest contractions are more likely to have symptomatic extramuscular involvement that includes retinal vascular disease, hearing loss, and, rarely, cognitive impairment or seizures.
- Facioscapulohumeral muscular dystrophy type 1 is caused by a deletion in the number of the macrosatellite repeat (D4Z4) elements on chromosome 4q35; this leads to decreased DNA methylation and opening of the chromatin structure.
- Facioscapulohumeral muscular dystrophy type 2 is caused by mutations in genes elsewhere in the genome that lead to decreased methylation in the same D4Z4 region on chromosome 4q35.
- The opening of the chromatic structure seen in both Facioscapulohumeral muscular dystrophy types 1 and 2 results in de-repression of the DUX4 gene, a transcriptional factor believed to cause disease through a toxic gain-of-function mechanism.
- The identification of a proposed disease mechanism opens the door to future disease-directed therapies.

INTRODUCTION

Facioscapulohumeral muscular dystrophy (FSHD), one of the most prevalent adult muscular dystrophies (1:15,000–1:20,000), is characterized by asymmetric and often descending weakness affecting the face, shoulder, and arms followed by weakness of the distal lower extremities and pelvic girdle.[1,2] FSHD is categorized as type 1 or

Support: MDA Clinical Research Training Grant (J.M. Statland); None (R. Tawil).
Disclosures: Both R. Tawil and J.M. Statland are consultants for Cytokinetics.
Department of Neurology, University of Rochester Medical Center, 265 Crittenden Boulevard, CU 420669, Rochester, NY 14642-0669, USA
* Corresponding author.
E-mail address: Jeffrey_Statland@URMC.Rochester.edu

Neurol Clin 32 (2014) 721–728
http://dx.doi.org/10.1016/j.ncl.2014.04.003
0733-8619/14/$ – see front matter © 2014 Elsevier Inc. All rights reserved.

type 2 based on the underlying genetic lesions. Approximately 95% of patients will have disease inherited in an autosomal dominant fashion associated with loss of part of a repeated sequence in the D4Z4 region on chromosome 4q35.[3,4] An additional 5% of patients will have disease with a variable inheritance pattern caused by a D4Z4 deletion-independent pathway.[5] Recent advances suggest both FSHD types 1 and 2 exert their effects through a common pathophysiologic pathway: de-repression of the retrogene *DUX4* believed to cause disease in a toxic-gain-of-function manner.[6] Studies have suggested FSHD1 and FSHD2 are clinically identical; although, the number of FSHD2 patients studied has been limited. Approximately 20% of FSHD patients greater than 50 years of age will require the use of a wheelchair.[2,7] FSHD1 patients with the largest contractions are more likely to have extramuscular manifestations of FSHD, which include symptomatic retinal vascular disease and hearing loss.[8,9] The elucidation of a proposed common molecular mechanism behind both FSHD types 1 and 2 has opened the door to research in potential disease-directed therapies.

CLINICAL FINDINGS

Both FSHD types 1 and 2 are clinically similar, characterized by:

- Symptom onset typically in the first or second decade of life but can present later in life
- Often marked side-to-side asymmetry
- Facial weakness seen as inability to squeeze the eyes shut or furrow the brow, a transverse smile, or flattening when puckering the lips
- Shoulder weakness often with scapular winging and flattening of the clavicles
- Arm weakness including the biceps and triceps often with forearm sparing
- Asymmetric abdominal weakness seen on examination as a positive Beevor's sign
- Usually distal lower extremity weakness before proximal, starting with a foot drop

FSHD can go on to affect most any skeletal muscle but typically spares extraocular muscles, cardiac muscles, and bulbar muscles. Debilitating paraspinal muscle weakness can develop, which can be an initial presentation.[10] Although the most common presentation is with facial and shoulder weakness and a descending pattern of progression, several initial presentations have been described, including bent spine and less-specific limb girdle patterns. The rate of progression has been evaluated in a large prospective natural history study, which found a loss of strength using combined quantitative strength testing and manual muscle testing of about 1% to 4% per year.[11] Although not life limiting, FSHD can cause significant lifetime morbidity.[2,7,12] The 6-year risk of wheelchair use overall is about 24%. Risk of wheelchair use shows a bimodal distribution: FSHD1 patients with the largest D4Z4 deletions (1–3 remaining repeats) have the highest risk, which peaks in the second and third decades, followed by a slow age-dependent increase in the risk. Respiratory involvement is seen in about 10% of patients, most commonly in the most severely affected or wheelchair-bound patients. Atrial arrhythmias are seen in about 5% of FSHD patients but are rarely symptomatic.

Extramuscular manifestations are also rarely symptomatic and include retinal vascular changes and hearing loss. Approximately half of FSHD patients show peripheral retinal vascular abnormalities on fluorescein angiography, but symptomatic retinal vasculopathy (Coat's syndrome) is only seen in approximately 1% of patients, typically patients with the largest D4Z4 deletions.[9,13,14] High-frequency hearing loss is reported in approximately half of FSHD patients; however, symptomatic hearing loss resulting in the need for hearing aids is almost exclusively seen in patients with the largest D4Z4 deletions.[8,15]

A more severe infantile form of FSHD has been described.[16,17] These patients typically:

- Have the largest deletions (1–3 D4Z4 repeats remaining)
- Have increased prevalence of symptomatic retinal vascular disease and hearing loss
- Have more severe disease with earlier wheelchair use
- Have, rarely, mental retardation or seizures

DIAGNOSIS

Clinical criteria for the diagnosis of FSHD include the presence of characteristic findings and the absence of other explanations.[18] FSHD is suggested by the presence of:

- Facial weakness
- Weakness of shoulder scapular stabilizers or foot dorsiflexors

The absence of:

- Ptosis, weakness of extraocular muscles, or bulbar weakness
- Electromyography in a patient or affected family member showing myotonia or neurogenic changes

Electromyography shows changes characteristic of a chronic myopathy, small polyphasic motor units, but may be normal or only show changes in limited muscles, like the serratus anterior or pectorals. Muscle biopsy is not required for diagnosis but can show nonspecific myopathic or dystrophic changes including variability in fiber size, rounded fibers, internal nuclei, necrotic or regenerating fibers, increased connective tissue, and fatty deposition. Up to one-third of muscle biopsies can show a primarily mononuclear inflammatory infiltrate.[19,20]

Muscle magnetic resonance imaging (MRI) is being used more frequently in the evaluation of patients with suspected muscular dystrophies, and although there are patterns of muscle involvement typical for FSHD, the role of MRI in diagnosis has yet to be determined.[21–23] Patterns of muscle involvement on MRI in FSHD include:

- Early involvement of trapezius, scapular girdle, and pectoral muscles
- Early involvement of the gastrocnemius and tibialis anterior
- Short tau inversion recovery–positive signal in structurally normal-appearing muscles, which may correspond to areas of inflammation in some patients

Ultimately, the diagnosis of FSHD is confirmed by genetic testing. Approximately 95% of patients meeting clinical criteria will turn out to have deletion of a key number of repetitive elements in the D4Z4 region of chromosome 4q35 (termed *FSHD1*). Normal individuals have greater than 10 repeats. Patients with FSHD1 have between 1 and 10 repeats.[3,4] An additional 5% of patients will have disease without a deletion in the number of D4Z4 repeats (termed *FSHD2*). Nevertheless, these patients have reduced methylation in the D4Z4 region of 4q35 as is seen in the contracted 4q35 allele in FSHD1.[5] Recently, up to two-thirds of patients with FSHD2 were discovered to have mutations in the gene SMCHD1, believed to have a role in chromatin inactivation.[24] Commercial genetic confirmation of FSHD2 is not yet available.

PATHOPHYSIOLOGY

Recent studies suggest that activation of a normally repressed transcriptional regulator, *DUX4*, contained within the D4Z4 repeat elements on chromosome 4q35 causes disease in FSHD via a toxic-gain-of-function fashion.[25]

In FSHD1, a key number of repeated sequences, each 3.3 kb long, are lost in the D4Z4 region on chromosome 4q35. Loss of the repetitive elements leads to decreased methylation and opening up of the chromatin structure. Contained in each D4Z4 repeat is a putative retrogene, *DUX4*, not normally expressed in adult muscle. Loss of the repetitive elements opens the chromatin structure allowing *DUX4* to be expressed from the most distal D4Z4 repeat. But that is not enough to cause disease in FSHD. In addition, patients must have a permissive genetic background; a certain polymorphism distal to the last repeat, known as the A variant, results in a polyadenylation sequence that is essential for the stability of nascent DUX4 transcripts, which would otherwise be degraded (**Fig. 1**).[6]

In FSHD2, patients do not have deletions in the D4Z4 region, and yet there is loss of methylation in the D4Z4 region of chromosome 4q35. Although the inheritance in FSHD1 is dominant (resulting from the occurrence of a contraction on one copy of 4q35 containing an A allele), the inheritance pattern in FSHD2 is more complex because it is a digenic disease. FSHD2 requires the inheritance of permissive A allele

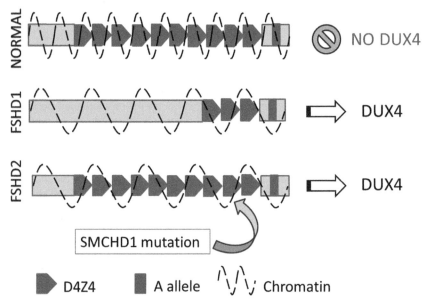

Fig. 1. Pathologic mechanism in FSHD. In normal individuals the chromatin is tightly wound keeping *DUX4* in a repressed state. In FSHD1, deletion of a critical number of D4Z4 repeats opens up the chromatin structure allowing *DUX4* to be expressed. However, this only occurs when the D4Z4 deletion occurs on a permissive genetic background, the A allele, which contains a polyadenylation sequence, which stabilizes the nascent *DUX4* transcripts. In FSHD2, patients do not have deletions in the D4Z4 region, but do have decreased methylation, which in approximately two-thirds of patients is associated with mutations in the SMCHD1 gene. Decreased methylation also causes an opening of chromatin structure, and when this occurs on a permissive genetic background containing the A allele, *DUX4* can be expressed. In both, expression of DUX4 is believed to cause disease in a toxic gain-of-function fashion.

and separate mutation in a gene that regulates chromatic structure (eg, SMCHD1 on chromosome 18). This loss of methylation in conjunction with a permissive genetic background also leads to expression of DUX4.[5] Recently, approximately two-thirds of patients with FSHD2 were found to have mutations in SMCHD1, a gene on chromosome 18 believed to have a role in chromatin inactivation (see **Fig. 1**).[24]

Several lines of evidence suggest that low levels of DUX4 expression interfere with myogenic differentiation, lead to apoptotic cell death, and make cells more susceptible to oxidative stress.[24,26–30]

Necessary for FSHD:

- Opening up of the chromatin structure in the D4Z4 region of chromosome 4q35, allowing the normally repressed *DUX4* gene to be expressed
- Stabilizing polymorphisms that prevent nascent *DUX4* mRNA from being degraded

THERAPEUTIC STRATEGIES

There currently are no FDA-approved treatments for FSHD. Several pharmacologic strategies have been tested to determine if they slow down or halt disease progression in FSHD: trials of anabolic agents, a myostatin inhibitor, creatine supplementation, and corticosteroids were either negative or inconclusive.[31–36] Future treatment strategies can be split into 2 categories: (1) therapies to increase muscle bulk or strength (anabolic agents, myostatin, or follistatin inhibitors) and (2) therapies to halt disease progression (molecular knock-down of DUX4 or downstream targets of DUX4).

A trial of exercise and albuterol, alone or in combination, showed improvement in isolated muscle strength with albuterol but was negative for individually trained muscles.[37] Strength training consisted of a progressive overload program that included dynamic and isometric exercises focusing on elbow flexors and ankle dorsiflexors. Patients receiving strength training did not do worse than those who did not pursue strength training, and dynamic strength improved in elbow flexors. Aerobic therapy is likely beneficial in FSHD, not only improving cardiovascular health but possibly increasing strength.[38]

Several observational studies and case series document improvement in shoulder function, shoulder range of motion, or improvement in scapular pain after scapular fixation.[39,40] Scapulodesis (the fixation of the scapula with screws, wires, or plates) with bone grafting is the preferred surgical procedure. Despite this fact, no randomized trials support the benefit seen in observational studies nor are there clear recommendations on which patients are most likely to benefit from this procedure or the optimal timing of surgery. Intuitively, patients considering surgery should have reasonable residual upper arm strength. The potential gain in range of motion from surgical fixation can be tested at the bedside by manual fixation of the scapula. Drawbacks to scapular fixation include postoperative immobilization, need for physiotherapy, and potential complications (breaks in the wire with consequent loss of the functional gain, brachial plexus injuries, or possible loss of respiratory forced vital capacity).

Although no prospective studies have determined the optimal surveillance strategy for use of orthotics or extramuscular manifestations of FSHD, we recommend:

- Baseline screening for retinal involvement with dilated ophthalmologic examination in all patients, then yearly in patients with the largest D4Z4 deletions (1–3 residual repeats)
- Baseline pulmonary function testing in patients with advanced disease, early pelvic girdle weakness, or significant kyphoscoliosis, then yearly follow-up

- Hearing test for all infantile-onset FSHD
- Yearly evaluation for need for orthotic devices for ambulation

SUMMARY AND FUTURE DIRECTIONS

Recent advances in our understanding of the molecular pathology of FSHD have identified potential molecular targets for future therapies. FSHD types 1 and 2 are clinically similar and share a final common pathway, suggesting that similar treatment strategies may prove successful for both. Future therapeutic strategies will likely include targeting the expression of DUX4 or its downstream targets and strategies geared toward increasing muscle bulk and strength.

REFERENCES

1. Mostacciuolo ML, Pastorello E, Vazza G, et al. Facioscapulohumeral muscular dystrophy: epidemiological and molecular study in a north-east Italian population sample. Clin Genet 2009;75(6):550–5.
2. Padberg GW, Frants RR, Brouwer OF, et al. Facioscapulohumeral muscular dystrophy in the Dutch population. Muscle Nerve 1995;2:S81–4.
3. van Deutekom JC, Wijmenga C, van Tienhoven EA, et al. FSHD associated DNA rearrangements are due to deletions of integral copies of a 3.2 kb tandemly repeated unit. Hum Mol Genet 1993;2(12):2037–42.
4. Wijmenga C, Hewitt JE, Sandkuijl LA, et al. Chromosome 4q DNA rearrangements associated with facioscapulohumeral muscular dystrophy. Nat Genet 1992;2(1):26–30.
5. de Greef JC, Lemmers RJ, Camano P, et al. Clinical features of facioscapulohumeral muscular dystrophy 2. Neurology 2010;75(17):1548–54.
6. van der Maarel SM, Tawil R, Tapscott SJ. Facioscapulohumeral muscular dystrophy and DUX4: breaking the silence. Trends Mol Med 2011;17(5):252–8.
7. Statland JM, Tawil R. Risk of functional impairment in facioscapulohumeral muscular dystrophy. Muscle Nerve 2013;49:520–7.
8. Lutz KL, Holte L, Kliethermes SA, et al. Clinical and genetic features of hearing loss in facioscapulohumeral muscular dystrophy. Neurology 2013;81(16):1374–7.
9. Statland JM, Sacconi S, Farmakidis C, et al. Coats syndrome in facioscapulohumeral dystrophy type 1: frequency and D4Z4 contraction size. Neurology 2013;80(13):1247–50.
10. Jordan B, Eger K, Koesling S, et al. Camptocormia phenotype of FSHD: a clinical and MRI study on six patients. J Neurol 2011;258(5):866–73.
11. FSH-DY. A prospective, quantitative study of the natural history of facioscapulohumeral muscular dystrophy (FSHD): implications for therapeutic trials. The FSH-DY Group. Neurology 1997;48(1):38–46.
12. Laforet P, de Toma C, Eymard B, et al. Cardiac involvement in genetically confirmed facioscapulohumeral muscular dystrophy. Neurology 1998;51(5):1454–6.
13. Fitzsimons RB, Gurwin EB, Bird AC. Retinal vascular abnormalities in facioscapulohumeral muscular dystrophy. A general association with genetic and therapeutic implications. Brain 1987;110(Pt 3):631–48.
14. Padberg GW, Brouwer OF, de Keizer RJ, et al. On the significance of retinal vascular disease and hearing loss in facioscapulohumeral muscular dystrophy. Muscle Nerve 1995;2:S73–80.

15. Trevisan CP, Pastorello E, Tomelleri G, et al. Facioscapulohumeral muscular dystrophy: hearing loss and other atypical features of patients with large 4q35 deletions. Eur J Neurol 2008;15(12):1353–8.
16. Funakoshi M, Goto K, Arahata K. Epilepsy and mental retardation in a subset of early onset 4q35-facioscapulohumeral muscular dystrophy. Neurology 1998; 50(6):1791–4.
17. Lunt PW, Jardine PE, Koch MC, et al. Correlation between fragment size at D4F104S1 and age at onset or at wheelchair use, with a possible generational effect, accounts for much phenotypic variation in 4q35-facioscapulohumeral muscular dystrophy (FSHD). Hum Mol Genet 1995;4(5):951–8.
18. Tawil R, McDermott MP, Mendell JR, et al. Facioscapulohumeral muscular dystrophy (FSHD): design of natural history study and results of baseline testing. FSH-DY Group. Neurology 1994;44(3 Pt 1):442–6.
19. Arahata K, Ishihara T, Fukunaga H, et al. Inflammatory response in facioscapulohumeral muscular dystrophy (FSHD): immunocytochemical and genetic analyses. Muscle Nerve 1995;2:S56–66.
20. Carpenter S, Karpati G. Pathology of skeletal muscle. 2nd edition. New York: Oxford University Press; 2001.
21. Friedman SD, Poliachik SL, Carter GT, et al. The magnetic resonance imaging spectrum of facioscapulohumeral muscular dystrophy. Muscle Nerve 2012; 45(4):500–6.
22. Kan HE, Scheenen TW, Wohlgemuth M, et al. Quantitative MR imaging of individual muscle involvement in facioscapulohumeral muscular dystrophy. Neuromuscul Disord 2009;19(5):357–62.
23. Masciullo M, Iannaccone E, Bianchi ML, et al. Myotonic dystrophy type 1 and de novo FSHD mutation double trouble: a clinical and muscle MRI study. Neuromuscul Disord 2013;23(5):427–31.
24. Lemmers RJ, Tawil R, Petek LM, et al. Digenic inheritance of an SMCHD1 mutation and an FSHD-permissive D4Z4 allele causes facioscapulohumeral muscular dystrophy type 2. Nat Genet 2012;44(12):1370–4.
25. Lemmers RJ, van der Vliet PJ, Klooster R, et al. A unifying genetic model for facioscapulohumeral muscular dystrophy. Science 2010;329(5999):1650–3.
26. Bosnakovski D, Daughters RS, Xu Z, et al. Biphasic myopathic phenotype of mouse DUX, an ORF within conserved FSHD-related repeats. PLoS One 2009; 4(9):e7003.
27. Kowaljow V, Marcowycz A, Ansseau E, et al. The DUX4 gene at the FSHD1A locus encodes a pro-apoptotic protein. Neuromuscul Disord 2007;17(8):611–23.
28. Snider L, Asawachaicharn A, Tyler AE, et al. RNA transcripts, miRNA-sized fragments and proteins produced from D4Z4 units: new candidates for the pathophysiology of facioscapulohumeral dystrophy. Hum Mol Genet 2009;18(13):2414–30.
29. Vanderplanck C, Ansseau E, Charron S, et al. The FSHD atrophic myotube phenotype is caused by DUX4 expression. PLoS One 2011;6(10):e26820.
30. Wuebbles RD, Long SW, Hanel ML, et al. Testing the effects of FSHD candidate gene expression in vertebrate muscle development. Int J Clin Exp Pathol 2010; 3(4):386–400.
31. Kissel JT, McDermott MP, Mendell JR, et al. Randomized, double-blind, placebo-controlled trial of albuterol in facioscapulohumeral dystrophy. Neurology 2001; 57(8):1434–40.
32. Payan CA, Hogrel JY, Hammouda EH, et al. Periodic salbutamol in facioscapulohumeral muscular dystrophy: a randomized controlled trial. Arch Phys Med Rehabil 2009;90(7):1094–101.

33. Rose MR, Tawil R. Drug treatment for facioscapulohumeral muscular dystrophy. Cochrane Database Syst Rev 2004;(2):CD002276.
34. Tawil R, McDermott MP, Pandya S, et al. A pilot trial of prednisone in facioscapulohumeral muscular dystrophy. FSH-DY Group. Neurology 1997;48(1):46–9.
35. Wagner KR, Fleckenstein JL, Amato AA, et al. A phase I/IItrial of MYO-029 in adult subjects with muscular dystrophy. Ann Neurol 2008;63(5):561–71.
36. Walter MC, Lochmuller H, Reilich P, et al. Creatine monohydrate in muscular dystrophies: a double-blind, placebo-controlled clinical study. Neurology 2000;54(9): 1848–50.
37. van der Kooi EL, Vogels OJ, van Asseldonk RJ, et al. Strength training and albuterol in facioscapulohumeral muscular dystrophy. Neurology 2004;63(4):702–8.
38. Olsen DB, Orngreen MC, Vissing J. Aerobic training improves exercise performance in facioscapulohumeral muscular dystrophy. Neurology 2005;64(6): 1064–6.
39. Orrell RW, Copeland S, Rose MR. Scapular fixation in muscular dystrophy. Cochrane Database Syst Rev 2010;(1):CD003278.
40. Van Tongel A, Atoun E, Narvani A, et al. Medium to long-term outcome of thoracoscapular arthrodesis with screw fixation for facioscapulohumeral muscular dystrophy. J Bone Joint Surg Am 2013;95(15):1404–8.

The Limb-Girdle Muscular Dystrophies

Matthew P. Wicklund, MD[a],*, John T. Kissel, MD[b]

KEYWORDS

- Limb-girdle muscular dystrophy • Calpain 3 • Dysferlin • Sarcoglycan
- Fukutin-related protein • Anoctamin 5 • Lamin A/C

KEY POINTS

- Limb-girdle muscular dystrophies (LGMDs) are genetic muscle diseases with onset after birth of progressive weakness and muscle atrophy predominantly affecting the hips, shoulders, and proximal extremity muscles.
- As a group, the LGMDs are the fourth most common genetic muscle condition, with a minimum prevalence of approximately 1 in 20,000.
- LGMDs stem from protein defects throughout the muscle fiber, including the nucleus, sarcoplasm, sarcomere, sarcolemma, and extracellular matrix.
- The most prevalent LGMD subtypes derive from defects in the following proteins in muscle: calpain, dysferlin, the sarcoglycans, fukutin-related protein, anoctamin 5, and lamins A and C.

INTRODUCTION

The most common presentation of muscle disease involves weakness in the hip girdle, thighs, shoulder girdle, and proximal arms. Many acquired and genetic muscle disorders present with this limb-girdle pattern (see the article by Barohn elsewhere in this issue). Of the 3 most common muscular dystrophies, the dystrophinopathies (see the article by Flanigan elsewhere in this issue) also have this proximal predominant limb-girdle pattern, whereas facioscapulohumeral muscular dystrophy (FSHD) (see the article by Statland and Tawil elsewhere in this issue) and myotonic dystrophy (see the article by Thornton elsewhere in this issue) have relatively unique phenotypes.

Funding Sources: Dr M.P. Wicklund: Penn State Hershey Medical Center, NIH, U.S. Food and Drug Administration, Lilly; Dr J.T. Kissel: NIH, MDA, Novartis.
Conflict of Interest: Nil.
[a] Departments of Neurology and Pediatrics, Penn State College of Medicine, Penn State University, EC037, 30 Hope Drive, Hershey, PA 17033, USA; [b] Departments of Neurology and Pediatrics, The Ohio State University Wexner Medical Center, 395 West 12th Avenue, 7th Floor, Columbus, OH 43210, USA
* Corresponding author.
E-mail address: mwicklund@hmc.psu.edu

Definition

The LGMDs are genetic muscle diseases with onset after birth of progressive weakness and muscle atrophy predominantly affecting the hips, shoulders, and proximal extremity muscles.

LGMDs are named based on a consensus nomenclature,[1,2] which divides LGMD by inheritance pattern into autosomal dominant (LGMD1) and autosomal recessive (LGMD2) subtypes. Overlaid on this division is an alphabetical lettering system that delineates the order of discovery of the chromosomal locus for each LGMD (LGMD1A was mapped prior to LGMD1B and so forth). Twenty-seven genetic muscle diseases are currently classified as LGMDs (**Table 1**) and the differential diagnosis for the LGMDs is broad. LGMDs derive from protein defects from all locations throughout the muscle fiber, including the nucleus, sarcoplasm, sarcomere, sarcolemma, and extracellular matrix (**Fig. 1**).

LGMD differential diagnosis

- Dystrophinopathies
- Bethlem myopathy
- X-linked Emery-Dreifuss muscular dystrophy (EDMD)
- Myofibrillar myopathies
- Metabolic myopathies
- Inclusion body myopathies
- Pompe disease
- FSHD (facial sparing)

This article discusses the diagnostic features of the 6 most prevalent LGMD subtypes: LGMD2A (calpain), LGMD2B (dysferlin), LGMD2C–F (α-, β-, γ-, and δ-sarcoglycans), LGMD2I (fukutin-related protein), LGMD2L (anoctamin 5), and LGMD1B (lamin A/C) (**Fig. 2**).[3]

LGMD2A—CALPAIN

LGMD2A, due to mutations in the calpain 3 gene, *CAPN3*, is the most common LGMD subtype in nearly all population studies to date, ranging from 15% to 40% of cases.[4] Mutations in *CAPN3* have also been reported in hyperCKemia and in children and adults with eosinophilic myositis.[5,6] Calpain is a muscle-specific calcium-activated neutral protease that binds to titin and is likely important for muscle regeneration during sarcomere remodeling.[7–9]

Clinical

Onset of weakness varies widely in reported cases (ie, 2–53 years) but most often begins in later childhood or young adulthood, with 75% of cases having onset prior to 20 years of age.[10] Hyperlordosis and a waddling gait are common. Proximal lower extremity muscles are weaker than shoulder girdle muscles from the outset. Hip extensor, knee flexor, and hip adductor muscles often display disproportionately severe weakness.[11] Facial muscles may be weak in early-onset and severe disease but oculomotor and velopharyngeal muscles are uniformly spared. Respiratory and cardiac dysfunction is essentially nonexistent, although asymptomatic reductions in forced vital capacity may occur 20 years into the course.[12] Abdominal laxity and scapular winging are common. Hip, knee, and elbow contractures develop after loss of ambulation. The disease

Table 1
The limb-girdle muscular dystrophies

LGMD	Gene	Protein	Usual Age at Onset (y)	Creatine Kinase Level
1A	*MYOT*	Myotilin	20–40	NL–15×
1B	*LMNA*	Lamin A/C	5–25	NL–20×
1C	*CAV3*	Caveolin 3	5–25	2×–30×
1D	*DNAJB6*	DNAJB6 protein	30–50	NL–5×
1E	*DES*	Desmin	15–50	NL–4×
1F	*TNPO3*	Transportin 3	10–40	NL–15×
1G	Unknown	Unknown	30–47	NL
1H	Unknown	Unknown	16–50	NL–10×
2A	*CAPN3*	Calpain 3	5–25	NL–60×
2B	*DYSF*	Dysferlin	10–30	2×–160×
2C–F	*SGCG, A, B, D*	γ-, α-, β-, δ-sarcoglycan	3–20	5×–120×
2G	*TCAP*	Telethonin	2–15	2×–25×
2H	*TRIM32*	TRIM32	5–30	NL–20×
2I	*FKRP*	Fukutin-related protein	1–40	5×–50×
2J	*TTN*	Titin	5–20	NL–5×
2K	*POMT1*	POMT1	<5	5×–40×
2L	*ANO5*	Anoctamin 5	20–50	NL–160×
2M	*FKTN*	Fukutin	<5	5×–30×
2N	*POMT2*	POMT2	<2	15×–30×
2O	*POMGnT1*	POMGnT1	12	10×–50×
2P	*DAG1*	α-Dystroglycan	3	10×–20×
2Q	*PLEC1*	Plectin	<5	20×–30×
2R	*DES*	Desmin	1–25	NL–2×
2S	*TRAPPC11*	TRAPPC11	5–10	2×–30×

Abbreviation: NL, normal.

progresses steadily with most patients no longer ambulatory 2 decades into their disease. Later onset of disease follows a milder course. Cases of LGMD2A have been confused with FSHD due to the prominent scapular winging, abdominal laxity, and occasional facial involvement.[13]

LGMD2A: Key diagnostic features

- Most common LGMD
- 75% onset 5–20 years of age
- Hip extensor, hip adductor, and knee flexor weakness
- Scapular winging
- Calf hypertrophy
- Abdominal laxity
- Achilles contractures
- Rare facial involvement
- Creatine kinase (CK) level = 500–20,000 U/L
- Lobulated fibers on biopsy
- Diagnosis via genetic testing

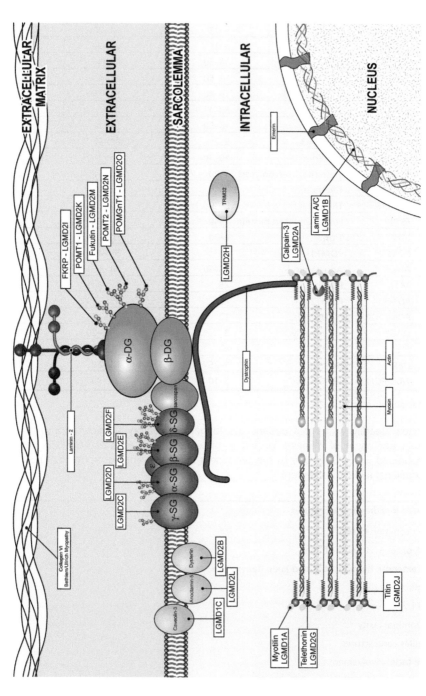

Fig. 1. Schematic diagram illustrating a muscle fiber and the associated LGMD proteins. DG, dystroglycan; SG, sarcoglycan.

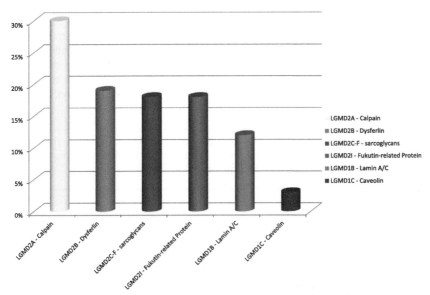

Fig. 2. Relative prevalence of the LGMD subtypes in the United States. This graph portrays the relative prevalence of LGMD subtypes. The data were derived from a US cohort with 488 genetically confirmed cases.[3] (Only the genes for these LGMDs were evaluated in this study, which was conducted prior to the discovery of *ANO5*, the gene for LGMD2L—anoctamin 5).

Laboratory

Evaluation reveals serum CK levels elevated 20-fold in typical patients with a range of 2 to 110 times the upper limit of normal.[14] Needle EMG yields abnormalities compatible with a myopathy. Although useful in documenting involvement of muscle in LGMD, muscle imaging (CT and MRI) is not reliable or accurate in discriminating one LGMD subtype from another.[15] Although rarely needed for diagnosis, muscle biopsy reveals variation in fiber size, internal nuclei, increased endomysial connective tissue, and necrotic and regenerating fibers, without inflammatory cells. Lobulated fibers can be seen in more than half of muscle biopsies (**Fig. 3**).[16]

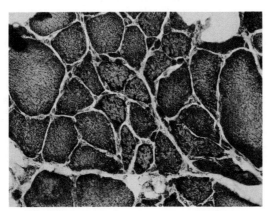

Fig. 3. Muscle biopsy with lobulated fibers from a patient with LGMD2A—calpainopathy. (NADH, original magnification 400×).

Diagnosis

Genetic testing is the diagnostic procedure of choice. Hundreds of mutations in CAPN3 have been delineated with no apparent hot spots.[17,18] Complicating matters is that in approximately one-fifth of cases with a typical phenotype and absent calpain-3 on Western blot, only a single mutation of CAPN3 is found. For this reason, many laboratories also test for deletions and duplications in this situation.

Treatment

No disease-specific treatment is available for calpainopathies. One 11-year-old girl with LGMD2A, however, presented with concurrent eosinophilic myositis and improved on immunosuppressive medications.[19]

Case 1

A 22-year-old young man presented with weakness. His motor development was equivalent to peers as a youth. At 13 years of age, he noted an awkward running style. Although his lower extremity weakness progressed, he continued to play basketball through high school. He was not as quick in his junior and senior years but was still used at the end of games for his incredible 3-point accuracy. At approximately his 19th birthday, proximal upper extremity weakness developed. Currently, he has trouble getting his arms over his head and must pull on a banister ascending stairs. He has always had large calves. There are no oculobulbar, respiratory, or cardiac symptoms. He has never had episodes of dark urine.

On examination, he had no facial weakness. There was marked bilateral scapular winging, very large calves, mild bilateral ankle contractures, and strength as follows—Medical Research Council (MRC) scale: upper extremities normal except shoulder abductors 5 3_ and elbow flexors 5 4; and in the lower extremities strength was hip flexors 5 41, hip extensors 5 2, hip abductors 5 5, hip abductors 5 0, knee extensors 5 5, and knee flexors 5 4_.

His CK level was 16,483 U/L. His nerve conduction study/electromyography (EMG) revealed a mostly nonirritable myopathy. His muscle biopsy when 15 years old revealed dystrophic features and 30% lobulated fibers. Genetic testing revealed 2 disease-associated mutations in CAPN3: n.245C>T; p.Pro82Leu and n.1465C>T; p.Arg489Trp.

This real-life case reveals all the key diagnostic features in LGMD2A.

LGMD2B—DYSFERLIN

LGMD2B is one phenotype associated with mutations in DYSF, the gene for dysferlin.[20] Dysferlin plays an important role in membrane trafficking, fusion, and, most notably, membrane repair.[21] Adeno-associated virus–mediated transfer of a mini-dysferlin or up-regulation of fetal myoferlin, however, correct this resealing function in a membrane laser wounding assay but do not rescue the histology in vivo. Thus, the pathogenesis of dysferlinopathies does not seem to be due exclusively to impaired membrane repair.[22] Dysferlin deficiency also reduces release of chemotactic cytokines resulting in an attenuated regeneration response.[23] Dysferlin additionally plays roles in myoblast differentiation and T-tubule system development.[24,25]

Clinical

LGMD2B is likely the second most prevalent subtype and responsible for 5% to 35% of cases.[26] Dysferlinopathies can present with numerous, often overlapping phenotypes: LGMD2B with proximal weakness, Miyoshi myopathy with distal weakness of calf muscles, early involvement of the anterior compartment muscles of the lower legs, a proximodistal pattern, biceps atrophy with deltoid hypertrophy, combination calf and deltoid hypertrophy, rigid spine syndrome, a pseudometabolic presentation, and asymptomatic hyperCKemia.[27–31] Heterozygous gene carriers may develop mild weakness later in life. In LGMD2B, onset generally occurs between 15 and 30 years of age, although congenital cases and symptomatic onset in the 70s have been reported.[32,33] Patients develop normally in cognitive and motor spheres, and some patients are actually gifted athletically when young.[30,31] Weakness begins in the legs in nearly all cases, the initial site of involvement determining the nomenclature. LGMD2B patients often show mild distal leg weakness and may have difficulty standing on their toes early in disease. Weakness progresses slowly over 10 to 20 years to wheelchair use in many. Occasional patients, however, report precipitous onset and progression with rapid loss of ambulation over 1 to 2 years, especially linked to pregnancy.[31] Upper limb weakness develops after onset of gait difficulties, but scapular winging is not a feature of this disorder. Cardiac or respiratory compromise in LGMD2B is uncommon, occurs late in life, and usually remains clinically silent.[34,35]

LGMD2B: Key diagnostic features

- Onset 15–35 years of age
- Legs affected first
- Some distal leg weakness in many
- Athletic prowess when young
- No facial weakness or dysphagia
- No clinical respiratory involvement
- No clinical cardiac involvement
- CK = 1000–40,000 U/L
- Inflammation on biopsy in approximately 40%
- Diagnosis via genetic testing

Laboratory

Serum CK levels may be substantially elevated, as great as 200-times normal. EMG frequently shows small, brief motor units with early recruitment, although long-duration polyphasic motor units with decreased recruitment often pop up in weak calf muscles. Muscle biopsies may reveal dystrophic features, vacuoles (a minor feature),[36] amyloid deposition (only with certain mutations and not in most cases),[37] and, importantly, endomysial and perivascular inflammatory infiltrates in more than 50% of biopsies in some series (mostly CD4$^+$ cells and macrophages).[38,39] This inflammation has been thought a secondary reaction to degeneration but has led to misdiagnosis of dysferlinopathies as treatment refractory polymyositis.[40]

Diagnosis

Immunostaining of muscle biopsies and protein-based monocyte assays are available for diagnosis. These modalities do not, however, detect all cases with *DYSF* mutations, and dysferlin deficiency can occur in other muscle disorders. Thus, genetic testing is the most appropriate and accurate methodology for diagnosis of LGMD2B.[41]

Treatment

Although there may often be inflammation on the muscle biopsy in dysferlinopathies, treatment with deflazacort (1) was associated with significant steroid side effects, (2) did not improve strength, and (3) perhaps worsened disease progression.[42] Genetic-based therapies are in phase 2 clinical trials.

Case 2

A 21-year-old young woman presented with weakness. Her motor development was normal as a child. In elementary school, she was actually faster and stronger than the other children. At 15 years of age, she noted that when she ran, she "just could not go." In high school softball, she could hit the ball very far but was slow running the bases. Over the ensuing 6 years, her leg weakness slowly progressed. Since at least age 16 years, she recalls she could not stand on her tiptoes. Her arms remain strong, and there are no oculobulbar, respiratory, or cardiac symptoms. She has never had cramps or episodes of dark urine.

On examination, she had diminished calf bulk but no facial weakness and no scapular winging. Her neck and upper extremity strength was normal. In her lower extremities, she had the following (MRC scale): hip flexors = 4+, hip extensors = 4+, hip abductors = 4+, hip adductors = 4+, knee extensors = 4−, knee flexors = 4+, ankle dorsiflexors = 5, ankle eversion = 4+, ankle inversion = 4+, and ankle plantar flexors = 4−. She had normal sensation and a mild Trendelenburg gait.

Her CK levels were 12,962 U/L, 8663 U/L, and 5575 U/L when checked on 3 successive years. Electrodiagnostic testing was not performed. A muscle biopsy showed mildly dystrophic features with diminished (but not absent) dysferlin immunostaining. Genetic testing revealed homozygous, known pathogenic, missense mutations in *DYSF* (c.5429G>A; p.Arg1810Lys).

This real-life case reveals many key diagnostic features in LGMD2B.

LGMD2C–F—α-, β-, γ-, AND δ-SARCOGLYCANS

Four sarcoglycans (γ, α, β, and δ) form a heterotetrameric complex spanning the sarcolemma in association with sarcospan, dystrophin, and the dystroglycans (see **Fig. 1**). This dystrophin-glycoprotein complex (DGC) provides a mechanical bridge between the extracellular basement membrane, the cytoskeleton, and the intracellular contractile mechanism of muscle fibers.[43] Additionally, the DGC facilitates cell signaling and trafficking in concert with neuronal nitric oxide synthase, dystrobrevin, and caveolin-3.[44] Muscular dystrophies due to mutations in the different sarcoglycan subunits yield similar clinical and laboratory characteristics. γ-Sarcoglycan was the first sarcoglycan gene locus discovered and is thus labeled LGMD2C. LGMD2D, -2E, and -2F correspond to α-, β-, and δ-sarcoglycan deficiencies, respectively.

Clinical

LGMD, due to mutations in one of the four sarcoglycans, comprise 10–20% of LGMD cases.[4,45] Onset is predominantly in childhood, most often between 5 and 10 years of age (range 1–30 years). Weakness starts in the pelvic girdle with decremental shoulder girdle strength a few years later. Proximal limb extensors (quadriceps and triceps brachii) are comparatively spared versus flexors (biceps brachii and hamstrings). Common examination features include calf hypertrophy, scapular winging, macroglossia, and lumbar hyperlordosis. Many patients are wheelchair dependent within 10 years.[46–48] Most patients' disease course mirrors a severe, Duchenne-like progression. Milder cases with slower progression and some with only exercise intolerance, myoglobinuria, or minimal muscle weakness dot the literature.[49–51] Additionally, a case of eosinophilic myositis was recently revealed to be due to mutations of γ-sarcoglycan.[52] As in Duchenne dystrophy, cardiac and respiratory dysfunction frequently afflicts patients. Symptomatic respiratory dysfunction along with arrhythmogenic, dilated, or hypertrophic cardiomyopathies are detected in one-third of patients 10 years into disease.[53,54]

LGMD2C–F: Key diagnostic features

- Usual onset 5–15 years of age
- Proximal leg weakness
- Scapular winging
- Calf hypertrophy
- Lumbar lordosis
- Cardiorespiratory dysfunction common 10–20 years into illness
- CK = 500–20,000 U/L
- Muscle biopsy usually has decreased immunostaining for all 4 sarcoglycans.
- Diagnosis via genetic testing

Laboratory

Serum CK values range from 5 to 120 times normal. Muscle biopsies show variability in fiber size, central nuclei, degenerating and regenerating fibers, and increased connective tissue, most often with normal immunostaining for dystrophin. Abnormal staining for all 4 skeletal muscle sarcoglycans occurs with mutations in any one particular sarcoglycan, and the staining pattern cannot be used to predict the genotype.[55] Cases exist of isolated immunostaining abnormalities for a single sarcoglycan (with preservation of staining for the other 3 sarcoglycans) in both γ-sarcoglycan[56] and α-sarcoglycan,[57] and in those cases the mutation analysis reflects the immunostaining pattern. Immunostaining and Western blot analysis for dystrophin may occasionally be simultaneously reduced in sarcoglycanopathies and tend to portend a more severe phenotype.[58]

Diagnosis

Muscle biopsy with immunostaining is often performed first, followed by genetic testing. Genetic testing is commercially available for the 4 sarcoglycan genes.

Case 3

A 12-year-old girl from Brazil presented in a wheelchair. She sat at 7 months and walked at 13 months. At 4 years of age, she preferred to be carried in the grocery store. At 6 years of age, she began to fall, had to pull on a banister to climb stairs, and could no longer run. By 10 years of age, she used a wheelchair fulltime.

On examination, there was mild, symmetric, bilateral scapular winging. Her calves were disproportionately large compared with her thighs. There was mild neck flexor weakness. Upper extremity strength was MRC grade 4 proximally. Lower extremity strength was 2 to 3 at the hips, 4− in the knee flexors and extensors, 4 in the ankle dorsiflexors, and 5 in the ankle plantar flexors. She had normal sensation.

Her CK levels were 17,006 U/L at age 6 years, 7993 U/L at age 10 years, and 4122 U/L at age 12 years. Her ECG demonstrated mild prolongation of the P–R interval. EMG revealed mild muscle membrane instability in most muscles along with small, myopathic motor units with early recruitment. A muscle biopsy showed a moderate to severe dystrophic pattern with diminished (but not absent) immunostaining for all γ-, α-, β-, and δ-sarcoglycans and for the N-terminal, rod, and C-terminal domains of dystrophin. Genetic testing revealed 2 heterozygous, disease-associated, missense mutations in the gene for α-sarcoglycan, *SGCA* and c.229C>T; p.Arg77Cys and c.850C>T; p.Arg284Cys.

This real-life case reveals many key diagnostic features in LGMD2D.

Treatment

Treatment requires attention to cardiac, respiratory, and orthopedic complications. A phase 1 human trial of gene therapy involved injection of α-sarcoglycan DNA via an adeno-associated virus vector into the extensor digitorum brevis muscle of 3 patients. This rescued treated muscles, demonstrating robust α-sarcoglycan gene expression at the sarcolemma of 57% to 69% of muscle fibers.[59] Further trials of this approach are in progress.

LGMD2I—FUKUTIN-RELATED PROTEIN

Expressed throughout human tissues, with highest levels in skeletal and cardiac muscle, fukutin-related protein (FKRP) demonstrates sequence similarities to a family of proteins involved in modifying cell surface glycoproteins and glycolipids. Mutations in *FKRP* are responsible for several phenotypes, including a congenital muscular dystrophy (MDC1C), milder patients with later-onset (LGMD2I), recurrent myoglobinuria, asymptomatic hyperCKemia, and isolated dilated cardiomyopathy.[60–64]

Clinical

Onset occurs over a broad range, from 1 to 50 years, but on average in the second decade of life. In Northern European neuromuscular centers, LGMD2I represents one of the most common LGMDs, constituting 20% to 40% of patients.[65,66] The prevalence in Southern Europe, however, is only approximately 5% and only 10% to 15% in North America.[3,67,68] Prominent respiratory and cardiac dysfunction may arise early in the clinical course and may not correlate with skeletal muscle involvement.[69,70] Strength may stabilize for years in patients, then progress once again. Often, patients walk well past the fourth decade. Initial pelvifemoral weakness subsequently spreads to the distal lower extremities and proximal upper extremities. Calf hypertrophy and lumbar lordosis are nearly universally present, sometimes leading to a misdiagnosis of Becker muscular dystrophy. Scapular winging, macroglossia, cognitive dysfunction, and MRI abnormalities are found in some cases.[71,72]

LGMD2I: Key diagnostic features

- Usual onset 10–20 years of age
- Proximal leg weakness
- Calf hypertrophy
- Lumbar lordosis
- Scapular winging
- Macroglossia
- Cardiorespiratory dysfunction
- 20%–30% May require bilevel positive airway pressure (BiPAP).
- CK = 500–20,000 U/L
- Muscle biopsy with decreased staining for α-dystroglycan
- Diagnosis via genetic testing

Laboratory

Serum CK ranges from 3 to 50 times normal but is nearly always more than 10 times the upper limit of normal. Myoglobinuria is common in patients with very high CK levels.[62] Echocardiography often reveals a dilated cardiomyopathy.[70] Forced vital capacity is reduced on pulmonary function testing in 30% to 50% of patients, and 20% to 30% of patients require BiPAP or ventilator support.[65,66] MRI of the pelvis and thigh often reveal disproportionate signal change (reflecting fibrosis and fatty infiltration) in the iliopsoas and thigh adductor muscles.[73] Muscle biopsies reveal dystrophic features (variability in fiber size, internal nuclei, degeneration, and regeneration with fatty and fibrous replacement) without distinctive features, such as rimmed vacuoles, inclusions, or inflammation.

Diagnosis

Biopsies reveal reduced or absent immunostaining for glycosylated α-dystroglycan. Confirmatory genetic testing is commercially available. There is a common mutation in the fukutin-related protein—*FKRP* 826C>A. Approximately two-thirds of patients are homozygous for this mutation, and these patients tend to have a milder clinical course.

Treatment

Of utmost importance in LGMD2I, monitoring of respiratory and cardiac function should take place in alternate years in asymptomatic patients and more frequently for those with previous testing abnormalities. Respiratory support with noninvasive ventilation and early treatment of cardiac dysfunction with medications, pacemakers, defibrillators, and transplantation improve quality of life.

Case 4

A 16-year-old young man from the north of England ran more slowly than other children since primary school. Lately, he has noted greater difficulties navigating stairs and arising from chairs and the floor. In his work at a pizza shop, he has trouble lifting pizzas out of the top ovens. At school, he has an individualized educational plan for mild learning difficulties.

On examination, there was no scapular winging, but he had large calves (**Fig. 4**). He had grade 4 strength proximally in his arms and legs, could not ascend steps 2 at a time, and was unable to run. On arising from a squat, he had a modified Gower sign.

His CK levels were 5683 U/L and 6084 U/L; his ECG, pulmonary function tests, and echocardiogram were normal; and his muscle biopsy showed a moderate to severe dystrophic pattern with absent immunostaining for glycosylated α-dystroglycan. Genetic testing revealed homozygous *FKRP* 826C>A mutations.

A 13-year-old, "asymptomatic" brother was not athletic. This brother's CK level was 9386 U/L, and he also harbored homozygous *FKRP* 826C>A mutations.

This real-life case reveals key diagnostic features in LGMD2I.

LGMD2L—ANOCTAMIN 5

LGMD2L due to mutations in *ANO5*, the gene for anoctamin 5, is a common LGMD subtype in Northern European populations, ranging from 15% to 40% of cases.[74] Its prevalence in the United States has not been determined. Anoctamin 5 is a putative calcium-activated chloride channel, but its exact function is not yet known. Dominant mutations in ANO5 can cause gnathodiaphyseal dysplasia.[75] Recessive mutations may lead to either LGMD2L or to a distal myopathy with predominant calf involvement, similar to Miyoshi myopathy.[76]

Clinical

Weakness in LGMD2L usually begins in adulthood between 20 and 50 years of age.[76] The pattern of weakness in LGMD2L was initially described as involving quadriceps

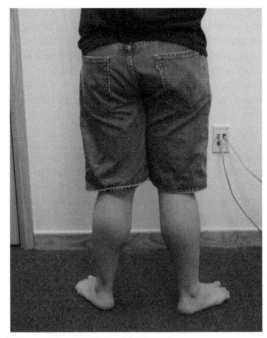

Fig. 4. A 16-year-old boy with LGMD2I and large calves.

and biceps atrophy.[77] Asymmetries were common. More recently, the phenotypic spectrum of ANO5-related genetic muscle disease has significantly expanded to include not only proximal upper and lower extremity weakness (limb-girdle pattern) but also a distal myopathy (Miyoshi-like with calf atrophy), proximal lower extremity weakness alone, proximal upper extremity weakness alone, proximodistal lower extremity weakness, isolated calf hypertrophy, and asymptomatic hyperCKemia.[78] Exercise intolerance and myalgias are common.[79] One-quarter of patients may require wheelchair use 10 to 20 years into disease. Cardiac and pulmonary involvement, however, has not been reported.

LGMD2L: Key diagnostic features

- Usual onset 20–50 years of age
- Proximal leg weakness
- Asymmetric weakness
- Early inability to stand on toes
- No cardiac or respiratory involvement
- CK = 2000–7000 U/L
- Muscle biopsy may have amyloid staining
- Diagnosis via genetic testing

Laboratory

CK levels tend to be elevated 10 to 40 times the upper limit of normal. On MRI of the lower limbs, the gracilis, sartorius, short head of the biceps femoris and tibialis anterior muscles tend to be spared.[80] Progression of muscle degeneration may be seen over a 3- to 7-year span on serial MRIs. Muscle biopsies reveal dystrophic features. Occasionally, Congo red staining may reveal amyloid deposits in the intramuscular blood vessel walls and within the interstitium.[79]

Diagnosis

Commercial genetic testing is available and is the only means to diagnose the condition.

Treatment

Supportive interventions, such as physical therapy, braces, and ambulatory aids, are the modalities available for this newly discovered entity. Gene-based interventions may be forthcoming in the future.

Case 5

A 45-year-old gentleman of Northern European heritage presented due to subjective weakness and hyperCKemia. He has noted a reduction in the size of his thighs over the past 1 to 2 years and only very occasionally has had difficulty arising from a kneeling position over the past year. A former heavy drinker, his aspartate aminotransferase and alanine aminotransferase were in the 400 range 5 years ago but remained elevated even after cessation of alcohol.

On examination, there was no scapular winging and no calf hypertrophy or atrophy. There was prominent quadriceps atrophy bilaterally, however. Facial, neck, and extremity strength was graded MRC grade 5 throughout.

His CK levels were 3753 U/L and 4684 U/L on repeat. ECG, stress test, echocardiogram, Holter monitor, and spirometry were normal. EMG revealed an irritable myopathy. He has 3 quadriceps muscle biopsies, each spaced a year apart. The first was normal, and the second showed minimal nonspecific changes. The third was dystrophic with marked variability in fiber size, copious fibers with internal nuclei, and endomysial fibrosis. There was no inflammation and a battery of immunostains for muscular dystrophies was negative. Genetic testing revealed homozygous mutations in *ANO5* (c.172C>T; p.Arg58Trp).

One year after diagnosis, his right leg was definitely weaker than his left, he was having more difficulty ascending and descending stairs, he was unable to arise from a squat, and he had a sensation his calves were constantly tight or stiff.

This real-life case reveals many key diagnostic features in LGMD2L.

LGMD1B—LAMIN A/C

Mutations in *LMNA*, the gene for lamins A and C, cause an array of human disease with numerous phenotypes. Five have skeletal muscle involvement. Nonskeletal muscle disorders include familial partial lipodystrophy, the Dunnigan-type (FPLD)[81]; autosomal recessive, axonal, peripheral polyneuropathy (Charcot-Marie-Tooth disease type 2A [AR-CMT2])[82]; autosomal dominant, axonal, peripheral polyneuropathy (Charcot-Marie-Tooth disease type 2 [AD-CMT2]) with or without leukonychia[83]; mandibuloacral dysplasia[84]; premature aging (Hutchinson-Gilford progeria syndrome)[85]; an isolated dilated cardiomyopathy[86]; heart-hand syndrome of the Slovenian type[87]; a fatal, infantile, restrictive dermopathy[88]; and the metabolic syndrome.[89] The syndromes with predominant skeletal muscle involvement include LGMD1B,[90] autosomal dominant[91] and recessive[92] EDMD (AD-EDMD), congenital muscular dystrophy,[93] and autosomal dominant dilated cardiomyopathy with atrioventricular block (CMD1A),[86] which on occasion also has clinically evident skeletal muscle weakness. The skeletal muscle phenotypes are overlapping syndromes exhibiting greater or lesser degrees of muscle weakness, joint contractures, and cardiac dysfunction. Nonpenetrance from generation to generation is not uncommon for the various laminopathy phenotypes.[94] LGMD1B makes up 5% to 10% of cases LGMD.

LGMD1B: Key diagnostic features

- Usual onset 2–25 years of age
- Variable penetrance generation to generation
- Limb-girdle or humeroperoneal pattern of weakness
- Joint contractures common
- Cardiac involvement by the second or third decade
- CK = 200–2000 U/L
- Diagnosis via genetic testing

Clinical

Onset may occur in the first decade and even as a congenital syndrome but can begin in the 20s, 30s, or 40s.[95] The pattern of weakness and atrophy tends to be humeroperoneal (biceps and below the knees) or limb girdle (proximal legs and arms). Calf hypertrophy and scapular winging occur infrequently. Joint contractures, although often subtle, are almost always present and can be helpful in suggesting the diagnosis, with elbow and neck flexors more so affected than ankle, knee, hip, and wrist joints. Although skeletal muscle weakness manifests from birth through the fourth decade, cardiac disease relatively uniformly begins in the second and third decades, independent of skeletal muscle involvement.[96] Cardiac manifestations include early dysrhythmias and conduction block. Dilated cardiomyopathy comes later in the course. Arrhythmias requiring pacemaker placement affect nearly all patients by the 20s, whereas progressive heart failure responds to cardiac transplantation.

Laboratory

CK values range up to 10-times normal. Needle EMG reveals myopathic motor units whereas nerve conduction studies remain normal. Muscle biopsies disclose variability in fiber size, increased internal nuclei, fiber splitting, and mild to moderate connective tissue replacement and fatty infiltration. Electron microscopy reveals abnormal distribution of heterochromatin in the nuclei of muscle fibers and satellite cells.[97,98]

Diagnosis

Muscle is not readily stained for lamin A/C; thus, DNA analysis is preferred for definitive diagnosis. Gene sequencing is commercially available from several sources.

Treatment

Currently, treatment remains supportive. Physical therapy enhances functional independence by augmenting range of motion and minimizing contractures. Monitoring cardiac involvement with cardiology consultations, ECGs, echocardiography, and Holter monitors can be lifesaving. For symptomatic patients, cardiac pacemakers, defibrillators, and transplantation should be considered early in the clinical course.

Case 6

A 28-year-old woman presented due to worsening weakness. She was never able to run or jump. She never could fully straighten her elbows. As a cheerleader, she was always reprimanded to straighten her elbows, and she could not. She currently works as a school bus driver and is having greater difficulties getting onto the bus. She states she walks just like her father, paternal aunt, and paternal grandmother. Her 6-year-old daughter cannot keep up with other children when running. The patient has had occasional palpitations.

On examination, there were 20° elbow flexor contractures. There was no scapular winging. Her strength was full except as follows (MRC scale): neck flexors 4, shoulder abductors 4+, elbow flexors 4−, elbow extensors 4+, hip flexors 4, hip extensors 3, hip abductors 4, hip abductors 4−, knee extensors 4+, and knee flexors 4. She had a mild Trendelenburg gait.

With testing, her CK level was 349 U/L. ECG was normal, but a Holter monitor revealed 5- to 40-second runs of a supraventricular tachycardia. EMG revealed a nonirritable myopathy. Genetic testing revealed the following mutation in *LMNA*: c.652A>C; p.Thr219Pro. This same mutation was found in her affected paternal aunt and her 6-year-old daughter.

This real-life case reveals many key diagnostic features in LGMD1B.

SUMMARY

When evaluating both men and women with limb-girdle weakness and a presumed genetic cause, clinicians should initially exclude dystrophinopathies and Pompe disease. For the LGMDs, there are 3 general diagnostic strategies. (1) Phenotype driven—if the clinical features, family history, examination, and creatine kinase level all point to a distinct diagnosis, many clinicians go directly to targeted genetic testing of a particular gene. Computer-based, smart algorithms are available to help guide to the most likely LGMD diagnosis (Jain Foundation Automated LGMD Diagnostic Assistant).[99] This tool is fairly adept at delineating the correct diagnosis in LGMDs with a common presentation. (2) Biopsy driven—if the phenotype approach does not yield an answer, or if the precise clinical diagnosis is unclear, muscle biopsy with immunostaining for a panel of muscular dystrophies is a reasonable next step. The results of the muscle biopsy can then direct further genetic testing. (3) Genetic testing driven—finally, if the first 2 strategies do not prove fruitful, genetic testing via gene panels or exome/genome sequencing is now available. Panels with 12, 50, or 163 muscle genes are available. The advantage of gene panels is they cast a broad net. The disadvantage is that often the results return with variants of unknown significance. Additionally, many of these panels only sequence genes and thus miss deletions, duplications, repeat sequences, and intronic mutations. The optimal strategy often depends on the comfort of the clinician, resources available, and insurance authorizations and may benefit from input from a geneticist or genetic counselor. As the technology improves and costs are reduced, direct genetic testing will probably assume a more prominent role in diagnosing LGMDs.

Using these strategies, a genetic diagnosis can be made in more than 60% of LGMD patients. The clinical features point to a correct diagnosis in approximately half the cases. Obtaining a precise genetic diagnosis in LGMD is important in defining the long-term prognosis, delineating other organ system involvement, clarifying the pattern of inheritance, avoiding unnecessary treatments (eg, immunosuppressants for dystrophies with inflammation on the biopsy), and providing proactive management of disease (eg, physical and occupational therapy, pacemaker-defibrillators for arrhythmias, and noninvasive positive airway pressure for ventilatory failure).

As a group, the LGMDs are the fourth most common genetic muscle condition, with a minimum prevalence of 3 to 5 per 100,000 (or approximately 1 in 20,000). This article highlights key features of what are widely thought the most common LGMDs. As knowledge of the genetic basis and pathophysiology of the LGMDs expands, the hopes of patients and families for effective treatments for these conditions may become a reality.

REFERENCES

1. Bushby KM. Diagnostic criteria for the limb-girdle muscular dystrophies: report of the ENMC consortium on limb-girdle dystrophies. Neuromuscul Disord 1995; 5:71–4.
2. Bushby KM, Beckmann JS. The limb-girdle muscular dystrophies – proposal for a new nomenclature. Neuromuscul Disord 1995;5:337–43.
3. Wicklund M, DiVincenzo C, Liaquat K, et al. Relative prevalence of limb girdle muscular dystrophies in the United States population. Neurology 2013;80. P07.030.
4. Norwood F, Harling C, Chinnery P, et al. Prevalence of genetic muscle disease in Northern England: in-depth analysis of a muscle clinic population. Brain 2009; 132:3175–86.
5. Krahn M, Lopez de Munain A, Streichenberger N, et al. CAPN3 mutations in patients with idiopathic eosinophilic myositis. Ann Neurol 2006;59:905–11.
6. Amato AA. Adults with eosinophilic myositis and calpain-3 mutations. Neurology 2008;70:730–1.
7. Richard I, Broux O, Allamand V, et al. Mutations in the proteolytic enzyme calpain 3 cause limb-girdle muscular dystrophy type 2A. Cell 1995;81:27–40.
8. Beckmann J, Spencer M. Calpain 3, the "gatekeeper" of proper sarcomere assembly, turnover and maintenance. Neuromuscul Disord 2008;18:913–21.
9. Hauerslev S, Sveen ML, Duno M, et al. Calpain 3 is important for muscle regeneration: evidence from patients with limb girdle muscular dystrophies. BMC Musculoskelet Disord 2012;13:43.
10. Fardeau M, Hillaire D, Mignard C, et al. Juvenile limb-girdle muscular dystrophy: clinical, histopathological and genetic data from a small community living in the Reunion Island. Brain 1996;119:295–308.
11. Pollitt C, Anderson LV, Pogue R, et al. The phenotype of calpainopathy: diagnosis based on a multidisciplinary approach. Neuromuscul Disord 2001;11:287–96.
12. Dirik E, Aydin A, Kurul S, et al. Limb girdle muscular dystrophy type 2A presenting with cardiac arrest. Pediatr Neurol 2001;24:235–7.
13. Leidenroth A, Sorte H, Gilfillan G, et al. Diagnosis by sequencing: correction of misdiagnosis of FSHD2 to LGMD2A by whole-exome analysis. Eur J Hum Genet 2012;20:999–1003.
14. Fanin M, Nascimbeni A, Fulizio L, et al. The frequency of limb girdle muscular dystrophy 2A in northeastern Italy. Neuromuscul Disord 2005;15:218–24.
15. ten Dam L, van der Kooi A, van Wattingen M, et al. Reliability and accuracy of skeletal muscle imaging in limb-girdle muscular dystrophies. Neurology 2012; 79:1716–23.
16. Nadaj-Pakleza A, Dorobek M, Nestorowicz K, et al. Muscle pathology in 31 patients with calpain 3 gene mutations. Neurol Neurochir Pol 2013;47:214–22.
17. Richard I, Roudaut C, Saenz A, et al. Calpainopathy – a survey of mutations and polymorphisms. Am J Hum Genet 1999;64:1524–40.
18. Kramerova I, Beckmann JS, Spencer MJ. Molecular and cellular basis of calpainopathy (limb girdle muscular dystrophy type 2A). Biochimica et Biophysica Acta 2007;1772:128–44.

19. Oflazer PS, Gundesli H, Zorludemir S, et al. Eosinophilic myositis in calpainop-athy: could immunosuppression of the eosinophilic myositis alter the natural course of the dystrophic disease? Neuromuscul Disord 2009;19:261–3.
20. Liu J, Aoki M, Illa I, et al. Dysferlin, a novel skeletal muscle gene, is mutated in Miyoshi myopathy and limb girdle muscular dystrophy. Nat Genet 1998;20: 31–6.
21. Bansal D, Miyake K, Vogel SS, et al. Defective membrane repair in dysferlin-deficient muscular dystrophy. Nature 2003;423:168–72.
22. Lostal W, Bartoli M, Roudaut C, et al. Lack of correlation between outcomes of membrane repair assay and correction of dystrophic changes in experimental therapeutic strategy in dysferlinopathy. PLoS One 2012;7:e38036.
23. Chiu Y, Hornsey M, Klinge L, et al. Attenuated muscle regeneration is a key factor in dysferlin-deficient muscular dystrophy. Hum Mol Genet 2009;18: 1976–89.
24. De Luna N, Gallardo E, Soriano M, et al. Absence of dysferlin alters myogenin expression and delays human muscle differentiation "In vitro". J Biol Chem 2006;281:17092–8.
25. Klinge L, Harris J, Sewry CA, et al. Dysferlin associates with the developing T-tubule system in rodent and human skeletal muscle. Muscle Nerve 2010;41: 166–73.
26. Guglieri M, Magri F, Grazia D'Angelo M, et al. Clinical, molecular, and protein correlations in a large sample of genetically diagnosed Italian limb girdle muscular dystrophy patients. Hum Mutat 2008;29:258–66.
27. Illa I, Serrano-Munuera C, Gallardo E, et al. Distal anterior compartment myop-athy: a dysferlin mutation causing a new muscular dystrophy phenotype. Ann Neurol 2001;49:130–4.
28. Nguyen K, Bassez G, Krahn M, et al. Phenotypic study in 40 patients with dys-ferlin gene mutations. Arch Neurol 2007;64:1176–82.
29. Krahn M, Béroud C, Labelle V, et al. Analysis of the DYSF mutational spectrum in a large cohort of patients. Hum Mutat 2008;30:E345–75.
30. Rosales X, Gastier-Foster J, Lewis S, et al. Novel diagnostic features of dysfer-linopathies. Muscle Nerve 2010;42:14–21.
31. Klinge L, Aboumousa A, Eagle M, et al. New aspects on patients affected by dysferlin deficient muscular dystrophy. J Neurol Neurosurg Psychiatry 2010; 81:946–53.
32. Paradas C, González-Quereda L, De Luna N, et al. A new phenotype of dysfer-linopathy with congenital onset. Neuromuscul Disord 2009;19:21–5.
33. Klinge L, Dean AF, Kress W, et al. Late onset dyferlinopathy widens the clinical spectrum. Neuromuscul Disord 2008;18:288–90.
34. Suzuki N, Takahashi T, Suzuki Y, et al. An autopsy case of a dysferlinopathy pa-tient with cardiac involvement. Muscle Nerve 2012;45:298–9.
35. Takahashi T, Aoki M, Suzuki N, et al. Clinical features and a mutation with late onset of limb girdle muscular dystrophy 2B. J Neurol Neurosurg Psychiatry 2013;84:433–40.
36. Shaibani A, Harati Y, Amato A, et al. Miyoshi myopathy with vacuoles. Neurology 1997;47(Suppl):A195.
37. Spuler S, Carl M, Zabojszcza J, et al. Dysferlin-deficient muscular dystrophy features amyloidosis. Ann Neurol 2008;63:323–8.
38. McNally EM, Ly CT, Rosenmann H, et al. Splicing mutation in dysferlin produces limb-girdle muscular dystrophy with inflammation. Am J Med Genet 2000;91: 305–12.

39. Gallardo E, Rojas-García R, de Luna N, et al. Inflammation in dysferlin myopathy: immunohistochemical characterization of 13 patients. Neurology 2001; 57:2136–8.
40. Vinit J, Samson M, Gaultier JB, et al. Dysferlin deficiency treated like refractory polymyositis. Clin Rheumatol 2010;29:103–6.
41. Nilsson ME, Laureano ML, Saeed M, et al. Dysferlin aggregation in limb-girdle muscular dystrophy type 2B/Myoshi myopathy necessitates mutational screen for diagnosis. Muscle Nerve 2013;47:740–7.
42. Walter MC, Reilich P, Thiele S, et al. Treatment of dysferlinopathy with deflazacort: a double-blind, placebo-controlled clinical trial. Orphanet J Rare Dis 2013;8:26.
43. Ervasti JM, Campbell KP. A role for the dystrophin-glycoprotein complex as a transmembrane linker between laminin and actin. J Cell Biol 1993;122:809–23.
44. Crosbie RH, Lim LE, Moore SA, et al. Molecular and genetic characterization of sarcospan: insights into sarcoglycan-sarcospan interactions. Hum Mol Genet 2000;9:2019–27.
45. Moore SA, Schilling CJ, Westra S, et al. Limb-girdle muscular dystrophy in the United States. J Neuropathol Exp Neurol 2006;65:995–1003.
46. Merlini L, Kaplan JC, Navarro C, et al. Homogeneous phenotype of the gypsy limb-girdle MD with the g-sarcoglycan C283Y mutation. Neurology 2000;54: 1075–9.
47. McNally EM, Passos-Bueno MR, Bönneman CG, et al. Mild and severe muscular dystrophy caused by a single γ-sarcoglycan mutation. Am J Hum Genet 1996; 59:1040–7.
48. Kefi M, Amouri R, Driss A, et al. Phenotype and sarcoglycan expression in Tunisian LGMD 2C patients sharing the same del521-T mutation. Neuromuscul Disord 2003;13:779–87.
49. Mongini T, Doriguzzi C, Bosone I, et al. Alpha-sarcoglycan deficiency featuring exercise intolerance and myoglobinuria. Neuropediatrics 2002;33:109–11.
50. Cagliani R, Comi GP, Tancredi L, et al. Primary beta-sarcoglycanopathy manifesting as recurrent exercise-induced myoglobinuria. Neuromuscul Disord 2001;11:389–94.
51. Pena L, Kim K, Charrow J. Episodic myoglobinuria in a primary gamma-sarcoglycanopathy. Neuromuscul Disord 2010;20:337–9.
52. Baumeister S, Todorovic S, Milić-Rasić V, et al. Eosinophilic myositis as presenting symptom in gamma-sarcoglycanopathy. Neuromuscul Disord 2009;19: 167–71.
53. Politano L, Nigro V, Passamano L, et al. Evaluation of cardiac and respiratory involvement in sarcoglycanopathies. Neuromuscul Disord 2001;11:178–85.
54. Fanin M, Melacini P, Boito C, et al. LGMD2E patients risk developing dilated cardiomyopathy. Neuromuscul Disord 2003;13:303–9.
55. Klinge L, Dekomien G, Aboumousa A, et al. Sarcoglycanopathies: can muscle immunoanalysis predict the genotype? Neuromuscul Disord 2008;18:934–41.
56. Vorgerd M, Glencik M, Mortier J, et al. Isolated loss of γ-sarcoglycan: diagnostic implications in autosomal recessive limb-girdle muscular dystrophy. Muscle Nerve 2001;24:421–4.
57. Vainzof M, Moreira ES, Canovas M, et al. Partial α-sarcoglycan deficiency with retention of the dystrophin-glycoprotein complex in a LGMD2D family. Muscle Nerve 2000;23:984–8.
58. Trabelsi M, Kavian N, Fatma D, et al. Revised spectrum of mutations in sarcoglycanopathies. Eur J Hum Genet 2008;16:793–803.

59. Mendell J, Rodino-Klapac L, Rosales-Quintero X, et al. Limb-girdle muscular dystrophy type 2D gene therapy restores α-sarcoglycan and associated proteins. Ann Neurol 2009;66:290-7.

60. Brockington M, Blake DJ, Prandini P, et al. Mutations in the Fukutin-related protein gene (FKRP) cause a form of congenital muscular dystrophy with secondary laminin α2 deficiency and abnormal glycosylation of α-dystroglycan. Am J Hum Genet 2001;69:1198-209.

61. Brockington M, Yuva Y, Prandini P, et al. Mutations in the Fukutin-related protein gene (FKRP) identify limb girdle muscular dystrophy 2I as a milder allelic variant of congenital muscular dystrophy MDC1C. Hum Mol Genet 2001;10:2851-9.

62. Mathews KD, Stephan CM, Laubenthal K, et al. Myoglobinuria and muscle pain are common in patients with limb-girdle muscular dystrophy 2I. Neurology 2011; 76:194-5.

63. Lindberg C, Sixt C, Oldfors A. Episodes of exercise-induced dark urine and myalgia in LGMD 2I. Acta Neurol Scand 2012;125:285-7.

64. Hanisch F, Grimm D, Zierz S, et al. Frequency of the FKRP mutation c.826C>A in isolated hyperCKemia and in limb girdle muscular dystrophy type 2 in German patients. J Neurol 2010;257:300-1.

65. Sveen ML, Schwartz M, Vissing J. High prevalence and phenotype-genotype correlations of limb girdle muscular dystrophy type 2I in Denmark. Ann Neurol 2006;59:808-15.

66. Stensland E, Lindal S, Jonsrud C, et al. Prevalence, mutation spectrum and phenotypic variability in Norwegian patients with limb girdle muscular dystrophy 2I. Neuromuscul Disord 2011;21:41-6.

67. Fanin M, Nascimbeni A, Aurino S, et al. Frequency of LGMD gene mutations in Italian patients with distinct clinical phenotypes. Neurology 2009;72:1432-5.

68. Kang P, Feener C, Estrella E, et al. LGMD2I in a North American population. BMC Musculoskelet Disord 2007;8:115.

69. Poppe M, Cree L, Bourke J, et al. The phenotype of limb-girdle muscular dystrophy type 2I. Neurology 2003;60:1246-51.

70. Wahbi K, Meune C, Hamouda EH, et al. Cardiac assessment of limb-girdle muscular dystrophy 2I patients: an echography, Holter ECG and magnetic resonance imaging study. Neuromuscul Disord 2008;18:650-5.

71. Bourteel H, Vermersch P, Cuisset JM, et al. Clinical and mutational spectrum of limb-girdle muscular dystrophy type 2I in 11 French patients. J Neurol Neurosurg Psychiatry 2009;80:1405-8.

72. Palmieri A, Manara R, Bello L, et al. Cognitive and MRI findings in limb-girdle muscular dystrophy 2I. J Neurol 2011;258:1312-20.

73. Fischer D, Walter MC, Kesper K, et al. Diagnostic value of muscle MRI in differentiating LGMD2I from other LGMDs. J Neurol 2005;252:538-47.

74. Hicks D, Sarkozy A, Muelas N, et al. A founder mutation in anoctamin 5 is a major cause of limb-girdle muscular dystrophy. Brain 2011;134:171-82.

75. Tsutsumi S, Kamata N, Vokes T, et al. The novel gene encoding a putative transmembrane protein is mutated in gnathodiaphaseal dysplasia (GDD). Am J Hum Genet 2004;74:1255-61.

76. Bolduc V, Marlow G, Boycott K, et al. Recessive mutations in the putative calcium-activated chloride channel anoctamin 5 cause proximal LGMD2L and distal MMD3 muscular dystrophies. Am J Hum Genet 2010;86:213-21.

77. Jarry J, Rioux M, Bolduc V, et al. A novel autosomal recessive limb-girdle muscular dystrophy with quadriceps atrophy maps to 11p13-p12. Brain 2007; 130:368-80.

78. Penttilä S, Palmio J, Suominen T, et al. Eight new mutations and the expanding phenotype variability in muscular dystrophy caused by *ANO5*. Neurology 2012; 78:897–903.

79. Milone M, Liewluck T, Winder T, et al. Amyloidosis and exercise intolerance in *ANO5* muscular dystrophy. Neuromuscul Disord 2012;22:13–5.

80. Sarkozy A, Deschauer M, Carlier RY, et al. Muscle MRI findings in limb girdle muscular dystrophy type 2L. Neuromuscul Disord 2012;22:S122–9.

81. Cao H, Hegele RA. Nuclear lamin A/C R482Q mutation in Canadian kindreds with Dunnigan-type familial partial lipodystrophy. Hum Mol Genet 2000;9:109–12.

82. De Sandre-Giovannoli A, Chaouch M, Kozlov S, et al. Homozygous defects in LMNA, encoding lamin A/C nuclear envelop proteins, cause autosomal recessive axonal neuropathy in human (Charcot-Marie-Tooth disorder type 2) and mouse. Am J Hum Genet 2002;70:726–36.

83. Goizet C, Ben Yaou R, Demay L, et al. A new mutation of the lamin A/C gene leading to autosomal dominant axonal neuropathy, muscular dystrophy, cardiac disease, and leukonychia. J Med Genet 2004;41:e29.

84. Novelli G, Muchir A, Sangiuolo F, et al. Mandibuloacral dysplasia is caused by a mutation in LMNA-encoding lamin A/C. Am J Hum Genet 2002;71:426–31.

85. Csoka AB, Cao H, Sammak PJ, et al. Novel lamin A/C gene (LMNA) mutations in atypical progeroid syndromes. J Med Genet 2004;41:304–8.

86. Fatkin D, MacRae C, Sasaki T, et al. Missense mutations in the rod domain of the lamin A/C gene as causes of dilated cardiomyopathy and conduction-system disease. N Engl J Med 1999;341:1715–24.

87. Renou L, Stora S, Ben Yaou R, et al. Heart-hand syndrome of Slovenian type: a new kind of laminopathy. J Med Genet 2008;45:666–71.

88. Navarro CL, De Sandre-Giovannoli A, Bernard R, et al. Lamin A and ZMPSTE24 (FACE-1) defects cause nuclear disorganization and identify restrictive dermopathy as a lethal neonatal laminopathy. Hum Mol Genet 2004;13:2493–503.

89. Decaudain A, Vantyghem MC, Guerci B, et al. New metabolic phenotypes in laminopathies: *LMNA* mutations in patients with severe metabolic syndrome. J Clin Endocrinol Metab 2007;92:4835–44.

90. Muchir A, Bonne G, van der Kooi AJ, et al. Identification of mutations in the gene encoding lamins A/C in autosomal dominant limb girdle muscular dystrophy with atrioventricular conduction disturbances (LGMD1B). Hum Mol Genet 2000;9: 1453–9.

91. Bonne G, Di Barletta MR, Varnous S, et al. Mutations in the gene encoding lamin A/C cause autosomal dominant Emery-Dreifuss muscular dystrophy. Nat Genet 1999;21:285–8.

92. Di Barletta MR, Ricci E, Galluzi G, et al. Different mutations in the LMNA gene cause autosomal dominant and recessive Emery-Dreifuss muscular dystrophy. Am J Hum Genet 2000;66:1407–12.

93. Quijano-Roy S, Mbieleu B, Bönnemann C, et al. De novo *LMNA* mutations cause a new form of congenital muscular dystrophy. Ann Neurol 2008;64:177–86.

94. Rankin J, Auer-Grumbach M, Bagg W, et al. Extreme phenotypic diversity and nonpenetrance in families with the LMNA gene mutation R644C. Am J Med Genet A 2008;146A:1530–42.

95. Benedetti S, Menditto I, Degano M, et al. Phenotypic clustering of lamin A/C mutations in neuromuscular patients. Neurology 2007;69:1285–92.

96. Bonne G, Mercuri E, Muchir A, et al. Clinical and molecular spectrum of autosomal dominant Emery-Dreifuss muscular dystrophy due to mutations of the lamin A/C gene. Ann Neurol 2000;48:170–80.

97. Sewry CA, Brown SC, Mercuri E, et al. Skeletal muscle pathology in autosomal dominant Emery-Dreifuss muscular dystrophy with lamin A/C mutations. Neuropathol Appl Neurobiol 2001;27:281–90.
98. Park YE, Hayashi YK, Goto K, et al. Nuclear changes in skeletal muscle extend to satellite cells in autosomal dominant Emery-Dreifuss muscular dystrophy/limb-girdle muscular dystrophy 1B. Neuromuscul Disord 2009;19:29–36.
99. Available at: http://www.jain-foundation.org/lgmd-subtyping-tool/.

Pompe Disease
Literature Review and Case Series

Majed Dasouki, MD[a,b,*], Omar Jawdat, MD[c], Osama Almadhoun, MD[d], Mamatha Pasnoor, MD[c], April L. McVey, MD[c], Ahmad Abuzinadah, MD[c], Laura Herbelin, BS[c], Richard J. Barohn, MD[c], Mazen M. Dimachkie, MD[c]

KEYWORDS

- Metabolic myopathy • Hypotonia • Autosomal recessive
- Enzyme replacement therapy • Newborn screening
- Lysosomal glycogen storage disease

KEY POINTS

- Pompe disease, also known as type II glycogenosis, is a progressive autosomal recessive glycogen storage disease caused by deficiency of lysosomal acid-α-glucosidase (GAA) primarily in skeletal and cardiac muscle with age of onset ranging from infancy through adulthood. Extramuscular phenotypes are also recognized.
- Recognized clinical presentations of Pompe disease include infantile (with/without cardiomyopathy) and late-onset (childhood, juvenile, and adult) forms. In addition to cardiomyopathy in the classic infantile form, musculoskeletal signs and symptoms are the most frequent.
- Excessive lysosomal glycogen storage and defects in autophagy are the main determinants of pathogenesis of Pompe disease.
- Diagnosis of symptomatic individuals, as well as screening in healthy newborns, is now possible by demonstrating low GAA enzyme activity in dried blood samples complemented by DNA mutation analysis.
- Diagnostic gaps in patients with Pompe disease across the disease spectrum continue.

Continued

Financial Disclosures and/or Conflicts of Interest: The following authors declare clinical trials support by Genzyme Corporation (M. Dasouki, R.J. Barohn, O. Almadhoun) and Amicus Therapeutics (M. Dasouki, M.M. Dimachkie); travel support by Genzyme Corporation (M. Dasouki, R.J. Barohn, M.M. Dimachkie) and honoraria by Genzyme Corporation (M.M. Dimachkie, R.J. Barohn).
This project was supported by an Institutional Clinical and Translational Science Award, National Institutes of Health/National Center for Advancing Translational Sciences Grant Number UL1TR000001. Its contents are solely the responsibility of the authors and do not necessarily represent the official views of the NIH.
[a] Department of Neurology, University of Kansas Medical Center, 3901 Rainbow Boulevard, Kansas City, KS 66160, USA; [b] Department of Genetics, King Faisal Specialist Hospital & Research Center, MBC-03-30, PO Box 3354, Riyadh 11211, Saudi Arabia; [c] Department of Neurology, University of Kansas Medical Center, Mailstop 2012, 3901 Rainbow Boulevard, Kansas City, KS 66160, USA; [d] Department of Pediatrics, University of Kansas Medical Center, Mailstop 4004, 3901 Rainbow Boulevard, Kansas City, KS 66160, USA
* Corresponding author. Department of Genetics, King Faisal Specialist Hospital & Research Center, MBC-03-30, PO Box 3354, Riyadh 11211, Saudi Arabia.
E-mail addresses: mdasouki@kumc.edu; madasouki@kfshrc.edu.sa

Continued

- In our cohort of patients, 3 with infantile and 9 with late-onset Pompe disease, we identi-fied 4 novel, potentially pathogenic *GAA* mutations and 1 pregnancy that was complicated by prenatal exposure to recombinant human GAA (rhGAA) and spontaneous miscarriage.
- In addition to supportive therapy, rhGAA enzyme replacement therapy is now available. Oral chaperone therapy, modified rhGAA, autophagy suppression, and gene transfer repre-sent potentially promising novel therapies that are being tested in clinical research trials.

INTRODUCTION

Pompe disease (GSD II) is an autosomal recessive disorder caused by deficiency of the lysosomal enzyme acid-α-glucosidase (GAA; EC 3.2.1.20), leading to generalized accumulation of lysosomal glycogen, especially in the heart, skeletal and smooth muscle, and the nervous system. Pompe disease was first described in a 7-month-old girl with severe muscle weakness who also had hypertrophic cardiomyopathy and generalized glycogen accumulation in various tissues throughout the body.[1] Bis-choff[2] and Putschar[3] also independently described the disease in the same year. Hers[4] identified alpha-glucosidase deficiency and localized the GAA enzyme activity to the lysosomes of liver, heart, and muscle tissues of 5 infants with classic Pompe disease and was the first to recognize impaired autophagy. Pompe disease is gener-ally classified based on the age of onset as infantile (IOPD) when it presents during the first year of life, and late onset (LOPD) when it presents afterward. Childhood, juvenile, and adult-onset Pompe disease are examples of the late-onset form. IOPD associated with cardiomyopathy is referred to as classic Pompe disease and, in the absence of cardiomyopathy, as nonclassic Pompe disease.[5–7] Similar to other lysosomal storage disorders, Pompe disease clinically presents as a continuum in its age of onset and multisystem involvement. The role of autophagy in the pathogenesis of Pompe dis-ease, especially the late-onset form, has increasingly become evident and may be clinically relevant. Autophagy (self-eating) is a highly complex, ubiquitously expressed, and evolutionarily conserved lysosomal degradative process, which is controlled by a multigene network (http://autophagy.lu/index.html). Its main function is to recycle obsolete cellular constituents and eliminate damaged organelles and protein aggre-gates. It involves dynamic membrane rearrangement for sequestration of cytoplasm and its delivery into the vacuole/lysosome. Basal autophagy plays a role in cellular development and differentiation,[8] innate and adaptive immunity,[9] and is induced in response to various stress conditions, such as nutrient limitation, heat, and oxidative stress. Ammonia derived from the deamination of glutamine via glutaminolysis sup-ports basal autophagy and protects cells from tumor necrosis factor alpha–induced cell death.[10] As a result, basic metabolites are released into the cytoplasm for new synthesis or as sources for energy. Autophagy also is implicated in a wide range of disorders, such as neurodegeneration, cancer, and aging, and now various lysosomal storage diseases, especially Pompe disease.[11–14]

Clinically, infants with classic Pompe disease typically present during the first few weeks of life with hypotonia, progressive weakness, macroglossia, hepatomegaly, and hypertrophic cardiomyopathy. With this typical clinical presentation, diagnosis is usually straightforward. The natural history of IOPD is that most of these infants die by their first birthday. On the other hand, the diagnosis of Pompe disease in older children and adults can be more challenging, as these patients generally present with slowly pro-gressive limb girdle–type weakness and respiratory insufficiency without significant cardiomyopathy.[5–7,15] Cardiac involvement in late-onset Pompe disease manifests as Wolff-Parkinson-White syndrome, left ventricular hypertrophy, and dilatation of the ascending aorta. Rigid spine syndrome (a progressive limitation of the neck and trunk), scoliosis, and low body weight also have been reported in a subset of patients with LOPD with onset in adolescence and resulting in postural anomalies.[16] The diagnosis of Pompe disease is usually made based on typical clinical presentation followed by the demonstration of deficiency of GAA enzyme activity in muscle, skin fibroblasts, or, more recently, dried blood spots (DBS), as well as *GAA* mutation analysis.[5,6] Diagnosis of Pompe disease through newborn screening is now possible. Pompe disease is still considered to be a rare inborn error of metabolism, with an estimated frequency of about 1 in 40,000 and a higher incidence in certain populations, such as African American (1/14,000), Northern European of Dutch origin, and South East Asian populations. However, early results of newborn screening pilot studies from Taiwan and the United States indicated a higher incidence. Interest in Pompe disease has grown significantly since the approval by the Food and Drug Administration of the first specific enzyme replacement therapy (ERT) with recombinant human GAA (rhGAA) (alglucosidase alfa) for this metabolic myopathy in 2006. Glycosylated alglucosidase alfa is targeted to the lysosomes through uptake via the mannose-6-phosphate receptors. Clinical experience with alglucosidase alfa showed more dramatic improvement of cardiac pathology compared with skeletal myopathy and especially in children more than adults. Abnormal autophagy in Pompe disease results in abnormal recycling of the cation-independent mannose-6-phosphate receptors, which may explain the less satisfactory clinical response of skeletal muscles.[17,18] Therefore, correction of abnormal autophagy in individuals with Pompe disease may improve therapeutic response to ERT.

In this report, we describe our experience with 12 patients with classic infantile (1 child), nonclassic infantile (2 siblings), juvenile (1), and adult-onset (8) Pompe disease, one of whom had a first trimester miscarriage while receiving ERT. We also report 4 potentially pathogenic, novel *GAA* gene variants in this group and review the recent advances in the pathogenesis, diagnosis, and treatment of individuals with Pompe disease.

Genetic Etiology and Prevalence

Pompe disease also is considered a polyglucosan vacuolar myopathy that results from absence or partial deficiency of the lysosomal GAA activity due to recessive mutations in the autosomal *GAA* gene. *GAA* (NM_000152.3) is approximately 18.3 kb long and contains 20 exons (**Fig. 1**). Its cDNA has 2859 nucleotides of coding sequence that encode the immature 952 amino acid enzyme. GAA is synthesized as a membrane-bound, catalytically inactive precursor that is sequestered in the endoplasmic reticulum (ER). It undergoes sugar chain modification in the Golgi complex, followed by transport into the (minor) secretory pathway, or into lysosomes, where it is trimmed in a stepwise process at both the amino- and carboxyl-termini.[19,20] Phosphorylation of mannose residues ensures efficient transport of the enzyme to the lysosomes via the mannose 6-phosphate receptor. GAA catalyzes the hydrolysis of $\alpha 1 \rightarrow 4$ glucosidic linkages in glycogen at acid pH. Specificity for the natural substrate (glycogen) is gained during its maturation. The activity of mature (76/70-kDa) GAA for its natural (glycogen) substrate is considerably more robust than its activity toward the artificial substrate (4-methylumbelliferyl-α-D-glucopyranoside4 [4-MU]), which is frequently used in in vitro assays.[20] However, 4-MU also is a substrate for several other enzymes, including "leukocyte" neutral isoenzymes, glucosidase II (GANAB) and neutral α-glucosidase C (GANC), and maltase glucoamylase (MGAM). Muscle tissue and cultured fibroblasts do not contain MGAM, allowing measurement of GAA (as the activity ratio of neutral to acid glucosidase, GANAB + GANC/GAA)

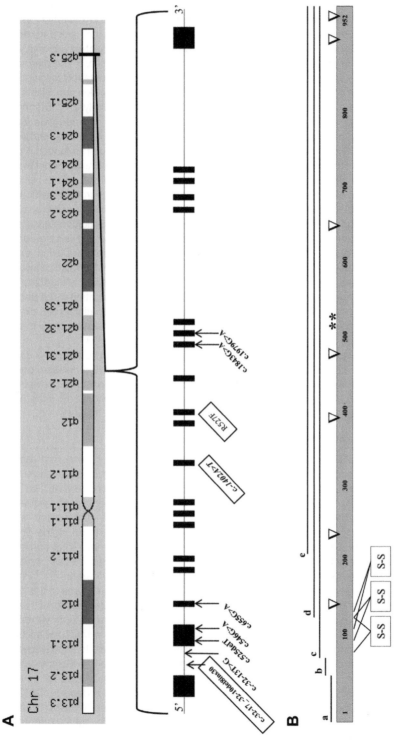

Fig. 1. Schematic representations of *GAA* genomic location and structure (*A*) and its protein structure (*B*). *GAA* maps to chr17q25.3 and consists of 20 (19 coding) exons that encode 952 amino acids. Mutations (DNA variants) identified in this study are shown according to their respective genomic position. Novel variants are boxed. GAA has 4 isoforms (a–d), 2 catalytically active sites (*asterisk*), 3 disulfide bonds (s-s), and 7 N-linked glycosylation sites (∇).

without interference. Because MGAM is expressed in neutrophils, not in lymphocytes, the same activity ratio determined in purified lymphocytes also has been used for the diagnosis of GSD II, which is not possible in DBSs. Using maltose or acarbose as an inhibitor of MGAM activity, the measurement of GAA activity in DBS samples with minimal interference by other α-glucosidases was accomplished, which now serves as the basis for newborn screening and the noninvasive diagnosis for Pompe disease.[21–23] As a result, multiplex newborn screening for Pompe disease and other lysosomal storage disorders using fluorometric, digital microfluidic and tandem mass spectrometry–based GAA enzyme activity assays had been developed.[24–27] In addition to qualitative and quantitative assessments of the disease burden, and clinical measures of the impact of Pompe disease on various affected systems, urinary glucose tetrasaccharide (Glc4), a biomarker of glycogen storage, with 94% sensitivity and 84% specificity for Pompe disease, is frequently used in monitoring the response of patients to ERT and as an adjunct to GAA activity measurements.[28] Also, in addition to the traditional 1-dimensional thin layer chromatography for urine oligosaccharide analysis, a new matrix-assisted laser desorption/ionization–time-of-flight/time-of-flight mass spectrometry–based assay of urinary free oligosaccharides useful for the diagnosis of Pompe disease and other lysosomal storage diseases is now available.[29]

Infants with Pompe disease are considered as cross-reactive immunologic material (CRIM)-positive if they have residual GAA enzyme activity, and CRIM-negative if no residual GAA activity is detected. Based on pooled clinical studies data, 28% of Pompe disease cases are infantile-onset, of which about 85% are classic infantile-onset and three-quarters of those are CRIM positive (http://www.hrsa.gov/advisorycommittees/mchbadvisory/heritabledisorders/nominatecondition/reviews/pompereport2013.pdf). CRIM status is usually determined by Western blot analysis in cultured skin fibroblasts, a process that can take a few weeks, and more recently via a blood-based CRIM assay that can yield results within 48 to 72 hours.[30] rhGAA was first produced in dihydrofolate reductase–deficient Chinese hamster ovary cells, was targeted to heart muscle, and corrected glycogen accumulation in fibroblasts from patients with Pompe disease.[31] Before the initiation of ERT, rapid determination of CRIM status in patients with IOPD who are at risk of developing neutralizing antibodies against rhGAA is extremely important.

Many normal allelic variants exist in GAA and are responsible for the 3 known alloenzymes (GAA1, GAA2, and GAA4). More than 450 mutations in GAA have been reported in individuals with Pompe disease. Nonsense mutations, large and small gene rearrangements, and splicing defects have been observed with some mutations being potentially specific to families, geographic regions, or ethnicities (http://www.pompecenter.nl/). Combinations of mutations that result in complete absence of GAA enzyme activity are seen more commonly in individuals with infantile-onset disease, whereas those combinations that allow partial enzyme activity typically have a later-onset presentation.[32] GAA mutations result in mRNA instability and/or severely truncated GAA or an enzyme with markedly decreased activity. By means of homology modeling, and using the crystal structure of the N-terminal subunit of human intestinal MGAM as a template, analysis of the 3-dimensional models of human GAA encompassing 27 relevant amino acid substitutions causing a processing or transport defect responsible for Pompe disease showed that they were widely spread over all of the 5 domains of GAA from the core to the surface of the enzyme and the predicted structural changes varied from large to very small.[33]

The c.1726 G>A (p.G576S) variant in cis with c.2065 G>A (p.E689K), also known as the c.[1726A; 2065A] pseudodeficiency allele, causes low GAA activity in healthy individuals and is relatively common in Asian populations.[34,35] About 3.9% of apparently healthy Japanese were reported to be homozygous for this pseudodeficiency allele that may complicate newborn screening and result in a high false-positive rate in such populations.[36] In their newborn screening pilot program in Taiwan, Labrousse and colleagues[37] identified 36 infants (0.027% screened) who had no pathogenic *GAA* mutation but were homozygous for the c.[1726A;2065A] pseudodeficiency allele. In the United States, the prevalence of Pompe disease is approximately 1 in 28,000, with the prevalence of pseudodeficiency being less than 1% as confirmed by genetic analysis of healthy individuals with low GAA enzyme activity level.[38]

CLINICAL PRESENTATION

Diagnosis of Pompe disease can be made clinically based on a typical clinical presentation, as in infantile cases or suspected in a young child or adult with limb weakness, difficulty walking, or limb girdle dystrophy. In combination with the clinical diagnosis, a histologic diagnosis can be confirmed in a muscle biopsy, which shows typical intramyofibrillar cytoplasmic membrane–bound glycogen, periodic acid-Schiff (PAS)-positive vacuolar myopathic abnormalities, and acid phosphatase–positive vacuoles (**Fig. 2**).[39–43] Low GAA activity in muscle, skin fibroblasts, and, more recently, DBSs confirms the diagnosis even in the absence of diagnostic histologic findings that are not regularly detected in patients with LOPD. Patients presenting with either a limb-girdle syndrome or dyspnea secondary to diaphragm weakness should undergo

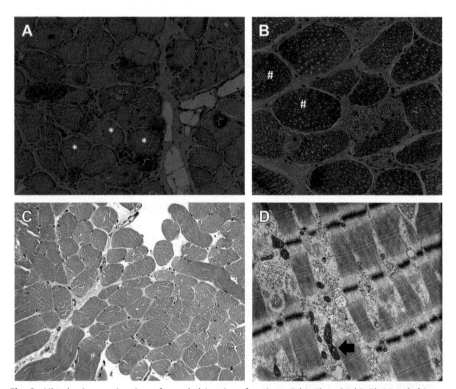

Fig. 2. Histologic examination of muscle biopsies of patients 9 (*A, B*) and 4 (*C, D*). Muscle biopsy stained with hematoxylin-eosin (H&E) (*A*) from patient 9 shows extensive vacuolar changes (*asterisk*) and (*B*) positive acid phosphatase aggregates (#). The H&E-stained muscle biopsy (*C*) from patient 4 is essentially unremarkable, whereas the muscle electron micrograph (*D*) shows membrane-bound glycogen deposits and (*arrow*) mildly distorted mitochondrial morphology.

further testing. A blood-based GAA enzyme activity assay is the recommended tool to screen for GAA enzyme deficiency, confirmed by a second test: either a second GAA enzyme activity assay in another tissue (such as lymphocytes, fibroblasts, or muscle) or *GAA* gene sequencing.[44] Deficient GAA enzyme activity leads to generalized tissue lysosomal glycogen accumulation, especially in skeletal, cardiac, and smooth muscles.[45,46] Typically, affected newborns present with hypotonia, upper and low limb weakness, macroglossia, hepatomegaly, failure to thrive, progressive hypertrophic cardiomyopathy, and cardiorespiratory insufficiency leading (if untreated) to early death. Generalized glycogen storage has been identified in autopsy material from fetal tissues and adults with IOPD and LOPD, respectively.[47–56] On the other hand, older children and adults usually present with slowly progressive limb girdle weakness, respiratory deterioration, rigid spine syndrome, scoliosis, and low body mass.[54,57] A growing number of large series of patients with LOPD had been described in the literature and were reviewed recently.[58–65] As a result, the clinical presentation in LOPD has been expanded to include ptosis, bulbar palsy, and urinary incontinence. Taken together, the pathologic accumulation of glycogen in several tissues identified on autopsy examination and clinical experience with patients with Pompe disease revealed the following clinical correlations:[66,67]

- Diaphragm and intercostal muscles: respiratory failure
- Proximal skeletal muscle: progressive limb-girdle myopathy
- Genioglossus: tongue weakness
- Extraocular muscles: unilateral or bilateral ptosis
- Smooth muscle: abdominal pain/nausea/vomiting/diarrhea/urinary incontinence
- Cerebral vasculature: cerebral aneurysm.

However, the following associations do not seem to have clinical correlates:

- Broadened cerebral gyri
- Increased number of cerebral and cerebellar astrocytes
- Lipofuscin deposits in neurons and astrocytes of the spinal cord and cerebellum
- Fibrillary gliosis and anterior horn cell degeneration
- Glycogen vacuoles in the Schwann cells surrounding myelinated and unmyelinated axons of peripheral nerves.

PATHOGENESIS OF POMPE DISEASE

In Pompe disease, it is well established that the initial insult is due to the accumulation of the intralysosomal glycogen. However, recent studies showed that multiple other cellular abnormalities occur and that the pathophysiology of Pompe disease is far more complex than appreciated previously. In particular, the central role of autophagy is becoming more important now.[68–79] Hers[4] was the first to describe the histologic features of autophagy, which were then explicitly demonstrated using light and electron microscopic examination of skeletal muscle and confirmed by Engel and Dale.[78,79] Large pools of autophagic debris in skeletal muscle cells, especially in type II fibers, were seen in both the mouse *GAA* knockout model and patients with Pompe disease.[71–74] MAP1LC3, often referred to as LC3, and its membrane-bound isoform (LC3-II) is commonly used as a specific marker of autophagosomes.[77] Skin fibroblasts from patients with Pompe disease had been shown to have abnormal morphology with abnormal mannose-6-phosphate receptor trafficking that secondarily impaired rhGAA uptake in these cells. By electron microscopy, various features of enhanced autophagy, such as the accumulation of multivesicular bodies, expansion of Golgi apparatus, abnormal intracellular distribution of cation-independent mannose-6-phosphate receptor (CI-MPR), and reduced availability of the receptor at the plasma membrane were identified. These abnormalities resulted in less efficient rhGAA uptake, processing, and correction.[72] Accumulation of autophagosomes is a key pathologic finding in skeletal muscle fibers and skin fibroblasts from patients with Pompe disease and is implicated in the poor response to ERT.[80] Mutant GAA initiates autophagy via the induction of ER stress, as well as Akt inactivation (ER stress-independent) using mammalian target of rapamycin suppression. Treatment with insulin, which activates Akt signaling, restored phosphorylation of both Akt and p70S6 kinase and suppressed autophagy in patient fibroblasts. Also, combination therapy using rhGAA and insulin enhanced correct colocalization of the enzyme with lysosomes.[81] On the other hand, suppression of autophagy in the whole organism by knocking out critical autophagic genes (Atgs), such as Atg5 or Atg7 is lethal.[75,76]

Metabolic abnormalities in tissues and body fluids of GAA2/2 mice and humans, respectively, had also been identified. Abnormal glycogen metabolism (suppressed phosphorylase activity, elevated glycogen synthase, glycogenin, hexokinase activities, and glucose-6-phosphate) in the heart, skeletal muscles, and liver from GAA2/2 mice was demonstrated.[82,83] The effect of GAA deficiency in muscles of patients with Pompe disease extends to various vesicle systems linked to lysosomes, including the early endosomes (rab5), recycling endosomes (transferrin receptor) and trans-Golgi network, as they all showed increased immunoreactivity.[84] Expression of the insulin-responsive glucose transporter 4 was also markedly increased and partially colocalized with all vesicular markers, a phenomenon that may contribute to its abnormal homeostasis. In addition, abnormal energy metabolism, diminished plasma methylation capacity, and elevated insulinlike growth factor binding protein 1 (IGFBP1) and IGFBP3 levels were found in patients with LOPD.[85] Low-carbohydrate and high-protein calorie diet was beneficial.

NEWBORN SCREENING FOR POMPE DISEASE

Over several decades and since the inception of the universal newborn screening programs for inborn errors of metabolism, the number of disorders and the laboratory assays used to detect them continued to be limited. However, the introduction of tandem mass spectrometry in the late 1990s resulted in a significant and rapid expansion of the number of such disorders, some of which may not fulfill the classical inclusion criteria of Wilson and Junger.[86] Once again, tandem mass spectrometry–based GAA enzyme activity assays had been shown recently to be potentially useful in newborn screening for Pompe disease and other lysosomal storage diseases using DBS (see **Table 5**). Newborn screening efforts for Pompe disease started in Taiwan in 2005. Recently, the US Secretary of the Department of Health and Human Services' Discretionary Advisory Committee for Heritable Disorders in Newborns and Children recommended universal newborn screening for Pompe disease, an effort that started in some states-based newborn screening laboratories. Few other newborn screening pilots were conducted in other countries around the world (see **Table 5**).[38,87–97] It is unclear how asymptomatic cases destined to have LOPD but detected on newborn screening should be followed and managed.[65] Although newborn screening for lysosomal storage diseases, including Pompe disease, is gaining acceptance, some investigators and ethicists recommended that screening for these conditions should be performed only in the research context with institutional review board approval and parental permission.[98]

THE UNIVERSITY OF KANSAS MEDICAL CENTER CASE SERIES

We performed a retrospective review of all patients diagnosed with IOPD and LOPD at the University of Kansas Medical Center between 2000 and 2013 (**Tables 1–4**). Muscle

Table 1
Symptoms characteristics in patients with infantile and late-onset Pompe disease

Patient	Family History	Sex	Age, y	1st	Age, y	2nd	Age, y	3rd	Sign/Symptom	Age, y	At Diagnosis, y	At Last Visit, y	Time from 1st Symptom-Diagnosis
									Presentation		Age		
					Manifestation Sequence								
1	Yes (brother)	F	0	PD	0	RD	0	MG	PD	0	PD	2	0
2	Yes (sister)	M	5/12	SOB	6/12	My	2	DW	RF	5	7	12	2
3	No	M	2/12	GW	4/12	CM	4/12	MG	GW	4/12	4/12	8.5	2/12
4	No	F	10	My	12	LBP	16	LW	My	10	19	22	9
5	Yes (brother)	M	15	AW	17	Fatigue	—	—	AW	19	19	20	5
6	Yes (brother)	M	15	AW	17	My	17	Fatigue	AW	19	19	25	4
7	No	F	9	LGW	16	My	21	Fatigue	LGW	23	21	26	12
8	No	M	2	LW	4	My	4	LGW	LGW	6	6	34	4
9	Yes (sister)	M	38	Weight loss	39	SOB	40	LGW	LGW	40	40	41	2
10	Yes (sister)	F	37	My	38	LGW	39	SOB	LGW	40	40	50	3
11	Yes (sister)	F	36	LBP	38	LGW	38	SOB	LGW	40	38	53	2
12	Yes (sister)	M	10	LW	30	Abnormal LFT	32	AMW[a]	AMW	32	32	52	22

Abbreviations: AMW, axial muscle weakness; AW, arm weakness; CM, cardiomyopathy; DW, delayed walking; F, female; GW, generalized weakness; LBP, low back pain; LFT, liver function test; LGW, limb girdle weakness; LW, leg weakness; M, male; MG, macroglossia; My, myalgia; PD, prenatal diagnosis; RD, respiratory distress; RF, respiratory failure; SOB, shortness of breath.

[a] With scoliosis.

Table 2
Summary of neurologic motor examination in patients with infantile and late-onset Pompe disease at last follow-up

Patient	CK Level, IU/L	Enlarged Tongue	Tongue Weakness	Scapular Winging	Trendelenburg Gait	Leg Weakness	Arm Weakness	Ankle Weakness	Hand Weakness
1	699	Yes	No	No	NA	+	+	+	+
2	1173	No	No	No	Yes	−	−	−	−
3	889	Yes	Yes	NA	NA	+	+	+	+
4	59	No	No	No	No	+	−	−	−
5	529	No	No	No	No	−	+	−	−
6	1684	No	No	No	No	−	−	−	−
7	1039	No	No	No	Yes	+	+	+	+
8	396	No	No	No	Yes	+	+	−	+
9	732	No	No	No	Yes	+	+	+	−
10	329	No	No	No	Yes	+	+	−	−
11	169	No	No	No	Yes	+	+	+	+
12	107	No	No	Yes	Yes	+	+	−	−

Abbreviations: CK, creatine kinase; NA, not applicable; +, present; −, absent.

Table 3
Respiratory status in patients with infantile and late-onset Pompe disease

Patient	FVC, L	Ventilatory Support, Onset in Years
1	—	—
2	0.96	Tracheostomy/5
3	—	Tracheostomy/0.5
4	4.6	—
5	—	—
6	5.08	—
7	3.8	—
8	4.06	—
9	1.7	BiPAP/39
10	3.15	—
11	2.00	BiPAP/48
12	4.14	—

In this group of patients, 4 (33%) of 12 needed assistive ventilation, including invasive ventilation in the 2 patients with infantile Pompe disease.
Abbreviations: BiPAP, bi-level positive air pressure; FVC, forced vital capacity; L, liter.

biopsies, *GAA* mutation analysis, and GAA enzyme activity of muscle, skin fibroblasts, amniocytes, and DBSs were performed at various medical centers and reference clinical laboratories using standard techniques. The Medline database was searched for reports of large series of patients with IOPD and LOPD, autopsies performed on patients with IOPD and LOPD and abortuses/abortions, as well as those reports that describe new diagnostic techniques related to Pompe disease.

We identified 3 patients with IOPD (1 classical and 2 siblings with nonclassical), and 9 patients with LOPD (1 patient with juvenile and 8 with adult) Pompe disease. The male:female ratio was 1.4:1.0 and the average age of onset was 17.7 years (0–39). In this group, all 3 patients with IOPD (cases 1, 2, 3) had varying degrees of hypertrophic cardiomyopathy, which was most severe in patient 3. Unlike patients 1 and 2 (**Fig. 3**A, B), patient 3 (see **Fig. 3**C) appeared to have classical Pompe disease with severe hypotonia and minimal strength in the upper and lower limbs. Overall, the presenting symptom was limb girdle weakness in 43%, whereas 25% presented with shortness of breath and 17% had myalgia. Delay from first symptom to diagnosis was 6 years (range: 1–22). In LOPD cases, shortness of breath affected 3 of 7 cases, presenting within 1 to 2 years of the first symptoms. Besides limb weakness, scapular winging was evident on presentation in 8% and 4 (57%) of 7 had Trendelenburg gait. Low back pain was reported in 1 LOPD patient (patient 12) in whom back surgery was done. Magnetic resonance image examination showed lower limb muscle fatty infiltration and edema (patient 4) and dilated cerebral (circle of Willis) vessels (patient 8). Echocardiography revealed septal hypertrophy in 2 patients, left ventricular hypertrophy in 1 patient, and hypertrophic cardiomyopathy in the child with classical IOPD. Urinary tetrasaccharide (Hex4) level was elevated in 2 patients (patients 3 and 8) and normal in 3 other patients with LOPD (patients 4, 7, and 9). Creatine kinase level ranged from 59 to 1684 IU/L (mean 878) and electromyography showed evidence of myotonia in 1 of 4 studied patients, with fibrillation and myopathic motor unit action potential (MUAP) present in this and another patient (patients 6 and 7). The other 2 cases were either normal (episodic severe myalgia) or revealed myopathic MUAPs. DBS-GAA enzyme activity was less than 40% of the lower normal limit

Table 4
GAA mutations and enzyme activities in various tissues in patients with Pompe disease

Patient	GAA Mutation		GAA Enzyme Activity			Order of Diagnostic Studies	Maximum Anti-Lumizyme IgG Antibody Titer[a]
	Allele 1	Allele 2	Muscle	Skin	DBS (Normal)	1st-2nd-3rd	
1	c.1979G>A (p.R660H)	VUS [c.-32-17_-32-10del8ins30]	ND	ND	<2.5 (>7.5)	Amniocytes GAA activity-DBS-DNA	Negative
2	c.1979G>A (p.R660H)	VUS [c.32-17_32-10del8ins30]	0.023 (0.42 ± 0.2)	ND	1.9 (10-49)	MBx-DBS-DNA	Negative
3	c.1843G>A (p.Gly615Arg)	c.1843G>A p.Gly615Arg	Low	Low	0[b]	DBS-MBx-DNA	1:1600
4	VUS [c.-1402A>T (p.I468F)]	Unknown (negative GAA deletion/duplication)	0.08 (0.42 ± 0.2)	88.77 (260 ± 82.2)	4.8 (10-49)	Skin fibroblast GAA MBx Muscle GAA -DBS-DNA	NA
5	ND	ND	ND	ND	2.8 (10-49)	DBS	NA
6	c.655G>A (p.G219R), exon 3	c.546G>A (p.T182T), exon 2 (splice site)	ND	ND	2.9 (10-49)	MBx-DBS-DNA	NA
7	c.-32-13T>G (IVS1-13T>G)	Multiple VUS (R527F)	ND	ND	4 (10-49)	MBx-DBS-DNA	1:1600
8	ND	ND	ND	ND	2.85 (10-49)	MBx-DBS	1:1600
9	c.-32-13T>G (IVS1-13T>G)	VUS [c.1402A>T (p.I468F)]	ND	ND	<2.5 (10-49)	MBx-DBS-DNA	ND
10	ND	ND	29.23 (260 ± 82.2)	ND		MBx-Muscle GAA	1:12,800
11	ND	ND	38.54 (260 ± 82.2)	38.54 (177.8-342.2)		MBx-Muscle GAA-Skin fibroblast	1:200
12	ND	ND	17.7 (63-123)	ND		MBx-Muscle GAA-DNA	1:1600

Four novel mutations (predicted to be pathogenic) were identified including "p.I468F," which was found in 2 unrelated individuals. Amniocytes in patient 1 showed undetectable GAA activity, which predicts severe classical infant-onset Pompe disease, whereas postnatal DBS showed detectable but markedly reduced GAA activity.

Units: GAA enzyme activity in muscle/skin fibroblasts (μmol/min/g tissue), DBS (pmol/h/punch).

Abbreviations: DBS, dried blood spot; GAA, acid-α-glucosidase; Ig, immunoglobulin; MBx, muscle biopsy; NA, not applicable; ND, not done; VUS, variant of unknown significance.

[a] Anti-Lumizyme antibody titers were reported by Genzyme Corporation, Cambridge, MA.

[b] GAA activity was measured in blood lymphocytes (mean 35 nmol/h/mg protein).

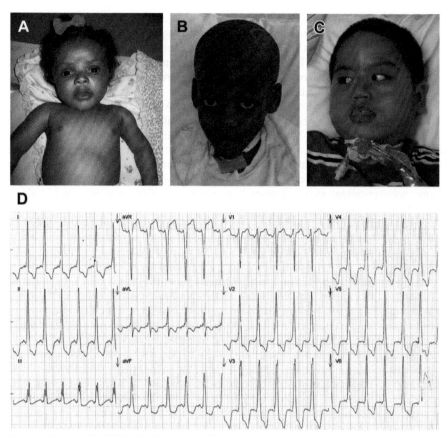

Fig. 3. Patients with IOPD. The sibling pair (A, B; patients 1 and 2, respectively) have nonclassical IOPD, whereas patient 3 (C) has classical IOPD with macroglossia, tracheostomy, and severe hypotonia. (D) Abnormal electrocardiogram of patient 3 shows sinus tachycardia, short PR interval, ST segment and T wave abnormalities, and left ventricular hypertrophy.

(10 pmol/punch/h) in 7 of 9 patients and in the other 2 was in the borderline range of 40% to 50% of normal lower limit.

Most patients (8 of 12) had muscle biopsy as their first test followed by DBS-GAA activity level as a confirmatory test. Of 3 IOPD cases, 2 underwent muscle biopsy; patient 2 showed vacuoles and microaggregates of glycogen on PAS confirmed to consist of abundant membrane-bound glycogen on ultrastructural analysis (and markedly reduced muscle GAA enzyme activity), and patient 3 had vacuoles in 50% of muscle fibers and accumulation of glycogen in less-vacuolated fibers that was also seen in smooth muscle fibers of erector pili muscles on skin biopsy. Altogether all 9 LOPD cases underwent muscle biopsy, except for patient 5; 7 of 8 muscle biopsies were suspicious for Pompe disease and the eighth biopsy showed nonspecific myopathic changes. Vacuoles were seen in 5 patients with LOPD, along with abnormal glycogen deposition on PAS stain, whereas the other 2 patients showed abnormal glycogen deposition without vacuolation. Hematoxylin and eosin–stained muscle tissue showed rimmed vacuoles in 2 patients and nonrimmed in an additional 2 patients. In one of these patients, rimmed vacuoles could not be confirmed on modified Gomori trichrome stain, but in patient 4 (severe episodic myalgia), there were nonrimmed vacuoles seen only on trichrome. Acid phosphatase positive vacuolar aggregates were seen in 2 of 5 vacuolated muscle biopsies. Abnormal glycogen deposition on PAS was present in 7 cases and was the only finding in 2 of 7 biopsies suggestive of Pompe.

Ten patients received ERT and reported subjective improvement, although this was not measurable on clinical examination except in patient 2 with nonclassical IOPD (see later in this article) and patient 9 in whom objective improvement in proximal arm strength was noted 4 months after the start of ERT. Anti-rhGAA antibody titers were elevated in 6 patients and negative in 2 patients (see **Table 4**). In this cohort, all patients are still alive except patient 11, who was intolerant of ERT and died at 53 years of age due to progressive and severe respiratory insufficiency. *GAA* mutation analysis was done in 8 of 12 patients and a total of 12 mutations and 4 variants of unknown significance were identified. All patients with identifiable mutations were compound heterozygotes, except patient 3 with classical IOPD who was "c.1843G>A; p.Gly615Arg" homozygote. Two unrelated patients were heterozygous for the common "IVS1-13T>G/c.-32-13t>g" mutation. The novel (heterozygous) mutation (c.-1402A>T p.I468F) was identified in 2 unrelated patients, whereas another novel splice site (c.546G>A) mutation was found in patient 6. Both novel alleles are predicted in silico to be pathogenic. In this series, family history was positive in 3 sibling pairs (patients 1 and 2, 5 and 6, 10 and 11). Next, we describe 4 patients in this cohort in more detail.

Patients 1 and 2 (see **Fig. 3**A, B) are an African American sibling pair. The older brother was diagnosed with hypertrophic cardiomyopathy at 2 months of age when he was also found to be carnitine deficient. Cardiomyopathy did not resolve despite carnitine supplementation. At 5 years of age, he presented with skeletal muscle weakness and respiratory failure triggered by influenza pneumonia for which a tracheostomy was placed. He then became ventilator dependent. Membrane-bound glycogen was abundant on muscle biopsy and muscle and DBS-GAA enzyme activity were markedly reduced. Approximately 18 months after the initiation of ERT, daytime ventilation was discontinued and muscle strength improved significantly. His younger sister was diagnosed prenatally with infantile Pompe disease via amniocentesis. GAA activity in amniocytes was undetectable. However, postnatal GAA activity in DBS was detectable but reduced. She had mild macroglossia (see **Fig. 3**B) and her echocardiogram showed septal hypertrophy only. She is doing quite well despite the delay in starting her ERT at 10 months of age. Both siblings maintain negative anti-rhGAA antibody titer. CRIM status was not tested in either sibling because they had significant residual GAA activity and by definition would be CRIM positive.

Patient 3 is 8.5-year-old Vietnamese boy (see **Fig. 3**A) with severe, classical, infantile Pompe disease and severe hypertrophic cardiomyopathy. His diagnosis was made at 4 months of age and he received ERT almost immediately. CRIM testing of his skin fibroblasts by Western blot analysis was positive (Duke University). He continues to be ventilator dependent with minimal muscle power in both upper and lower limbs. He maintained a negative anti-rhGAA antibody titer until 1 year ago when he developed a non-neutralizing low titer at 1:200.

Patient 4 had a muscle biopsy at 10 years of age when she presented with severe recurrent myalgia. A provisional diagnosis of "atypical" dermatomyositis was made for which she was treated with steroids and hydroxychloroquine. Numerous other laboratory studies were uninformative. A second muscle biopsy was done at 18 years of age and showed membrane-bound glycogen. Low GAA enzyme activity was detected in muscle tissue and skin fibroblasts, whereas DBS-GAA activity was borderline reduced at 4.8 (normal 10–49). Only one predicted to be pathogenic novel *GAA* mutation (c.1402A>T; p.I468F) was identified. Deletion/duplication analysis using exon array (GeneDx, Gaithersburg, MD) was negative as well.

Patient 7 presented as a young adult with progressive skeletal muscle weakness. The diagnosis of Pompe disease was made based on abnormal findings in muscle biopsy. GAA activity in DBS was low and *GAA* mutation analysis revealed compound heterozygosity for the common mutation (IVS1-13T>G) and a novel, likely deleterious, variant (p.R527F). She became pregnant for the first time while she was receiving alglucosidase alfa. She suffered a spontaneous miscarriage at 10 weeks' gestation. Unfortunately, no pathologic examination of the abortus was done.

DISCUSSION, CURRENT MANAGEMENT, AND THERAPEUTIC OPTIONS

Our clinical experience with the 12 patients with Pompe disease that we report here is consistent with the literature. Findings in our case series suggest that a short latency between muscle symptoms and shortness of air should raise suspicion for LOPD. Muscle biopsy histopathology was done in 10 of the 12 patients and was the first test to yield suspicion for Pompe disease in 8 patients and the second test in 2 of the 4 remaining patients. DBS-GAA enzymatic activity was done in 9 of the 12 patients, being the first test in 2 patients, the second confirmatory test in 6 patients (in 5/6 after muscle biopsy), and the third test in patient 4 after skin fibroblast and muscle GAA analysis. Our only patient with classic IOPD who was CRIM positive still has profound muscle weakness and hypotonia despite early and adequate ERT and a very low non-neutralizing anti-rhGAA antibody titer, which suggests another mechanism for his suboptimal clinical response. Patient 11, an adult with LOPD, died due to progressive respiratory failure that was associated with a high anti-rhGAA antibody titer, an experience consistent with what Patel and colleagues[99] reported recently. Our 26-year old white woman (patient 7) who became pregnant for the first time while receiving alglucosidase alfa had a serious adverse event, as she suffered a spontaneous miscarriage at 14 weeks' gestation. Unfortunately, we did not have access to the product of conception and therefore we were unable to determine the genotype. Her fetus may or may not have been affected with Pompe disease. Although recombinant ERT is generally thought to be safe during pregnancy, a possible direct/indirect detrimental effect on that pregnancy could not be excluded. In addition, the maternal anti-rhGAA antibodies may have played a role as well. Although high sustained antibody titers in infantile and more recently LOPD correlate with poor outcome, their potential effect in pregnancy had not be reported yet.[99] On the other hand, there are only 2 reports in the literature that describe a normal outcome in 2 infants whose mothers with Pompe disease were successfully and safely treated with alglucosidase alfa throughout their pregnancies.[100,101] More clinical experience with the prenatal use of alglucosidase alfa is needed to establish its safety.

Since the recognition that maltose and acarbose inhibit neutral α-glucosidase activity, reliable measurement of acid GAA activity in DBS became feasible and was quickly adopted as a noninvasive alternative to skin fibroblasts and muscle biopsies, which are invasive, more expensive, and take longer time to process. Preisler and colleagues[15] used this approach to identify 3 patients with LOPD among 38 patients with unclassified limb-girdle muscular dystrophy (8%). Also, as newborn screening for metabolic disorders uses blood collected on dried filter papers (DBS), various platforms to measure GAA activity in DBS were developed. They include tandem mass spectrometry, and fluorometric and microfluidics-based enzyme assays **(Table 5)**. Emerging evidence from these studies suggests a higher incidence of Pompe disease (1/28,000) compared with lower estimates reported previously. In addition, GAA pseudodeficiency (<1% in white and up to 3.9% in Asians) was recognized, which prompted an adjustment of the newborn screening algorithms.[37]

Table 5
Newborn screening studies for Pompe disease

Country	Newborns Screened	Screening Method/Criteria	Outcome	Ref.
USA-Washington	111,544	MS/MS; cutoff of <2.60 mmol/h/L (<15% of mean)	4 PD cases (1/27, 800), 3 carriers with an additional pseudodeficiency allele, 6 were heterozygotes for a pseudodeficiency allele only; PPV 0.24; FPR 1/8600	87
	5055	MS/MS; cutoff: <20% daily mean activity	5 with low GAA activity	88
USA-Missouri	27,724	Digital microfluidics	3 PD cases (1/8657): 1 classic, 1 nonclassic IOPD and 1 LOPD; 3 false-positive results (carrier status unknown), 1 pseudodeficiency, 2 carriers, 2 pending cases	38
USA-Illinois	8012	Digital microfluidics	2 false positive	89
Taiwan	344,056 (2005–2009)	Fluorescence assay, NAG/GAA >60 and GAA inhibition by acarbose >80%, 2nd tier: lymphocyte GAA activity <5% of normal mean and GAA activity in skin fibroblasts, GAA sequencing	13 LOPD (1/26,466) and 6 IOPD cases	90
	473,738 (2005–2011)	Fluorescence assay, NAG/GAA ratio ≥100	9 IOPD and 19 LOPD cases; NAG/GAA cutoff ratio ≥60 (PPV) of 63.4%	91

Country	Sample	Method	Results	Ref.
Japan	496 healthy controls, 29 PD cases, and 5 PD carriers (530 DBS)	GAA activity <8% of normal mean and % GAA inhibition >60% and NAG/GAA ratio >30	5 healthy pseudodeficiency homozygotes and 1 obligate carrier	92
Italy	3403	Fluorescent GAA activity; cutoff: <35% of average control activities	3 cases with low GAA activity (final status not confirmed)	93
Hungary	40,024	MS/MS followed by molecular confirmation	9 PD cases	94
Germany	3251 944 (symptomatic individuals)	MS/MS and fluorometric assays; repeat testing in <0.5% of DBS samples	No PD cases 14 PD cases and 8 GAA carriers	95
Colombia	4700 (DBS samples from symptomatic, high-risk individuals; 3 mo–73 y old)	Fluorometric microfluidic, molecular GAA analysis (some)	16 PD cases	96
Austria	34,736 (January–July, 2010)	ESI-MS/MS	4 confirmed by GAA mutation analysis (1/8684). Most GAA missense mutations were LOPD; PPV 80%; 1 false-positive case (FPR 30 per million)	97

Abbreviations: ESI, electrospray ionization; FPR, false-positive rate; GAA, acid glucosidase; IOPD, infantile-onset Pompe disease; LOPD, late-onset Pompe disease; MS/MS, tandem mass spectrometry; NAG, neutral alpha-glucosidase; PD, Pompe disease; PPV, positive predictive value; Ref., reference number.

Based on a pooling of clinical studies, 28% of Pompe disease cases are infantile onset, of which about 85% are classic infantile onset and 75% of those are CRIM positive.[30,102,103] CRIM-negative patients with classic IOPD very likely will develop neutralizing antibodies on exposure to rhGAA. Such antibodies limit the efficacy of ERT. Induction of immune tolerance using various regimens, such as rituximab with plasma exchange or alternatively the combination of rituximab and methotrexate with or without intravenous gamma-globulin, is an important therapeutic intervention that should be accomplished before initiation of ERT in such naïve patients.[102–106] The recent development of a blood-based assay for determining CRIM status is expected to facilitate this process in a timely manner.

The growing literature on Pompe disease reveals significant clinical variability in the age of onset of symptoms among patients with LOPD, which can be only partially predicted by their *GAA* genotype. Recently, expert opinion–based guidelines about newborn screening, confirmatory and symptomatic diagnostic testing, and management of patients with Pompe disease have been published.[7,107,108] The international Pompe disease registry (https://www.registrynxt.com/Pompe/), as well as country-based registries, have been established.[38,88–92] Recent reports from these registries indicate that diagnostic delay for patients with Pompe disease is still significant; fewer than two-third of muscle biopsies done in French patients showed specific features of Pompe disease, thus confirming the importance of GAA enzymatic assessment, and high prevalence of scoliosis (33%), especially among patients with IOPD.[109–113] Systematic analysis of data collected from the Pompe Registry will help improve recognition of the disease, and enhance understanding of its variable course and the effect of direct interventions, such as current ERT and other potential future therapies.

The literature contains 29 autopsy examination reports of patients with Pompe disease, including 9 in the non-English literature and 8 reports of autopsies of fetuses affected with Pompe disease. Collectively, these studies demonstrated the extensive and generalized accumulation of lysosomal glycogen in various organs, including the brain, well beyond the liver, heart, and skeletal muscles. In the brain, the cytoplasm of Schwann cells, but not neurons, was shown to accumulate glycogen. This observation suggests that progressive neurodegeneration of the brain is not expected. Although glycogen deposition also was demonstrated in the spinal cord and peripheral nerves, there is no clinical correlate to this finding, as peripheral neuropathy had not been demonstrated clinically, by electromyography, or by histologic examination of muscle. These observations are consistent with the report of better than expected cognitive outcomes in a small group of 10 children with classic infantile Pompe disease treated with alglucosidase alfa. They were evaluated prospectively, both developmentally and by neuroimaging.[114] Cognitive development at school age improved and ranged between normal and mildly delayed. Periventricular white matter abnormalities were found in 4 children. Although treatment with alglucosidase alfa had been demonstrated to significantly increase survival in patients with IOPD, and because Pompe disease affects many tissues, including the brain, rhGAA is not expected to have beneficial effects on the central nervous system, as it does not cross the blood-brain barrier.

The new insights into the complex pathogenesis of Pompe disease explain, at least partially, the suboptimal clinical response in patients with LOPD and some patients with IOPD. As a result, novel therapies, including modified ERT, are being investigated. Novel experimental modified rhGAA therapies include glycosylation-independent lysosomal targeting of GAA (rhGAA-GILT), ICAM-1–targeted nanocarriers, which aim to enhance delivery of α-glucosidase and muscle glycogen clearance, and neo-GAA.[115–117] The neo-rhGAA is a carbohydrate-remodeled enzyme with higher affinity for the cation-independent mannose 6-phosphate receptor and improved delivery to muscles of Pompe mice. Because patients with IOPD who are CRIM negative are likely to develop neutralizing anti-rhGAA antibodies, early identification of their CRIM status and initiation of immunomodulation tolerance therapy using various approaches are very important for these patients. Coadministration of the pharmacologic chaperone, Duvoglustat hydrochloride (AT2220), with alglucosidase alfa in Pompe disease fibroblasts, blood cell lines, and in vivo appears to stabilize the enzyme and enhance its activity.[117–119] A bacterial glycosidase that enables mannose-6-phosphate modification also improves cellular uptake of yeast-produced recombinant human lysosomal enzymes.[120]

Additional potentially promising investigational therapeutic approaches include autophagy suppression, gene therapy using modified single-stranded oligonucleotides, short hairpin ribonucleic acids, transcription factors, AAV1-CMV-hGAA, hematopoietic stem cell transplantation, and induced pluripotent stem cells.[120–134] GILT-tagged rhGAA (BMN 701), Duvoglustat hydrochloride (AT2220), neo-rhGAA and AAV1-CMV-hGAA are currently in clinical trials.

SUMMARY AND FUTURE DIRECTIONS

Pompe disease is the first metabolic myopathy for which corrective targeted ERT was developed. Besides limb-girdle weakness and scoliosis in patients with LOPD, shortness of breath affected nearly half of our cases and led to early presentation within the first 2 years of symptom onset. The most common first diagnostic test to raise Pompe suspicion was muscle biopsy and confirmation was often with DBS assay. DBS-GAA enzymatic activity levels in the borderline 40% to 50% range warrants further investigation. The efficacy of the current form of ERT is generally variable and unpredictable, especially in patients with LOPD given the long diagnostic delay. There is a need for improved early recognition and therapy for this disorder, which will be aided by improved understanding of its pathogenesis. Novel therapies based on improved understanding of the disease pathogenesis are already under study and some are in clinical trials. Early identification through newborn screening and more effective and specific therapies will likely significantly improve the outcome for all patients with Pompe disease.

ACKNOWLEDGMENTS

The authors thank all of our patients and their families for their kind support and interest in this study. We also thank Dawn Lockhart and all of the staff of the Clinical Trials Unit at the University of Kansas Medical Center for providing exemplary care for the patients and their families.

REFERENCES

1. Pompe JC. Over idiopatische hypertrophie van het hart. Ned Tijdschr Geneeskd 1932;76:304–12.
2. Bischoff G. Zum klinischen Bild der Glykogen-Speicherungs-Krankheit (Glykogenose). Z Kinderheilk 1932;52:722–5.
3. Putschar M. Uber angeborene Glykogenspeicher-Krankheit des herzens. "Thesaurismosis glycogenica" (v. Gierke). Biochem J 1932;90:222–31.
4. Hers HG. alpha-Glucosidase deficiency in generalized glycogen-storage disease (Pompe's disease). Biochem J 1963;86:11–6.

5. van den Hout HM, Hop W, van Diggelen OP, et al. The natural course of infantile Pompe's disease: 20 original cases compared with 133 cases from the literature. Pediatrics 2003;112:332–40.

6. Case LE, Beckemeyer AA, Kishnani PS. Infantile Pompe disease on ERT: update on clinical presentation, musculoskeletal management, and exercise considerations. Am J Med Genet C Semin Med Genet 2012;160C:69–79.

7. Cupler EJ, Berger KI, Leshner RT, et al. Consensus treatment recommendations for late-onset Pompe disease. Muscle Nerve 2012;45:319–33.

8. Levine B, Klionsky DJ. Development by self-digestion: molecular mechanisms and biological functions of autophagy. Dev Cell 2004;6:463–77.

9. Levine B, Deretic V. Unveiling the roles of autophagy in innate and adaptive immunity. Nat Rev Immunol 2007;7:767–77.

10. Eng CH, Yu K, Lucas J, et al. Ammonia derived from glutaminolysis is a diffusible regulator of autophagy. Sci Signal 2010;3:ra31.

11. Shintani T, Klionsky DJ. Autophagy in health and disease: a double-edged sword. Science 2004;306:990–5.

12. Huang J, Klionsky DJ. Autophagy and human disease. Cell Cycle 2007;6:1837–49.

13. Mizushima N, Levine B, Cuervo AM, et al. Autophagy fights disease through cellular self-digestion. Nature 2008;451:1069–75.

14. Nixon RA. The role of autophagy in neurodegenerative disease. Nat Med 2013; 19:983–97.

15. Preisler N, Lukacs Z, Vinge L, et al. Late-onset Pompe disease is prevalent in unclassified limb-girdle muscular dystrophies. Mol Genet Metab 2013;110:287–9.

16. Schüller A, Wenninger S, Strigl-Pill N, et al. Toward deconstructing the phenotype of late-onset Pompe disease. Am J Med Genet C Semin Med Genet 2012;160:80–8.

17. Meikle PJ, Yan M, Ravenscroft EM, et al. Altered trafficking and turnover of LAMP-1 in Pompe disease-affected cells. Mol Genet Metab 1999;66:179–88.

18. Platt FM, Boland B, van der Spoel AC. The cell biology of disease: lysosomal storage disorders: the cellular impact of lysosomal dysfunction. J Cell Biol 2012;199:723–34.

19. Kornfeld S. Trafficking of lysosomal enzymes in normal and disease states. J Clin Invest 1986;77:1–6.

20. Wisselaar HA, Kroos MA, Hermans MM, et al. Structural and functional changes of lysosomal acid alpha-glucosidase during intracellular transport and maturation. J Biol Chem 1993;268:2223–31.

21. Chamoles NA, Niizawa G, Blanco M, et al. Glycogen storage disease type II: enzymatic screening in dried blood spots on filter paper. Clin Chim Acta 2004;347:97–102.

22. Niizawa G, Levin C, Aranda C, et al. Retrospective diagnosis of glycogen storage disease type II by use of a newborn-screening card. Clin Chim Acta 2005; 359:205–6.

23. Zhang H, Kallwass H, Young SP, et al. Comparison of maltose and acarbose as inhibitors of maltase-glucoamylase activity in assaying acid alpha-glucosidase activity in dried blood spots for the diagnosis of infantile Pompe disease. Genet Med 2006;8:302–6.

24. Sista RS, Wang T, Wu N, et al. Multiplex newborn screening for Pompe, Fabry, Hunter, Gaucher, and Hurler diseases using a digital microfluidic platform. Clin Chim Acta 2013;424:12–8.

25. Metz TF, Mechtler TP, Orsini JJ, et al. Simplified newborn screening protocol for lysosomal storage disorders. Clin Chem 2011;57:1286–94.

26. Spáčil Z, Elliott S, Reeber SL, et al. Comparative triplex tandem mass spectrometry assays of lysosomal enzyme activities in dried blood spots using fast liquid chromatography: application to newborn screening of Pompe, Fabry, and Hurler diseases. Anal Chem 2011;83:4822–8.

27. Mechtler TP, Metz TF, Müller HG, et al. Short-incubation mass spectrometry assay for lysosomal storage disorders in newborn and high-risk population screening. J Chromatogr B Analyt Technol Biomed Life Sci 2012;908:9–17.

28. Young SP, Piraud M, Goldstein JL, et al. Assessing disease severity in Pompe disease: the roles of a urinary glucose tetrasaccharide biomarker and imaging techniques. Am J Med Genet C Semin Med Genet 2012;160C:50–8.

29. Xia B, Asif G, Arthur L, et al. Oligosaccharide analysis in urine by MALDI-TOF mass spectrometry for the diagnosis of lysosomal storage diseases. Clin Chem 2013;59:1357–68.

30. Wang Z, Okamoto P, Keutzer J. A new assay for fast, reliable CRIM status determination in infantile-onset Pompe disease. Mol Genet Metab 2014;111:92–100.

31. Van Hove JL, Yang HW, Wu JY, et al. High-level production of recombinant human lysosomal acid alpha-glucosidase in Chinese hamster ovary cells which targets to heart muscle and corrects glycogen accumulation in fibroblasts from patients with Pompe disease. Proc Natl Acad Sci U S A 1996;93:65–70.

32. Nascimbeni AC, Fanin M, Tasca E, et al. Molecular pathology and enzyme processing in various phenotypes of acid maltase deficiency. Neurology 2008;70: 617–26.

33. Sugawara K, Saito S, Sekijima M, et al. Structural modeling of mutant alpha-glucosidases resulting in a processing/transport defect in Pompe disease. J Hum Genet 2009;54:324–30.

34. Kroos MA, Mullaart RA, Van Vliet L, et al. p.[G576S; E689K]: pathogenic combination or polymorphism in Pompe disease? Eur J Hum Genet 2008;16: 875–9.

35. Tajima Y, Matsuzawa F, Aikawa S, et al. Structural and biochemical studies on Pompe disease and a "pseudodeficiency of acid alpha-glucosidase." J Hum Genet 2007;52:898–906.

36. Kumamoto S, Katafuchi T, Nakamura K, et al. High frequency of acid alpha-glucosidase pseudodeficiency complicates newborn screening for glycogen storage disease type II in the Japanese population. Mol Genet Metab 2009; 97:190–5.

37. Labrousse P, Chien YH, Pomponio RJ, et al. Genetic heterozygosity and pseudodeficiency in the Pompe disease newborn screening pilot program. Mol Genet Metab 2010;99:379–83.

38. Kemper AR. The Condition Review Workgroup. Evidence report: newborn screening for pompe disease. Available at: http://www.hrsa.gov/advisorycommittees/mchbadvisory/heritabledisorders/nominatecondition/reviews/pompereport2013.pdf. Accessed June 3, 2013.

39. Costin-Kelly N. Histological analysis of a muscle biopsy. The biomedical scientist. 2008:1063–70.

40. Werneck LC, Lorenzoni PJ, Kay CS, et al. Muscle biopsy in Pompe disease. Arq Neuropsiquiatr 2013;71:284–9.

41. Vissing J, Lukacs Z, Straub V. Diagnosis of Pompe disease: muscle biopsy vs blood-based assays. JAMA Neurol 2013;70:923–7.

42. Winkel LP, Kamphoven JH, van den Hout HJ, et al. Morphological changes in muscle tissue of patients with infantile Pompe's disease receiving enzyme replacement therapy. Muscle Nerve 2003;27:743–51.

43. Prater SN, Patel TT, Buckley AF, et al. Skeletal muscle pathology of infantile Pompe disease during long-term enzyme replacement therapy. Orphanet J Rare Dis 2013;8:90.

44. Al-Lozi MT, Amato AA, Barohn RJ, et al, American Association of Neuromuscular & Electrodiagnostic Medicine. Diagnostic criteria for late-onset (childhood and adult) Pompe disease. Muscle Nerve 2009;40:149–60.

45. van der Beek NA, de Vries JM, Hagemans ML, et al. Clinical features and predictors for disease natural progression in adults with Pompe disease: a nationwide prospective observational study. Orphanet J Rare Dis 2012;7:88.

46. Hobson-Webb LD, Jones HN, Kishnani PS. Oropharyngeal dysphagia may occur in late-onset Pompe disease, implicating bulbar muscle involvement. Neuromuscul Disord 2013;23:319–23.

47. Bruni CB, Paluello FM. A biochemical and ultrastructural study of liver, muscle, heart and kidney in type II glycogenosis. Virchows Arch B Cell Pathol 1970;4: 196–207.

48. Libert J, Martin JJ, Ceuterick C, et al. Ocular ultrastructural study in a fetus with type II glycogenosis. Br J Ophthalmol 1977;61:476–82.

49. Nakamura Y, Tanimura A, Yasuoka C, et al. An autopsy case of type II glycogenosis. Kurume Med J 1979;26:349–54.

50. Pokorny KS, Ritch R, Friedman AH, et al. Ultrastructure of the eye in fetal type II glycogenosis (Pompe's disease). Invest Ophthalmol Vis Sci 1982;22: 25–31.

51. Margolis ML, Howlett P, Goldberg R, et al. Obstructive sleep apnea syndrome in acid maltase deficiency. Chest 1994;105:947–9.

52. Teng YT, Su WJ, Hou JW, et al. Infantile-onset glycogen storage disease type II (Pompe disease): report of a case with genetic diagnosis and pathological findings. Chang Gung Med J 2004;27:379–84.

53. Phupong V, Shuangshoti S, Sutthiruangwong P, et al. Prenatal diagnosis of Pompe disease by electron microscopy. Arch Gynecol Obstet 2005;271: 259–61.

54. Kobayashi H, Shimada Y, Ikegami M, et al. Prognostic factors for the late onset Pompe disease with enzyme replacement therapy: from our experience of 4 cases including an autopsy case. Mol Genet Metab 2010;100:14–9.

55. Hobson-Webb LD, Proia AD, Thurberg BL, et al. Autopsy findings in late-onset Pompe disease: a case report and systematic review of the literature. Mol Genet Metab 2012;106:462–9.

56. Fuller DD, ElMallah MK, Smith BK, et al. The respiratory neuromuscular system in Pompe disease. Respir Physiol Neurobiol 2013;189:241–9.

57. Zamanifekri B, Barohn RJ, Herbelin L, et al. Tongue weakness in a patient with myopathy. J Clin Neuromuscul Dis 2013;14(S1):19.

58. Güngör D, Kruijshaar ME, Plug I, et al. Impact of enzyme replacement therapy on survival in adults with Pompe disease: results from a prospective international observational study. Orphanet J Rare Dis 2013;8:49.

59. van der Ploeg AT, Barohn R, Carlson L, et al. Open-label extension study following the Late-Onset Treatment Study (LOTS) of alglucosidase alfa. Mol Genet Metab 2012;107:456–61.

60. Papadimas GK, Spengos K, Konstantinopoulou A, et al. Adult Pompe disease: clinical manifestations and outcome of the first Greek patients receiving enzyme replacement therapy. Clin Neurol Neurosurg 2011;113:303–7.

61. Herzog A, Hartung R, Reuser AJ, et al. A cross-sectional single-centre study on the spectrum of Pompe disease, German patients: molecular analysis of the

GAA gene, manifestation and genotype-phenotype correlations. Orphanet J Rare Dis 2012;7:35.

62. Güngör D, de Vries JM, Brusse E, et al. Enzyme replacement therapy and fatigue in adults with Pompe disease. Mol Genet Metab 2013;109:174–8.

63. Angelini C, Semplicini C. Enzyme replacement therapy for Pompe disease. Curr Neurol Neurosci Rep 2012;12:70–5.

64. Toscano A, Schoser B. Enzyme replacement therapy in late-onset Pompe disease: a systematic literature review. J Neurol 2013;260:951–9.

65. Chien YH, Hwu WL, Lee NC. Pompe disease: early diagnosis and early treatment make a difference. Pediatr Neonatol 2013;54:219–27.

66. Patel TT, Banugaria SG, Frush DP, et al. Basilar artery aneurysm: a new finding in classic infantile Pompe disease. Muscle Nerve 2013;47:613–5.

67. El-Gharbawy AH, Bhat G, Murillo JE, et al. Expanding the clinical spectrum of late-onset Pompe disease: dilated arteriopathy involving the thoracic aorta, a novel vascular phenotype uncovered. Mol Genet Metab 2011;103:362–6.

68. DiMauro S, Spiegel R. Progress and problems in muscle glycogenoses. Acta Myol 2011;30:96–102.

69. Oldfors A, DiMauro S. New insights in the field of muscle glycogenoses. Curr Opin Neurol 2013;26:544–53.

70. Malicdan MC, Nishino I. Autophagy in lysosomal myopathies. Brain Pathol 2012; 22:82–8.

71. Raben N, Wong A, Ralston E, et al. Autophagy and mitochondria in Pompe disease: nothing is so new as what has long been forgotten. Am J Med Genet C Semin Med Genet 2012;160C:13–21.

72. Cardone M, Porto C, Tarallo A, et al. Abnormal mannose-6-phosphate receptor trafficking impairs recombinant alpha-glucosidase uptake in Pompe disease fibroblasts. Pathogenetics 2008;1:6.

73. Fukuda T, Ewan L, Bauer M, et al. Dysfunction of endocytic and autophagic pathways in a lysosomal storage disease. Ann Neurol 2006;59:700–8.

74. Seppälä EH, Reuser AJ, Lohi H. A nonsense mutation in the acid α-glucosidase gene causes Pompe disease in Finnish and Swedish Lapphunds. PLoS One 2013;8:e56825.

75. Kuma A, Hatano M, Matsui M, et al. The role of autophagy during the early neonatal starvation period. Nature 2004;432:1032–6.

76. Komatsu M, Waguri S, Ueno T, et al. Impairment of starvation-induced and constitutive autophagy in Atg7-deficient mice. J Cell Biol 2005;169:425–34.

77. Kabeya Y, Mizushima N, Ueno T, et al. LC3, a mammalian homologue of yeast Apg8, is localized in autophagosome membranes after processing. EMBO J 2000;19:5720–8.

78. Engel AG, Dale AJ. Autophagic glycogenosis of late onset with mitochondrial abnormalities: light and electron microscopic observations. Mayo Clin Proc 1968;43:233–79.

79. Engel AG. Acid maltase deficiency in adults: studies in four cases of a syndrome which may mimic muscular dystrophy or other myopathies. Brain 1970; 93:599–616.

80. Nascimbeni AC, Fanin M, Masiero E, et al. Impaired autophagy contributes to muscle atrophy in glycogen storage disease type II patients. Autophagy 2012;8:1697–700.

81. Nishiyama Y, Shimada Y, Yokoi T, et al. Akt inactivation induces endoplasmic reticulum stress-independent autophagy in fibroblasts from patients with Pompe disease. Mol Genet Metab 2012;107:490–5.

82. Taylor KM, Meyers E, Phipps M, et al. Dysregulation of multiple facets of glycogen metabolism in a murine model of Pompe disease. PLoS One 2013; 8:e56181.
83. Raben N, Danon M, Gilbert AL, et al. Enzyme replacement therapy in the mouse model of Pompe disease. Mol Genet Metab 2003;80:159–69.
84. Orth M, Mundegar RR. Effect of acid maltase deficiency on the endosomal/lysosomal system and glucose transporter 4. Neuromuscul Disord 2003;13:49–54.
85. Pascual JM, Roe CR. Systemic metabolic abnormalities in adult-onset acid maltase deficiency: beyond muscle glycogen accumulation. JAMA Neurol 2013;70:756–63.
86. Wilson JM, Jungner G. Principles and practice of mass screening for disease. Bol Oficina Sanit Panam 1968;65:281–393.
87. Scott CR, Elliott S, Buroker N, et al. Identification of infants at risk for developing Fabry, Pompe, or mucopolysaccharidosis-I from newborn blood spots by tandem mass spectrometry. J Pediatr 2013;163:498–503.
88. Orsini JJ, Martin MM, Showers AL, et al. Lysosomal storage disorder 4+1 multiplex assay for newborn screening using tandem mass spectrometry: application to a small-scale population study for five lysosomal storage disorders. Clin Chim Acta 2012;413:1270–3.
89. Burton BK. Newborn screening for Pompe disease: an update, 2011. Am J Med Genet C Semin Med Genet 2012;160C:8–12.
90. Chien YH, Lee NC, Huang HJ, et al. Later-onset Pompe disease: early detection and early treatment initiation enabled by newborn screening. J Pediatr 2011; 158:1023–7.
91. Chiang SC, Hwu WL, Lee NC, et al. Algorithm for Pompe disease newborn screening: results from the Taiwan screening program. Mol Genet Metab 2012;106:281–6.
92. Oda E, Tanaka T, Migita O, et al. Newborn screening for Pompe disease in Japan. Mol Genet Metab 2011;104:560–5.
93. Paciotti S, Persichetti E, Pagliardini S, et al. First pilot newborn screening for four lysosomal storage diseases in an Italian region: identification and analysis of a putative causative mutation in the GBA gene. Clin Chim Acta 2012;413:1827–31.
94. Wittmann J, Karg E, Turi S, et al. Newborn screening for lysosomal storage disorders in Hungary. JIMD Rep 2012;6:117–25.
95. Lukacs Z, Nieves Cobos P, Keil A, et al. Dried blood spots in the diagnosis of lysosomal storage disorders–possibilities for newborn screening and high-risk population screening. Clin Biochem 2011;44:476.
96. Uribe A, Giugliani R. Selective screening for lysosomal storage diseases with dried blood spots collected on filter paper in 4,700 high-risk Colombian subjects. JIMD Rep 2013;11:107–16.
97. Mechtler TP, Stary S, Metz TF, et al. Neonatal screening for lysosomal storage disorders: feasibility and incidence from a nationwide study in Austria. Lancet 2012;379:335–41.
98. Ross LF. Newborn screening for lysosomal storage diseases: an ethical and policy analysis. J Inherit Metab Dis 2012;35:627–34.
99. Patel TT, Banugaria SG, Case LE, et al. The impact of antibodies in late-onset Pompe disease: a case series and literature review. Mol Genet Metab 2012; 106:301–9.
100. de Vries JM, Brugma JD, Ozkan L, et al. First experience with enzyme replacement therapy during pregnancy and lactation in Pompe disease. Mol Genet Metab 2011;104:552–5.

101. Zagnoli F, Leblanc A, Blanchard C. Pregnancy during enzyme replacement therapy for late-onset acid maltase deficiency. Neuromuscul Disord 2013;23: 180–1.

102. Messinger YH, Mendelsohn NJ, Rhead W, et al. Successful immune tolerance induction to enzyme replacement therapy in CRIM-negative infantile Pompe disease. Genet Med 2012;14:135–42.

103. Banugaria SG, Prater SN, Patel TT, et al. Algorithm for the early diagnosis and treatment of patients with cross reactive immunologic material-negative classic infantile pompe disease: a step towards improving the efficacy of ERT. PLoS One 2013;8:e67052.

104. Kishnani PS, Goldenberg PC, DeArmey SL, et al. Cross-reactive immunologic material status affects treatment outcomes in Pompe disease infants. Mol Genet Metab 2010;99:26–33.

105. Deodato F, Ginocchio VM, Onofri A, et al. Immune tolerance induced using plasma exchange and rituximab in an infantile Pompe disease patient. J Child Neurol 2013;29:850–4.

106. Elder ME, Nayak S, Collins SW, et al. B-Cell depletion and immunomodulation before initiation of enzyme replacement therapy blocks the immune response to acid alpha-glucosidase in infantile-onset Pompe disease. J Pediatr 2013; 163:847–54.

107. Wang RY, Bodamer OA, Watson MS, et al. Lysosomal storage diseases: diagnostic confirmation and management of presymptomatic individuals. Genet Med 2011;13:457–84.

108. Byrne BJ, Kishnani PS, Case LE, et al. Pompe disease: design, methodology, and early findings from the Pompe Registry. Mol Genet Metab 2011;103:1–11.

109. Roberts M, Kishnani PS, van der Ploeg AT, et al. The prevalence and impact of scoliosis in Pompe disease: lessons learned from the Pompe Registry. Mol Genet Metab 2011;104:574–82.

110. Kishnani PS, Amartino HM, Lindberg C, et al. Timing of diagnosis of patients with Pompe disease: data from the Pompe registry. Am J Med Genet A 2013; 161:2431–43.

111. Martins AM, Kerstenezky M, Linares A, et al. Utility of rare disease registries in Latin America. JIMD Rep 2011;1:111–5.

112. Hundsberger T, Rohrbach M, Kern L, et al. Swiss national guideline for reimbursement of enzyme replacement therapy in late-onset Pompe disease. J Neurol 2013;260:2279–85.

113. Laforêt P, Laloui K, Granger B, et al. The French Pompe registry. Baseline characteristics of a cohort of 126 patients with adult Pompe disease. Rev Neurol (Paris) 2013;169:595–602.

114. Ebbink BJ, Aarsen FK, van Gelder CM, et al. Cognitive outcome of patients with classic infantile Pompe disease receiving enzyme therapy. Neurology 2012;78: 1512–8.

115. Maga JA, Zhou J, Kambampati R, et al. Glycosylation-independent lysosomal targeting of acid α-glucosidase enhances muscle glycogen clearance in Pompe mice. J Biol Chem 2013;288:1428–38.

116. Hsu J, Northrup L, Bhowmick T, et al. Enhanced delivery of α-glucosidase for Pompe disease by ICAM-1-targeted nanocarriers: comparative performance of a strategy for three distinct lysosomal storage disorders. Nanomedicine 2012;8:731–9.

117. Zhu Y, Li X, McVie-Wylie A, et al. Carbohydrate-remodelled acid alpha-glucosidase with higher affinity for the cation-independent mannose

6-phosphate receptor demonstrates improved delivery to muscles of Pompe mice. Biochem J 2005;389:619–28.

118. Khanna R, Flanagan JJ, Feng J, et al. The pharmacological chaperone AT2220 increases recombinant human acid α-glucosidase uptake and glycogen reduction in a mouse model of Pompe disease. PLoS One 2012;7:e40776.

119. Flanagan JJ, Rossi B, Tang K, et al. The pharmacological chaperone 1-deoxynojirimycin increases the activity and lysosomal trafficking of multiple mutant forms of acid alpha-glucosidase. Hum Mutat 2009;30:1683–92.

120. Porto C, Cardone M, Fontana F, et al. The pharmacological chaperone N-butyldeoxynojirimycin enhances enzyme replacement therapy in Pompe disease fibroblasts. Mol Ther 2009;17:964–71.

121. Tiels P, Baranova E, Piens K, et al. A bacterial glycosidase enables mannose-6-phosphate modification and improved cellular uptake of yeast-produced recombinant human lysosomal enzymes. Nat Biotechnol 2012;30:1225–31.

122. Richard E, Douillard-Guilloux G, Caillaud C. New insights into therapeutic options for Pompe disease. IUBMB Life 2011;63:979–86.

123. Raben N, Hill V, Shea L, et al. Suppression of autophagy in skeletal muscle uncovers the accumulation of ubiquitinated proteins and their potential role in muscle damage in Pompe disease. Hum Mol Genet 2008;17:3897–908.

124. Raben N, Schreiner C, Baum R, et al. Suppression of autophagy permits successful enzyme replacement therapy in a lysosomal storage disorder–murine Pompe disease. Autophagy 2010;6:1078–89.

125. Lu IL, Lin CY, Lin SB, et al. Correction/mutation of acid alpha-D-glucosidase gene by modified single-stranded oligonucleotides: in vitro and in vivo studies. Gene Ther 2003;10:1910–6.

126. Douillard-Guilloux G, Raben N, Takikita S, et al. Modulation of glycogen synthesis by RNA interference: towards a new therapeutic approach for glycogenosis type II. Hum Mol Genet 2008;17:3876–86.

127. Feeney EJ, Spampanato C, Puertollano R, et al. What else is in store for autophagy? Exocytosis of autolysosomes as a mechanism of TFEB-mediated cellular clearance in Pompe disease. Autophagy 2013;9:1117–8.

128. Spampanato C, Feeney E, Li L, et al. Transcription factor EB (TFEB) is a new therapeutic target for Pompe disease. EMBO Mol Med 2013;5:691–706.

129. Byrne BJ, Falk DJ, Pacak CA, et al. Pompe disease gene therapy. Hum Mol Genet 2011;20:R61–8.

130. Qiu K, Falk DJ, Reier PJ, et al. Spinal delivery of AAV vector restores enzyme activity and increases ventilation in Pompe mice. Mol Ther 2012;20:21–7.

131. Conlon TJ, Erger K, Porvasnik S, et al. Preclinical toxicology and biodistribution studies of recombinant adeno-associated virus 1 human acid α-glucosidase. Hum Gene Ther Clin Dev 2013;24:127–33.

132. Douillard-Guilloux G, Richard E, Batista L, et al. Partial phenotypic correction and immune tolerance induction to enzyme replacement therapy after hematopoietic stem cell gene transfer of alpha-glucosidase in Pompe disease. J Gene Med 2009;11:279–87.

133. van Til NP, Stok M, Aerts Kaya FS, et al. Lentiviral gene therapy of murine hematopoietic stem cells ameliorates the Pompe disease phenotype. Blood 2010;115:5329–37.

134. Kawagoe S, Higuchi T, Meng XL, et al. Generation of induced pluripotent stem (iPS) cells derived from a murine model of Pompe disease and differentiation of Pompe-iPS cells into skeletal muscle cells. Mol Genet Metab 2011;104:123–8.

Metabolic and Mitochondrial Myopathies

Lydia J. Sharp, MD[a,b], Ronald G. Haller, MD[a,b,c],*

KEYWORDS

- Metabolic myopathies • Mitochondrial myopathies • Glycogen storage diseases
- Fatty acid oxidation defects • Exercise intolerance

KEY POINTS

- Disorders that cause complete blocks in glycogenolysis or glycolysis such as muscle phosphorylase deficiency (McArdle disease) or muscle phosphofructokinase (PFK) deficiency cause exertional fatigue with moderate activity such as walking that is attributable to low oxidative capacity; this limitation in oxidative metabolism lowers the threshold for exertional muscle contractures and rhabdomyolysis caused by higher-intensity exercise that normally would be supported by high rates of glycogenolysis.
- Disorders of lipid metabolism include disorders that cause weakness and marked intramuscular lipid accumulation (systemic carnitine deficiency, neutral lipid storage myopathy, and multiple acyl-CoA dehydrogenase deficiency [MADD]) and those that cause episodic rhabdomyolysis triggered by fasting, infection/fever, or prolonged exercise (carnitine palmitoyltransferase [CPT]2, very-long-chain acyl-CoA dehydrogenase [VLCAD], trifunctional protein [TP], and LPIN1 mutations).
- Mitochondrial myopathies are caused by mutations in mitochondrial DNA (mtDNA) or nuclear DNA and have heterogeneous clinical manifestations. The hallmark of significant limitations in muscle oxidative phosphorylation is impaired use of available oxygen associated with muscle fatigue and lactic acidosis at low levels of physical activity.

INTRODUCTION

Metabolic myopathies are a group of genetic disorders that limit the ability of skeletal muscle to use fuels to generate ATP. These disorders can be classified either as disorders of glycogen/glucose metabolism or as disorders of lipid metabolism. Mitochondrial myopathies encompass disorders that impair both fat and carbohydrate metabolism and restrict oxidative phosphorylation. These disorders have diverse clinical manifestations but typically result in low exercise capacity. Although many

[a] Department of Neurology and Neurotherapeutics, University of Texas Southwestern Medical Center, 5323 Harry Hines Boulevard, Dallas, TX 75390, USA; [b] Neuromuscular Center, Institute for Exercise and Environmental Medicine, Texas Health Presbyterian Hospital, 7232 Greenville Avenue, Dallas, TX 75231, USA; [c] North Texas VA Medical Center, 4500 South Lancaster Road, Dallas, TX 75216, USA
* Corresponding author. North Texas VA Medical Center, 4500 South Lancaster Road, Dallas, TX 75216.
E-mail address: Ronald.Haller@UTSouthwestern.edu

Neurol Clin 32 (2014) 777–799
http://dx.doi.org/10.1016/j.ncl.2014.05.001
0733-8619/14/$ – see front matter © 2014 Elsevier Inc. All rights reserved.

patients with metabolic and mitochondrial myopathy have lifelong symptoms of exercise limitations, diagnosis is often delayed. Recognizing key manifestations of disorders of muscle metabolism leads to earlier diagnosis and improved patient management.

CASE REPORT

A 20-year-old woman presented with an elevated creatine kinase (CK) level. She attributed any exercise limitations to being out of shape. On detailed questioning, she admitted that her legs would give out while trying to play softball as a child. After hitting what should have been a home run, she was unable to run around all bases and was hardly moving by the time she passed second base. While in college, she was a waitress. By the end of 1 shift, she was unable to straighten her fingers in both hands. She also states that sometimes if she stops and rests after fatiguing with exercise, she is able to resume activity without difficulties. She denies ever experiencing dark urine.

On physical examination, muscle bulk and strength are normal. The remainder of the physical examination is within normal limits. Nonischemic forearm caused rapid fatigue, no increase in lactate, but an exaggerated increase in ammonia. With cycle exercise, there was a "second wind," marked by a decrease in heart rate and perceived exertion and increase in exercise capacity after 7 minutes of cycling. Serum CK levels at rest were 20 times the upper limit of normal. Muscle biopsy revealed myophosphorylase deficiency (McArdle disease).

This case illustrates the common presentation of a disorder of glycogenolysis with lifelong exercise intolerance, contractures, and the second wind phenomenon. Frequently, pointed questioning is needed to establish the history of exercise intolerance, because patients may view themselves as just being not athletic or out of shape.

CARBOHYDRATE DISORDERS CAUSING EXERCISE-INDUCED SYMPTOMS
Muscle Phosphorylase Deficiency (McArdle Disease, Glycogen Storage Disease Type V)

Pathophysiology
Virtually all of the more than 100 causative mutations in the PGYM gene result in a complete loss of phosphorylase enzyme function and thus a complete block in glycogen breakdown (**Fig. 1**). Forceful muscle contractions, which normally would be supported by anaerobic glycogenolysis, are responsible for severe episodes of exertional muscle contracture and injury. Glycogen is also necessary for normal oxidative metabolism, and the resulting substrate-limited oxidative phosphorylation accounts for low capacity for moderate exercise as well as the characteristic variation in exercise capacity as illustrated by the classical second wind phenomenon that is attributable to increased uptake of glucose and combustion of fatty acids.[1,2] Importantly, mutations that preserve a minor degree of residual phosphorylase activity (~2% of normal) normalize oxidative capacity.[3]

Clinical features
Maximal effort muscle contraction in lifting or pushing heavy objects, performing sit-ups, or running the bases in softball or baseball rapidly cause fatigue, and if continued, lead to muscle contractures, pain, and rhabdomyolysis that may result in myoglobinuria and renal failure. Patients also experience fatigue, tachycardia, and sometimes shortness of breath with sustained moderate activity such as walking, especially uphill, and must routinely slow their pace or stop to rest after a few minutes. Patients often invent excuses to disguise this fatigability, such as checking a cell phone, tying a shoe, or looking in a window. On resuming activity, patients may experience a second wind with enhanced exercise capacity. Formal exercise testing indicates that the second

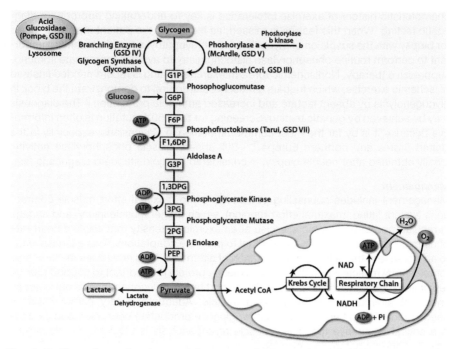

Fig. 1. Outline of muscle glycogen/glucose metabolism indicating defects that impair glycogen/glucose breakdown and glycogen synthesis. For the most common muscle glycogen storage diseases, glycogen storage disease (GSD) designations (GSD types II, III, V, and VII) eponyms are provided. Note that glycogen and glucose are metabolized anaerobically (with ATP generated by substrate-level phosphorylation and pyruvate reduced to lactate) as well as aerobically (with pyruvate metabolized to acetyl CoA with ATP produced via oxidative phosphorylation). PEP, phosphoenolpyruvate; PG, phosphoglycerate; DPG, diphosphoglycerate; G3P, glyceraldehyde-3-phosphate; F1 6 DP, fructose1 6 diphosphate; F6P, fructose-6-phosphate; G6P, glucose-6-phosphate.

wind reliably occurs after 6 to 8 minutes of exercise and is associated with a decrease in exercise heart rate that is proportional to an increase in muscle oxidative capacity.

Most patients experience muscle contractures, especially in the finger flexors after carrying bags or luggage. These are not necessarily painful, and patients often do not consider them cramps. The affected muscle is locked, and unlike common neural cramps, they cannot be relieved by stretching; attempting to do so causes pain. More than 50% of patients report one or more episodes of pigmenturia, which typically occurs the first time they urinate after exertional muscle injury.[4] About 10% of these patients have experienced renal failure.[5–7] Typically, patients have normal strength, but permanent muscle weakness occurs in up to 25% of patients with McArdle disease, most often affecting patients have who are more than 40 years old.[5–8]

Diagnosis

Despite symptoms of exercise intolerance from early childhood, the diagnosis is almost never made in the first decade of life; in approximately 50% of cases, the diagnosis is delayed until the fourth decade or later.[5] Generally, diagnostic testing is undertaken only after a sentinel event, such as an episode of rhabdomyolysis and myoglobinuria or after the discovery of an otherwise unexplained elevated serum CK level, which commonly is 5 to 10 times the upper limit of normal.[6] Recognition of the characteristic history of exercise intolerance is key to undertaking appropriate diagnostic testing. When this feature is missed, as it often is, the patient may be referred for biopsy with the suspicion of myositis or other myopathy, a fact that makes it important to perform routine phosphorylase histochemistry to avoid inappropriate immunosuppressive therapy. Nonischemic forearm exercise testing is recommended (instead of ischemic exercise, which triggers a muscle contracture) to demonstrate the block in glycogenolysis by absent lactate and increased ammonia production.[9] The diagnosis may be achieved by genetic testing. Screening for the R50X mutation is often informative because it is by far the most common mutation in Caucasians, especially in the United States and northern Europe.[5–7] Still absent muscle phosphorylase activity, ideally obtained after needle biopsy, is considered the gold standard diagnostic test.

Management
Management includes counseling patients to avoid maximal effort muscle contractions (weight lifting, maximal effort running), which trigger muscle injury, and engage in regular moderate, aerobic exercise at an exercise intensity that elicits a heart rate of no more than 60% to 70% of maximal to promote adaptations. This exercise leads to an increase in the delivery and utilization of alternative fuels and raises the threshold for exertional muscle injury.[10] Adequate dietary protein is important to support muscle repair and regeneration and possibly to support hepatic gluconeogenesis but is not an important alternative fuel for working muscle. Adequate dietary carbohydrate is needed to maintain hepatic glycogen for glucose production because blood glucose is a critical alternative fuel when muscle glycogenolysis is blocked. Simple sugars ingested shortly before exercise increase exercise capacity but must be used sparingly to avoid weight gain.[11]

Phosphorylase b Kinase Deficiency (Glycogen Storage Disease Type IX)

Pathophysiology
Phosphorylase b kinase (PhK) is a homotetramer with each tetramer containing 4 subunits, α, β, γ, and δ, with tissue-specific isoforms of all but the β subunit. Selective skeletal muscle PhK deficiency is an X-linked disorder caused by mutations in the PHAK1 gene, which encodes the muscle isoform of the α subunit, a regulatory component of the enzyme. PhK phosphorylates specific serine residues of glycogen phosphorylase, converting it from the inactive b form to the active a form.[12] However, phosphorylase can also be activated by AMP, inosine monophosphate, and inorganic phosphate. It has been hypothesized that deficiency of muscle PhK impairs glycogen breakdown by insufficient activation of muscle phosphorylase to cause a less severe form of muscle phosphorylase deficiency; but recent physiologic assessments of genetically proven muscle PhK deficiency have found little evidence of significant limitations in glycogen metabolism during exercise.

Clinical features
A host of neuromuscular manifestations have been attributed to muscle PhK deficiency including exertional muscle pain and muscle cramps, with or without myoglobinuria,[13–18] progressive proximal or distal weakness,[14,15,19] and otherwise asymptomatic hyperCKemia.[20,21] However, only 7 patients have had genetic confirmation of mutations in the PHKA1 gene[17,18,21–24]; serum CK and muscle glycogen levels have been reported as normal or elevated. Three patients with muscle PhK deficiency and confirmed PHKA1 mutations had minor and inconsistent limitations in lactate production with ischemic or cycle exercise testing.[21] From these reports and their own experience, the authors conclude that muscle PhK deficiency attributable to PHKA1 mutations does not cause clinically significant exercise limitations.

Diagnosis
Muscle biopsy may reveal elevated levels of subsarcolemmal glycogen, and muscle glycogen levels are typically elevated with biochemical assessment. Diagnosis is achieved by enzymatic analysis of muscle tissue or by genetic testing.

Management
Because there is little evidence that glycogen metabolism during exercise is significantly limited in this condition, it is unlikely that exercise-related symptoms are the direct result of this metabolic defect.

Muscle PFK Deficiency (Tauri Disease, Glycogen Storage Disease Type VII)

Pathophysiology
PFK enzyme catalyzes the rate-limiting step of glycolysis. There are 3 isoforms of PFK: muscle (M), liver (L), and platelet (P). PFK is a tetramer, and in muscle, the tetramer consists exclusively of the M isoform. Erythrocytes contain both the M and L isoforms.[25] Deficiency of the M isoform leads to a complete block of glycolysis in muscles and a partial block in red blood cells. Like McArdle disease, PFK deficiency results in impaired anaerobic and oxidative metabolism.[26] Unlike McArdle disease, glucose administration cannot bypass the block in glycolysis.

Clinical features
The clinical manifestations of PFK deficiency closely mirror those of McArdle disease, with lifelong low exercise capacity and muscle contractures and rhabdomyolysis provoked by brief maximal effort muscle contractions. Patients also have low oxidative capacity and develop fatigue, tachycardia, and shortness of breath, often associated with nausea, with modest aerobic exercise. In contrast to patients with McArdle disease, patients do not experience a second wind, because exogenous glucose cannot bypass the block in glycolysis.[26] Carbohydrate ingestion lowers exercise and oxidative capacity in PFK deficiency by inhibiting lipolysis and lowering blood levels of fatty acids.[27] In addition, these patients have compensated hemolytic anemia. Patients from multiple different ethnic backgrounds have been affected, but the disease is especially prevalent in people of Ashkenazi Jewish descent.[28] A severe infantile variant as well as a late-onset form with progressive weakness have been described.

Diagnosis
The diagnosis of PFK deficiency is suspected in cases of exercise intolerance with a compensated hemolytic anemia (increased reticulocytes and bilirubin levels). Forearm exercise testing shows no lactate and exaggerated ammonia production. [31]Phosphorus magnetic resonance spectroscopy undertaken during exercise shows no pH decrease in exercising muscle, as well as a phosphomonoester peak secondary to the accumulation of sugar phosphates behind the block in glycolysis. The diagnosis can be confirmed by absent PFK histochemical staining, by decreased PFK enzymatic activity, or by genetic testing. It should be emphasized that PFK is a highly labile enzyme with enzymatic activity easily lost by improper muscle handling. In fact most patients referred to the authors' center with alleged PFK deficiency have been proved to be incorrectly diagnosed related to loss of enzymatic activity by this mechanism.

Management
Management consists of patient counseling to avoid strenuous exercise and also avoidance of high carbohydrate intake immediately before exercise. Moderate aerobic exercise should be encouraged.

Phosphoglucomutase Deficiency

Pathophysiology

Phosphoglucomutase 1 (PGM1) catalyzes the interconversion of glucose-1-phosphate and glucose-6-phosphate and is the predominant isoform found in muscle and liver. In addition, PGM1 is critical for normal protein glycosylation.[29]

Clinical features

Deficiency of muscle PGM1 was first described in a 35-year-old man without congenital abnormalities who had exercise-induced muscle cramps, 2 episodes of pigmenturia, and CK levels that increased 10- to 20-fold after strenuous exercise. Exercise testing revealed an exaggerated increase in ammonia but a normal increase in lactate with both ischemic forearm exercise and cycle testing.[30] A second patient with a congenital glycosylation defect including first branchial arch syndrome had chronically elevated CK levels, fatigue with mild exercise, and no increase in lactate with forearm testing indicating that the severity of blocked glycogen breakdown and the presence of associated symptoms may vary widely.[31] A recent series of 19 patients that focused on the congenital glycosylation defect in this enzyme deficiency identified myopathy as a manifestation of approximately half of these patients.[32]

Management

Exercise testing in the originally described patient revealed a tendency to hypoglycemia and improved exercise capacity with glucose infusion, endorsing the need for adequate dietary carbohydrate.[33] Galactose supplementation was shown to improve glycosylation in cultured fibroblasts and in the serum of 6 patients who had received this treatment[32]; 2 patients reported to have recurrent rhabdomyolysis had no further episodes while on this therapy.

Distal Glycolytic Defects

Pathophysiology

Distal glycolytic defects include phosphoglycerate kinase (PGK), phosphoglycerate mutase (PGM), and lactate dehydrogenase (LDH) deficiencies. These defects typically preserve a fraction of enzymatic activity that is sufficient to produce a 2-fold (in contrast to a normal 4- to 5-fold) increase in lactate levels with forearm exercise. Symptoms of fatigue, muscle contractures, and rhabdomyolysis are triggered by maximal effort muscle contractions that require peak rates of glycolysis. Because relatively modest rates of pyruvate production are sufficient to support glycogen-dependent oxidative metabolism, oxidative capacity is relatively preserved in these disorders and is not affected by variations in fuel availability related to diet or exercise as in muscle phosphorylase and PFK deficiencies.

Clinical features

PGK is encoded by a single gene on Xq13 in all tissues but testes. The clinical manifestations of PGK deficiency are heterogeneous. Nonspherocytic hemolytic anemia alone or with central nervous system (CNS) involvement (including mental retardation, seizures, tremor, or behavioral abnormalities) is seen in approximately one-third of cases. Another third has an isolated myopathy with muscle cramps, pain, and pigmenturia triggered by high-intensity exercise. Other presentations include myopathy with CNS involvement, anemia with myopathy, or involvement of all 3 systems. Responsible mutations are diverse with differing clinical manifestations postulated to relate to differences in protein stability, catalytic activity, or both.[34]

PGM has 2 isoforms, M (muscle) and B (brain), and functions as a dimer. In muscle, 95% of the enzyme activity is attributable to the MM homodimer, whereas MB or BB isoforms predominate in other tissues. Mutations in the M isoform cause a pure myopathy characterized by exertional fatigue, contractures, and myoglobinuria. Of the 15 cases, 10 described to date affected African Americans in whom a common W78X mutation was most often responsible. Tubular aggregates are often present in the muscle biopsy.[35]

LDH is a tetrameric enzyme containing muscle (LDH-A), heart (LDH-B), or both subunits. A deficiency was first described in Japan and subsequently identified in 2 families from North America. The disorder is purely a defect in anaerobic glycolysis. Nicotinamide adenine dinucleotide phosphate formed in glycolysis via glyceraldehyde phosphate dehydrogenase (GADPH) and normally oxidized by LDH builds up with levels of exercise that normally would result in accelerated lactate formation and ultimately blocks glycolysis at the level of GADPH. Rapid fatigue, contractures, and rhabdomyolysis with myoglobinuria accompany maximal effort exercise. Affected patients sometimes have an associated dermatitis because LDH-A is the dominant isoform expressed in skin.

Diagnosis

Forearm exercise testing reveals a blunted lactate level and an exaggerated ammonia increase indicating a relative block in glycolysis. ^{31}P magnetic resonance spectroscopy detects an exercise-induced increase in a phosphomonoester peak related to sugar phosphates that accumulate behind the metabolic block to confirm a defect in glycolysis. Diagnosis is made by enzyme analysis of muscle.

Management

Patients should be counseled to avoid the high-intensity exercise that can lead to muscle damage and myoglobinuria. More moderate, regular aerobic exercise may increase aerobic fitness and exercise capacity and raise the threshold for exercise-induced muscle symptoms.

Other Rare Defects

There are 3 isoforms of aldolase (A, B, C) encoded by 3 different genes. The A isoform is the sole form in muscle and red blood cells. Aldolase A deficiency causes hemolytic anemia, and in 2 patients, it has been reported to cause hemolytic anemia and myopathy.[36,37] In these patients, hemolytic anemia and rhabdomyolysis were triggered by a febrile illness, attributable to the thermolability of the mutant enzyme.

Beta-enolase deficiency has been described in a single patient with exercise-induced muscle pain and fatigability without pigmenturia.[38] Enolase is a dimeric enzyme composed potentially of 3 isoforms coded by separate genes, alpha (ubiquitous), beta (muscle), and gamma (brain). The beta isoform is found exclusively in muscle. The affected patient had 5% of normal enolase in muscle and a blunted lactate response to ischemic forearm exercise.

To date, 5 patients from 3 families have been described with muscle glycogen synthase deficiency (GYS1).[39–41] Of the 5 patients, 2 died of sudden cardiac arrest in childhood. All 5 patients have had evidence of cardiac involvement. Of the 5 patients, 2 also experienced recurrent generalized tonic-clonic seizures. Results of muscle biopsy have shown decreased glycogen content, type I fiber predominance, and mitochondrial proliferation.

There has also been a report of 1 patient with a missense mutation in the gene encoding the muscle primer glycogenin-1 (GYG1), resulting in failure of glycogenin to autoglycosylate, a crucial step for the initiation of glycogen synthesis.[42] The clinical phenotype was similar to glycogen synthase deficiency with exercise intolerance and cardiomyopathy. Results of muscle biopsy showed absent glycogen with marked type 1 fiber predominance and mitochondrial proliferation.

CARBOHYDRATE DISORDERS CAUSING MUSCLE WEAKNESS
Debrancher Deficiency (Cori Disease, Glycogen Storage Disease Type III)

Pathophysiology

Debrancher is a single protein with 2 separate enzymatic domains: one is an oligo-1,4-1,4-glucantransferase and the other is an amylo-1,6-glucosidase. Once the peripheral chains of glycogen have been shortened by phosphorylase to 4 glycosyl units, these stubs are removed by debrancher in 2 steps. First, a maltotriosyl unit is transferred from a donor to an acceptor chain (transferase activity) leaving behind a single glycosyl unit. Second, the remaining glycosyl unit is hydrolyzed by the amylo-1,6-glucosidase, liberating a molecule of glucose. Debrancher is encoded by a single gene, although expression of the enzyme varies in a tissue-dependent manner by alternative splicing.[43] Clinical symptoms result from impaired glycogen breakdown and glycogen accumulation in the liver and variable impairment of the degradation of glycogen in skeletal and cardiac muscles. To date, more than 100 mutations have been reported.[43] In 85% of cases (glycogen storage disease [GSD] type IIIa), debrancher deficiency affects liver and muscle; less commonly (15% of cases), debrancher deficiency affects liver only (GSD type IIIb).

Clinical features

In GSD type IIIa, disease manifestations begin in infancy and childhood with symptoms predominately secondary to hepatic involvement and include hepatomegaly, hypoglycemia, ketosis, hyperlipidemia, and short stature. These symptoms typically improve with age; however, there are reports of liver disease progressing to cirrhosis, hepatic adenoma formation, or hepatocellular carcinoma.[44] Patients may also develop left ventricular hypertrophy, which can progress to symptomatic hypertrophic cardiomyopathy and arrhythmias, and even necessitate cardiac transplant.[45] There have even been cases in which cardiac involvement was suspected as the cause for sudden death.[46]

Skeletal muscle symptoms may begin in childhood with delayed motor milestones, but weakness typically develops in the third or fourth decade of life with a course that is generally slowly progressive, and not debilitating.[47] Patients may have symmetric, predominantly proximal, or more generalized weakness. Another manifestation is distal weakness and atrophy, suggesting the diagnosis of Charcot-Marie-Tooth or motor neuron disease.[48] In contrast to patients with muscle phosphorylase deficiency, exertional muscle contractures, recurrent rhabdomyolysis, and pigmenturia are not typical of this disorder despite the fact that patients commonly have blunted lactate and exaggerated ammonia increase with forearm exercise similar to glycolytic disorders with such exercise-induced symptoms. However, a recent cycle exercise study revealed low work and oxidative capacity compared with those of control subjects, which were improved by glucose infusion implying the presence of substrate-limited oxidative metabolism.[49]

Diagnosis

Elevated serum aspartate aminotransferase, alanine aminotransferase, and CK levels in a patient with hepatomegaly and ketotic hypoglycemia should raise the possibility of debrancher deficiency. Electromyography may show both neurogenic and myopathic features.[50] Muscle histochemistry shows abnormal glycogen accumulation, and biochemistry may identify glycogen with short outer branches.[44] The diagnosis can be confirmed by enzymatic testing on muscle or liver or by genetic testing.[44]

Management
Infants and children should be managed with avoidance of fasting and frequent feedings. Cornstarch may be used to maintain euglycemia. There are also reports of improvement in myopathy and cardiomyopathy with high-protein diet.[51–53] Adults are advised to adopt a high-protein diet with complex carbohydrates favored over simple sugars. Patients with GSD type IIIa should be monitored with echocardiogram every 12 to 24 months and electrocardiogram every other year. Liver function tests should be monitored every 6 to 12 months, and hepatic ultrasonography should be performed every 12 to 24 months.[44]

Glycogen Branching Enzyme Deficiency (Andersen Disease, GSD Type IV)

Pathophysiology
Glycogen branching enzyme (GBE) participates in the synthesis of glycogen by transferring alpha-1,4-linked glucosyl units from the outer end of a glycogen chain to an alpha-1,6 position, leading to branched glycogen with increased solubility and decreased osmotic strength.[54] GBE deficiency, an autosomal recessive disorder, results in the accumulation of glycogen with few branch points (resembling amylopectin) in all tissues to variable degrees.[55] To date, 40 mutations in the gene encoding GBE have been described.[56] The relationship between genotype and phenotype remains poorly understood.

Clinical features
There is considerable variation in the presentation of branching enzyme deficiency, with variable involvement of the liver, heart, skeletal muscle, and the CNS. The classic form of the disease presents in childhood with liver disease, leading to cirrhosis and death by 5 years of age. However, some patients have a milder form of the disease and can reach adulthood without progression of liver disease.[57] There is also significant variation in the degree of neuromuscular involvement, ranging from a severe perinatal presentation with fetal akinesia deformation sequence, consisting of multiple congenital contractures, hydrops fetalis, and perinatal death, to an isolated myopathy with or without cardiomyopathy presenting in childhood or adulthood.[55] Adult polyglucosan body disease, caused by intracellular accumulation of abnormal amylopectin-like glycogen in both the central and peripheral nervous systems, presents with neurogenic bladder, spastic paraplegia, and axonal neuropathy.[58]

Diagnosis
Results of muscle, liver, or nerve biopsies may demonstrate accumulations of abnormal glycogen, polyglucosan bodies. The diagnosis can be confirmed by analysis of GBE activity in liver, muscle, or fibroblasts. Gene sequencing can also be performed to confirm the diagnosis.

Management
No guidelines currently exist for management of GBE deficiency. Liver function tests, abdominal ultrasonography, and echocardiogram should be performed, with frequency depending on the severity of the disease. Transplant can be considered for severe liver or cardiac disease.[56]

LIPID METABOLISM DISORDERS CAUSING MUSCLE WEAKNESS AND LIPID ACCUMULATION

Primary Carnitine Deficiency

Pathophysiology
Primary carnitine deficiency is an autosomal recessive disorder caused by mutations in the gene encoding the high-affinity, sodium-dependent plasma membrane carnitine

transporter, OCTN2, causing impaired muscle carnitine transport across the plasma membrane of cells and impaired reabsorption of the filtered carnitine by the kidney (**Fig. 2**).[59] Carnitine is required for the transport of long-chain fatty acids into the mitochondrial matrix, where fatty acid oxidation takes place.

Clinical features

The most severe presentation occurs in infants, and is characterized by hypotonia and episodes of metabolic crisis triggered by fasting or infections with hypoketotic hypoglycemia, elevated ammonia, hepatomegaly, and hepatic encephalopathy. A childhood onset form presents with muscle weakness, elevated levels of CK, and cardiomyopathy. At the other end of the spectrum, some adults may only present with complaints of easy fatigability.[60] Affected women may decompensate during pregnancy.

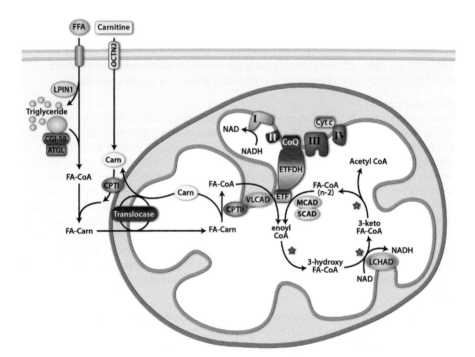

Fig. 2. Overview of fat utilization in skeletal muscle indicating sites of genetic defects that impair fat metabolism. OCTN2, carnitine transporter; FFA, free fatty acid; LPIN1, protein involved in triglyceride synthesis; ATGL, adipose triglyceride lipase; GCI-58, protein involved in activation of ATGL; Carn, carnitine; CPT1, carnitine palmitoyl transferase 1; translocase, the carnitne, fatty acylCo-A transferase; CPT2, carnitine palmitoyl transferase 2; VLCAD, very long chain acyl Co-A dehydrogenase; MCAD and SCAD, medium and short chain acylCo-A dehydrogenase; ETF, electron transfer flavoprotein (receives electrons from the dehydrogenase reaction catalyzed by VLCAD, MCAD and SCAD); ETFDH, electron transfer flavoprotein dehydrogenase (receives electrons from ETF, transfers them to coenzyme Q10 for oxidation via respiratory chain complexes III and IV); enolyl CoA, 3-hydroxy FA-CoA, 3 keto FA-CoA are intermediates in beta oxidation ultimately yielding acetyl-CoA (for oxidation by the TCA cycle and a fatty acylCoA (FA-CoA) shortened by two carbons for further beta oxidation; LCHAD, long chain hydroxy-acylCo-A dehydrogenase, one of the three enzymatic reactions (indicated by stars) catalyzed by mitochondrial trifunctional proten. NADH produced in the reaction catalyzed by LCHAD is oxidized via complex I of the respiratory chain.

Diagnosis

Primary carnitine deficiency causes increased intramuscular lipid deposition predominantly in type 1 muscle fibers. Diagnosis is suggested by severe deficiency (<10% of normal) of free carnitine and acylcarnitines in plasma, muscle, and other tissues and may be confirmed by the demonstration of impaired carnitine uptake in lymphocytes or fibroblasts of patients.[60]

Management

Patients should be monitored for cardiomyopathy and arrhythmias with echocardiogram and electrocardiogram. L-Carnitine supplementation should be initiated as soon as possible, and lifelong compliance results in a favorable prognosis.[60]

Neutral Lipid Storage Disease

Pathophysiology

Neutral lipid storage disease (NLSD) is caused by mutations in neutral lipases necessary for the liberation of fatty acids from triglyceride stores in skeletal muscle, adipocytes, and other tissues. Adipocyte triglyceride lipase (ATGL), activated by the protein CGI-58, catalyzes the first step in triglyceride hydrolysis. Mutations in the gene encoding CGI-58, ABHD5, cause NLSD with icthyosis (NLSDI) or Chanarin-Dorfman syndrome.[61] NLSD with myopathy (NLSDM) is caused by mutations in the gene encoding ATGL, PNPLA2.[62] Both fatty acid mobilization and use during exercise seem to be impaired in this disorder.[63]

Clinical features

Patients with NLSDI typically have mild weakness associated with marked lipid accumulation in skeletal muscle and other tissues in conjunction with the characteristic dermatologic feature of icthyosis.[64] Patients with NLSDM may be asymptomatic despite elevated CK levels and marked lipid accumulation in muscle, heart, and other tissues. These patients commonly develop muscle weakness usually around the third decade, sometimes associated with dilated cardiomyopathy.[65]

Diagnosis

Patients with NLSD have a characteristic accumulation of lipid droplets within leukocytes on peripheral blood smear, a finding that is known as Jordans anomaly. Results of muscle biopsy show massive lipid accumulation especially in type I muscle fibers.[66]

Management

There are no established treatments for these conditions.

MADD

Pathophysiology

MADD is caused by mutations in electron transfer flavoprotein (ETF) A or B or to mutations in electron transfer flavoprotein dehydrogenase (ETFDH, ETF:ubiquinone oxidoreductase).[67] These proteins function to transfer electrons from multiple dehydrogenases involved in fatty acid oxidation to coenzyme Q10 in the respiratory chain.

Clinical features

The clinical presentation can range from a fatal infantile form with multisystem disease with or without congenital malformations to a milder disease with later onset. Late-onset disease may cause proximal limb and axial weakness (especially neck weakness), dysphagia, exercise intolerance, hepatomegaly, and episodes of encephalopathy, myoglobinuria, vomiting, and hypoglycemia, which may be triggered by infections, fasting, or surgery.[68,69] The late-onset variant has been found to be most commonly associated with ETFDH mutations.[68]

Diagnosis

Serum CK levels may be elevated. Acylcarnitine profiles show elevated concentrations of acylcarnitines of all lengths. Serum carnitine levels may be decreased. Organic aciduria with excretion of hydroxyglutaric, ethymalonic, and dicarboxylic acids is also characteristic.[70] Respiratory chain complexes may also show decreased activity in some patients.[71] Results of muscle biopsy demonstrate increased lipid deposition.

Management

Riboflavin has been shown to improve symptoms in a group of patients, known as riboflavin responsive MADD (RR-MADD). Patients with RR-MADD have been shown to have mutations in the ETFDH gene.[68] A secondary deficiency of coenzyme Q may be associated with MADD because of ETFDH mutations, and coenzyme Q (CoQ) supplementation is appropriate for these patients.[72] Patients should also be counseled to avoid fasting.[73]

LIPID METABOLISM DISORDERS CAUSING RECURRENT MYALGIA, RHABDOMYOLYSIS, AND MYOGLOBINURIA
CPT2 Deficiency

Pathophysiology

CPT2 deficiency is the most common disorder of fatty acid oxidation and the most common metabolic cause of recurrent rhabdomyolysis and myoglobinuria. The CPT proteins are involved in the transport of long-chain fatty acids into the mitochondrial matrix, where fatty acid oxidation takes place.[74] CPT1 is located in the outer mitochondrial membrane, whereas CPT2 is located in the inner aspect of the inner mitochondrial membrane.

Clinical features

A severe neonatal form presents with encephalopathy, congenital malformations, hepatomegaly, and cardiomegaly and is rapidly fatal. An infantile form presents with recurrent liver failure, hypoketotic hypoglycemia, and seizures. Episodes can be triggered by infections, fever, or fasting. The common adult myopathic form presents with recurrent muscle pain, rhabdomyolysis, and myoglobinuria. These episodes can also be triggered by fever, fasting, or prolonged submaximal exercise (especially when activity is undertaken while fasting). In contrast to patients with glycolytic disorders, these patients are able to easily tolerate brief maximal exercise. The more severe neonatal and infantile forms of the disease correlate with more severely reduced CPT2 enzyme activity than the mutations associated with the milder myopathic adult form of the disease.[75] In the myopathic form, the presence of residual enzyme activity may be adequate to support fat oxidation at rest but is not sufficient for normal fat oxidation during exercise.[76] Patients with haploinsufficiency of the CPT2 gene may also experience limited fat oxidation during exercise.[76]

Diagnosis

Diagnosis is suggested by increased long-chain acylcarnitines (C-18, 18:1, 16) in blood after an overnight fast or in fibroblasts incubated with long-chain fatty acids. Enzyme activity can be measured in fibroblasts, lymphocytes, or skeletal muscle. Genetic testing can also be used to confirm pathogenic mutations in the CPT2 gene.[67] The common Ser113Leu missense mutation accounts for about 70% of mutant alleles.[77]

Management

Patients should be instructed to avoid fasting and to eat sufficient carbohydrates, with carbohydrate-rich snacks between meals and when patients are physically active. An alternative source of fuel is medium-chain triglycerides, which are a source of medium-chain fatty acids that can diffuse into the mitochondrial matrix independent of the carnitine shuttle. Bezafibrate, a peroxisome proliferator-activated receptor agonist, has been shown to increase CPT2 messenger RNA and protein levels, leading to increased long-chain fatty acid oxidation. A 3-year study of 6 patients treated with bezafibrate resulted in improvement in the patients' perceived function, level of physical activity, and muscle pain.[78]

VLCAD Deficiency

Pathophysiology

VLCAD localizes to the inner mitochondrial membrane and catalyzes the first step in oxidation of long-chain fatty acids after importation into the mitochondrial matrix and metabolism by CPT2.[79]

Clinical features

Null mutations in VLCAD cause severe, often fatal multisystem disease in infancy, whereas missense mutations that retain some residual enzyme activity cause recurrent rhabdomyolysis and myoglobinuria that mimics adult CPT2 deficiency. Exercise, fasting, and cold exposure may trigger episode of rhabdomyolysis.[80]

Diagnosis

Key to diagnosis is the assessment of fasting plasma acylcarnitines that reveals an accumulation of long-chain acylcarnitines with tetradecenoylcarnitine (C14:1) as the predominant acylcarnitine.[81] Responsible mutations are diverse.

Management

Management is similar to that of CPT2 deficiency, with avoidance of fasting; a high-carbohydrate, low-fat diet; and medium-chain triglyceride supplementation. Bezafibrate may also be beneficial in VLCAD deficiency as in CPT2 deficiency.[82]

TP/Long-Chain 3-Hydroxyacyl-CoA Dehydrogenase Deficiency

Pathophysiology

Trifunctional protein (TP) encompasses 3 enzyme reactions involved in long-chain fatty acid oxidation, enoyl-CoA hydratase, long-chain 3-hydroxyacyl-CoA dehydrogenase (LCHAD), and acyl thiolase (see **Fig. 2**), and yields acetyl CoA and an acyl CoA shorted by 2 carbons, which becomes the substrate of a new β-oxidation cycle. Mutations can affect all subunits of the enzyme, although most commonly LCHAD.[67]

Clinical features

TP mutations affecting all enzyme activities or predominantly LCHAD produce severe, infantile or adult forms. The adult form manifests with recurrent rhabdomyolysis, triggered by exercise, fasting, or infection. Rhabdomyolysis is often associated with respiratory failure. TP mutations are often associated with an axonal sensorimotor peripheral neuropathy and pigmentary retinopathy, distinguishing this condition from CPT2 and VLCAD deficiencies.[67]

Diagnosis

Between episodes of rhabdomyolysis, the acylcarnitine profile may be normal. However, elevated hydroxyacylcarnitine levels and 3-hydroxydicarboxylic aciduria accompany episodes of rhabdomyolysis.[67] A gly510gln missense mutation accounts for 90% of mutant alleles in LCHAD deficiency.

Management
As in other long-chain fatty acid defects, avoidance of fasting, adequate carbohydrate, and medium-chain triglyceride supplements are common approaches to therapy.

Lipin-1 Deficiency

Pathophysiology
The LPIN1 gene encodes lipin-1, which has 2 functions: (1) a phosphatidic acid phosphatase to convert phosphatidic acid to diacylglycerol, which is involved in triglyceride and phospholipid synthesis, and (2) a transcriptional coactivator to regulate genes involved in fatty acid oxidation and mitochondrial biosynthesis.[83] The exact mechanism by which LPIN1 mutations cause recurrent rhabdomyolysis remains poorly understood.

Clinical features
LPIN1 gene mutations are a major cause of severe recurrent episodes of rhabdomyolysis in childhood almost always triggered by febrile illnesses, occasionally by fasting. The first episode of rhabdomyolysis typically begins before the age of 6 years (mean age of onset 30 months).[84] However, at least 1 adult has been described with an LPIN1 mutation, with the first episode of rhabdomyolysis occurring at the age of 42 years.[84]

Diagnosis
Muscle biopsy may show increased lipid accumulation. Diagnosis is confirmed by genetic testing.[84]

Management
Management currently involves supportive care during episodes of rhabdomyolysis.

Mitochondrial Myopathies

Mitochondrial myopathies are conventionally considered to be genetic defects that predominate in skeletal muscle and impair the synthesis, assembly, or maintenance of components the respiratory chain (**Fig. 3**). The number of defects responsible is experiencing exponential growth and now includes myopathies caused by (1) primary mtDNA mutations; (2) nuclear mutations that disrupt the replication or maintenance of mtDNA leading to multiple mtDNA deletions or/and mtDNA depletion; (3) nuclear mutations that directly impair the synthesis of individual respiratory chain subunits, alter the synthesis of critical prosthetic groups, or impair the function of critical assembly factors; and (4) nuclear mutations that impair mitochondrial protein synthesis.[85]

mtDNA Mutations

Pathophysiology
mtDNA mutations are classically heteroplasmic with impairment of respiratory chain function when the percentage of mutant mtDNA reaches a critical threshold.

Clinical
The first class of mtDNA mutations recognized to cause mitochondrial myopathy were heteroplasmic, single large-scale deletions. Affected patients characteristically have chronic progressive external ophthalmoplegia (CPEO) with or without a more generalized myopathy, or a multisystem syndrome (Kearns-Sayre syndrome) with CPEO, pigmentary retinopathy, cardiac conduction defects, and CNS dysfunction. Another

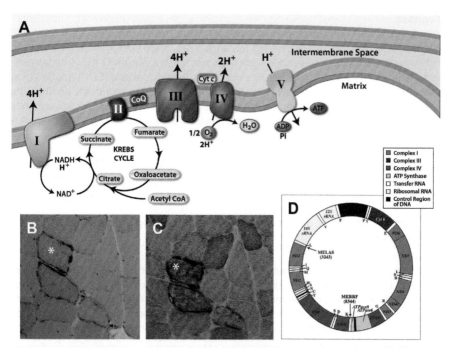

Fig. 3. Cartoon illustrating mitochondrial respiratory chain complexes (*A*) and mitochondrial DNA (*D*) indicating transfer RNA genes (letters) and coding subunits that are components of complexes I, III, IV, and V. Note that subunits of complex II are exclusively nuclear encoded, so expression of complex II (succinate dehydrogenase) is preserved and typically enhanced in proportion to mitochondrial proliferation with mitochondrial DNA mutations. (*B*) and (*C*) are serial sections of muscle from a patient with a heteroplasmic mtDNA mutation. Muscle fibers with a high abundance of mutant mtDNA show subsarcolemmal mitochondrial proliferation resulting in ragged red fibers (*asterisk*) with Gomori trichrome (*B*); the same fibers stain blue with combined cytochrome c oxidase (complex IV) and succinate dehydrogenase (complex II) stain (*C*). CoQ, coenzyme Q; MELAS, mitochondrial encephalomyopathy, lactic acidosis, and strokelike episodes; MERRF, myoclonus epilepsy with ragged red fibers.

class of pathogenic mtDNA defects is represented by point mutations that are maternally inherited or sporadic and affect transfer RNA (tRNA) or coding region genes. Muscle weakness and/or exercise intolerance commonly accompanies multisystem mitochondrial disease, including classic maternally inherited mitochondrial encephalomyopathies caused by the m.3243A>G mutation in tRNA$^{leu(UUR)}$, the most common cause of mitochondrial encephalomyopathy, lactic acidosis, and strokelike episodes and the m.8344A>G mutation in tRNA^{lys}, the typical cause of myoclonus epilepsy with ragged red fibers. Pure myopathy, often characterized by marked exercise intolerance, has been associated with heteroplasmic mutations in tRNA or protein-coding genes, especially the cytochrome b gene. Most mutations in protein-coding genes are sporadic and apparently de novo. Although pathogenic mtDNA mutations that cause mitochondrial myopathy are typically heteroplasmic; homoplasmic mutations are sometimes responsible. Notably, the reversible cytochrome c oxidase (COX) deficiency (also known as reversible respiratory chain deficiency) of infancy is caused by a maternally inherited homoplasmic m.14674T>C mutation in tRNA^{glu}.[86]

Diagnosis
Muscle fibers harboring large percentages of mutant mtDNA exhibit subsarcolemmal mitochondrial proliferation, appearing as ragged red fibers with the modified Gomori trichrome stain. Usually these fibers lack COX histochemical activity (COX-negative fibers), whereas they stain intensely with succinate dehydrogenase (SDH) (ragged blue fibers). This muscle histology profile is typical of most mtDNA mutations and reflects deficiency of respiratory chain complexes that contain mtDNA-encoded subunits (especially complex IV) while preserving complex II (SDH), all subunits of which are nuclear encoded (see **Fig. 3**). Fibroblast growth factor 21 (FGF21) is upregulated in mitochondrial myopathies caused by mtDNA and other mutations, and plasma FGF21 levels is commonly increased in these patients.[87,88] Accordingly, FGF21 has been advanced as a potentially important diagnostic test in mitochondrial myopathy patients.

Mitochondrial Myopathy due to Nuclear Mutations Causing Multiple mtDNA Deletions or mtDNA Depletion

Pathogenesis
Mutations in nuclear genes necessary for mtDNA replication and maintenance generally result in adult-onset CPEO, usually dominantly inherited.[89] Most often, mutations in the catalytic subunit of the mtDNA polymerase, polymerase gamma (POLG) are responsible. However, mutations in other nuclear genes also cause CPEO and myopathy, including the mtDNA helicase; Twinkle, the muscle-heart isoform of the mitochondrial adenine nucleotide translocase (ANT1); and the ribonucleotide reductase, p53-R2 subunit (RRM2B). Phenotypes include not only CPEO and weakness but also CPEO with peripheral or CNS disorders and other symptoms. CPEO and multiple mtDNA deletions also may be seen in mitochondrial neurogastrointestinal encephalomyopathy, attributable to mutations in thymidine phosphorylase (TYMP).[90] POLG1, Twinkle, and TYMP mutations may also be associated with mtDNA depletion.[91] Among other defects responsible for mtDNA depletion, thymidine kinase 2 (TK2) defects are noteworthy. TK2 mutations cause a rapidly progressive myopathy of infancy or early childhood associated with elevated CK levels and muscle histology resembling muscular dystrophy or spinal muscular atrophy.[91]

Diagnosis
Mitochondrial myopathies attributable to these mutations typically cause varying abundance of COX-negative, SDH-positive fibers, which are best visualized with the combined COX/SDH stain; cytochrome b or complex I subunit mutations contain ragged red fibers that are COX positive. When the phenotype is CPEO, genetic testing to ascertain whether there are multiple mtDNA deletions is the appropriate next step, followed by genetic testing for genes known to cause these abnormalities.

Mitochondrial Myopathy due to Nuclear DNA Mutations Affecting Individual Subunits, Prosthetic Groups, or Respiratory Complex Assembly

Pathophysiology/Clinical
This class of mitochondrial disease encompasses a large array of defects. Most of the nuclear gene defects that have been identified to date affect subunits or assembly factors that result in deficiency of complexes I or IV and cause childhood encephalopathy. However several mitochondrial myopathies attributable to nuclear defects have been described. Myopathy with coenzyme Q deficiency has multiple causes. A common cause of secondary CoQ deficiency in association with weakness, exercise intolerance, CK level elevation, and muscle lipid accumulation have been shown to be

attributable to riboflavin-responsive mutations in ETFDH. Another form of myopathic CoQ deficiency was due to a mutation in CABC1, the human homolog of a gene necessary for ubiquinone synthesis in yeast.[92] Additional genetic mechanisms of myopathic CoQ deficiency remain to be discovered. Acyl-CoA dehydrogenase 9 (ACAD9), which closely resembles VLCAD, has been shown to be important for complex I assembly. Mutations in ACAD9 result in childhood onset, severe exercise intolerance, and riboflavin-responsive complex I deficiency[93]; other mutations in this gene may cause cardiomyopathy and encephalopathy.[94] Another interesting pure mitochondrial myopathy is attributable to a splice site mutation in the iron-sulfur (Fe-S) cluster scaffold (ISCU) gene resulting in ISCU deficiency and reduced levels of Fe-S cluster containing proteins including the tricarboxylic acid cycle enzymes aconitase and SDH and Fe-S subunits of respiratory chain complexes I and III.[95] Symptoms are lifelong severe exercise intolerance in which modest exercise causes fatigue, tachycardia, and shortness of breath with episodes of myoglobinuria. Detailed physiologic investigations performed in affected patients more than 40 years ago represent the first description of exercise pathophysiology in a severe mitochondrial myopathy showing dramatically impaired extraction of oxygen from blood and a hyperkinetic circulation in exercise with a marked mismatch between O_2 delivery and O_2 use.[96] Subsequent study has revealed that this exercise response is a consistent feature of all severe muscle oxidative defects.[97]

Mitochondrial Myopathy due to Defects in Mitochondrial tRNA Translation

Pathophysiology/Clinical
Mitochondrial protein synthesis requires a vast array of nuclear-encoded proteins including those involved in modifying mitochondrial tRNA bases; aminoacyl-tRNA synthetases that attach specific amino acids to tRNAs; ribosomal proteins and assembly factors; translation initiation, elongation, and release factors; and translational activators.[98] Most mutations result predominantly in CNS disease including Leigh syndrome, leukoencephalopathy, ataxia, and spastic paraplegia. However, mitochondrial myopathy is a central feature of myopathy, lactic acidosis, and sideroblastic anemia (MLASA) attributable to mutations in pseudouridine synthase 1, which converts urine to pseudouridine in the pseudouridine loop that is characteristic of tRNAs.[99] MLASA can also be caused by mutations in YARS2, the aminoacyl-tRNA synthetase that catalyzes the binding of tyrosine to its cognate tRNA.[100] Another tRNA-base-modifying gene, TRMU, most often causes a reversible infantile hepatopathy, but TRMU mutations have also been implicated as a cause of reversible infantile respiratory chain (also known as cytochrome oxidase) deficiency.[101] These abnormalities in mitochondrial protein synthesis mimic the biochemical and, often, the histologic features of primary mtDNA mutations (tRNA mutations, large-scale mtDNA deletions) and nuclear mutations that lead to multiple mtDNA deletions or mtDNA depletion. They result in variable deficiency of respiratory chain complexes that contain mitochondrial-encoded subunits (complex I, III, IV, and V) and mitochondrial proliferation that results in elevated levels of nuclear-encoded mitochondrial enzymes such as citrate synthase and SDH. Muscle histology may also reveal a checkerboard or more generalized pattern of cytochrome-oxidase-negative, SDH-positive muscle fibers.

Diagnosis
Serum testing may reveal elevated lactate levels or an elevated lactate to pyruvate ratio. Serum CK levels are typically normal. Cycle exercise testing shows reduced oxidative capacity, reduced arteriovenous oxygen difference, and hyperdynamic circulation

with increased cardiac output relative to oxygen use. Muscle biopsy may reveal muscle fibers with mitochondrial proliferation causing ragged red fibers on Gomori trichrome staining. Dual staining for SDH (nuclear encoded) and COX, encoded by both nuclear DNA and mtDNA may show COX-deficient fibers with intact SDH staining. However, normal aging causes a low frequency of SDH-positive, COX-negative fibers. Respiratory enzyme activity may also be measured on muscle tissue. Citrate synthetase activity is increased due to mitochondrial proliferation, so respiratory chain complex activities should be normalized to citrate synthetase when evaluating for deficient respiratory chain complexes. Definitive diagnosis can be made by genetic testing of the mitochondrial genome as well as nuclear genes known to be targeted to the mitochondria.

Management
A recent Cochrane review identified 12 randomized controlled trials without bias for treatments in mitochondrial disease. These studies included high-dose coenzyme Q10, creatine monohydrate, dichloroacetate, dimethylglycine, a whey-based supplement, and combination of coenzyme Q10, creatine monohydrate, and lipoic acid. This review concluded that there is no clear evidence supporting the use of these agents at this time. Aerobic training has been shown to increase oxidative capacity in patients with heteroplasmic mtDNA mutations.[102] In addition, resistance training in patients with single, large-scale mtDNA deletions has also been shown to increase strength and oxidative capacity.[103]

REFERENCES

1. Haller RG, Vissing J. Spontaneous "second wind" and glucose-induced second "second wind" in McArdle disease: oxidative mechanisms. Arch Neurol 2002; 59(9):1395–402.
2. Vissing J, Haller RG. Mechanisms of exertional fatigue in muscle glycogenoses. Neuromuscul Disord 2012;22(Suppl 3):S168–71.
3. Vissing J, Duno M, Schwartz M, et al. Splice mutations preserve myophosphorylase activity that ameliorates the phenotype in McArdle disease. Brain 2009; 132(Pt 6):1545–52.
4. Lucia A, Nogales-Gadea G, Perez M, et al. McArdle disease: what do neurologists need to know? Nat Clin Pract Neurol 2008;4(10):568–77.
5. Lucia A, Ruiz JR, Santalla A, et al. Genotypic and phenotypic features of McArdle disease: insights from the Spanish national registry. J Neurol Neurosurg Psychiatry 2012;83(3):322–8.
6. Quinlivan R, Buckley J, James M, et al. McArdle disease: a clinical review. J Neurol Neurosurg Psychiatry 2010;81(11):1182–8.
7. Vieitez I, Teijeira S, Fernandez JM, et al. Molecular and clinical study of McArdle's disease in a cohort of 123 European patients. Identification of 20 novel mutations. Neuromuscul Disord 2011;21(12):817–23.
8. Martin MA, Rubio JC, Buchbinder J, et al. Molecular heterogeneity of myophosphorylase deficiency (McArdle's disease): a genotype-phenotype correlation study. Ann Neurol 2001;50(5):574–81.
9. Kazemi-Esfarjani P, Skomorowska E, Jensen TD, et al. A nonischemic forearm exercise test for McArdle disease. Ann Neurol 2002;52(2):153–9.
10. Haller RG, Wyrick P, Taivassalo T, et al. Aerobic conditioning: an effective therapy in McArdle's disease. Ann Neurol 2006;59(6):922–8.
11. Vissing J, Haller RG. The effect of oral sucrose on exercise tolerance in patients with McArdle's disease. N Engl J Med 2003;349(26):2503–9.

12. Zander NF, Meyer HE, Hoffmann-Posorske E, et al. cDNA cloning and complete primary structure of skeletal muscle phosphorylase kinase (alpha subunit). Proc Natl Acad Sci U S A 1988;85(9):2929–33.

13. Abarbanel JM, Bashan N, Potashnik R, et al. Adult muscle phosphorylase "b" kinase deficiency. Neurology 1986;36(4):560–2.

14. Wilkinson DA, Tonin P, Shanske S, et al. Clinical and biochemical features of 10 adult patients with muscle phosphorylase kinase deficiency. Neurology 1994; 44(3 Pt 1):461–6.

15. Clemens PR, Yamamoto M, Engel AG. Adult phosphorylase b kinase deficiency. Ann Neurol 1990;28(4):529–38.

16. Carrier H, Maire I, Vial C, et al. Myopathic evolution of an exertional muscle pain syndrome with phosphorylase b kinase deficiency. Acta Neuropathol 1990; 81(1):84–8.

17. Bak H, Cordato D, Carey WF, et al. Adult-onset exercise intolerance due to phosphorylase b kinase deficiency. J Clin Neurosci 2001;8(3):286–7.

18. Orngreen MC, Schelhaas HJ, Jeppesen TD, et al. Is muscle glycogenolysis impaired in X-linked phosphorylase b kinase deficiency? Neurology 2008; 70(20):1876–82.

19. Wuyts W, Reyniers E, Ceuterick C, et al. Myopathy and phosphorylase kinase deficiency caused by a mutation in the PHKA1 gene. Am J Med Genet A 2005;133A(1):82–4.

20. Echaniz-Laguna A, Akman HO, Mohr M, et al. Muscle phosphorylase b kinase deficiency revisited. Neuromuscul Disord 2010;20(2):125–7.

21. Preisler N, Orngreen MC, Echaniz-Laguna A, et al. Muscle phosphorylase kinase deficiency: a neutral metabolic variant or a disease? Neurology 2012; 78(4):265–8.

22. Bruno C, Manfredi G, Andreu AL, et al. A splice junction mutation in the alpha(M) gene of phosphorylase kinase in a patient with myopathy. Biochem Biophys Res Commun 1998;249(3):648–51.

23. Burwinkel B, Hu B, Schroers A, et al. Muscle glycogenosis with low phosphorylase kinase activity: mutations in PHKA1, PHKG1 or six other candidate genes explain only a minority of cases. Eur J Hum Genet 2003;11(7): 516–26.

24. Wehner M, Clemens PR, Engel AG, et al. Human muscle glycogenosis due to phosphorylase kinase deficiency associated with a nonsense mutation in the muscle isoform of the alpha subunit. Hum Mol Genet 1994;3(11):1983–7.

25. Vora S, Seaman C, Durham S, et al. Isozymes of human phosphofructokinase: identification and subunit structural characterization of a new system. Proc Natl Acad Sci U S A 1980;77(1):62–6.

26. Haller RG, Vissing J. No spontaneous second wind in muscle phosphofructokinase deficiency. Neurology 2004;62(1):82–6.

27. Haller RG, Lewis SF. Glucose-induced exertional fatigue in muscle phosphofructokinase deficiency. N Engl J Med 1991;324(6):364–9.

28. Musumeci O, Bruno C, Mongini T, et al. Clinical features and new molecular findings in muscle phosphofructokinase deficiency (GSD type VII). Neuromuscul Disord 2012;22(4):325–30.

29. Timal S, Hoischen A, Lehle L, et al. Gene identification in the congenital disorders of glycosylation type I by whole-exome sequencing. Hum Mol Genet 2012;21(19):4151–61.

30. Stojkovic T, Vissing J, Petit F, et al. Muscle glycogenosis due to phosphoglucomutase 1 deficiency. N Engl J Med 2009;361(4):425–7.

31. Perez B, Medrano C, Ecay MJ, et al. A novel congenital disorder of glycosylation type without central nervous system involvement caused by mutations in the phosphoglucomutase 1 gene. J Inherit Metab Dis 2013;36(3):535–42.

32. Tegtmeyer LC, Rust S, van Scherpenzeel M, et al. Multiple phenotypes in phosphoglucomutase 1 deficiency. N Engl J Med 2014;370(6):533–42.

33. Preisler N, Laforet P, Echaniz-Laguna A, et al. Fat and carbohydrate metabolism during exercise in phosphoglucomutase type 1 deficiency. J Clin Endocrinol Metab 2013;98(7):E1235–40.

34. Spiegel R, Gomez EA, Akman HO, et al. Myopathic form of phosphoglycerate kinase (PGK) deficiency: a new case and pathogenic considerations. Neuromuscul Disord 2009;19(3):207–11.

35. Naini A, Toscano A, Musumeci O, et al. Muscle phosphoglycerate mutase deficiency revisited. Arch Neurol 2009;66(3):394–8.

36. Kreuder J, Borkhardt A, Repp R, et al. Brief report: inherited metabolic myopathy and hemolysis due to a mutation in aldolase A. N Engl J Med 1996; 334(17):1100–4.

37. Yao DC, Tolan DR, Murray MF, et al. Hemolytic anemia and severe rhabdomyolysis caused by compound heterozygous mutations of the gene for erythrocyte/ muscle isozyme of aldolase, ALDOA(Arg303X/Cys338Tyr). Blood 2004;103(6): 2401–3.

38. Comi GP, Fortunato F, Lucchiari S, et al. Beta-enolase deficiency, a new metabolic myopathy of distal glycolysis. Ann Neurol 2001;50(2):202–7.

39. Kollberg G, Tulinius M, Gilljam T, et al. Cardiomyopathy and exercise intolerance in muscle glycogen storage disease 0. N Engl J Med 2007;357(15):1507–14.

40. Cameron JM, Levandovskiy V, MacKay N, et al. Identification of a novel mutation in GYS1 (muscle-specific glycogen synthase) resulting in sudden cardiac death, that is diagnosable from skin fibroblasts. Mol Genet Metab 2009;98(4): 378–82.

41. Sukigara S, Liang WC, Komaki H, et al. Muscle glycogen storage disease 0 presenting recurrent syncope with weakness and myalgia. Neuromuscul Disord 2012;22(2):162–5.

42. Moslemi AR, Lindberg C, Nilsson J, et al. Glycogenin-1 deficiency and inactivated priming of glycogen synthesis. N Engl J Med 2010;362(13):1203–10.

43. Sentner CP, Vos YJ, Niezen-Koning KN, et al. Mutation analysis in glycogen storage disease type III patients in the Netherlands: novel genotype-phenotype relationships and five novel mutations in the AGL gene. JIMD Rep 2013;7:19–26.

44. Kishnani PS, Austin SL, Arn P, et al. Glycogen storage disease type III diagnosis and management guidelines. Genet Med 2010;12(7):446–63.

45. Moses SW, Wanderman KL, Myroz A, et al. Cardiac involvement in glycogen storage disease type III. Eur J Pediatr 1989;148(8):764–6.

46. Miller CG, Alleyne GA, Brooks SE. Gross cardiac involvement in glycogen storage disease type 3. Br Heart J 1972;34(8):862–4.

47. Cornelio F, Bresolin N, Singer PA, et al. Clinical varieties of neuromuscular disease in debrancher deficiency. Arch Neurol 1984;41(10):1027–32.

48. Moses SW, Gadoth N, Bashan N, et al. Neuromuscular involvement in glycogen storage disease type III. Acta Paediatr Scand 1986;75(2):289–96.

49. Preisler N, Pradel A, Husu E, et al. Exercise intolerance in glycogen storage disease type III: weakness or energy deficiency? Mol Genet Metab 2013;109(1): 14–20.

50. Hobson-Webb LD, Austin SL, Bali DS, et al. The electrodiagnostic characteristics of glycogen storage disease type III. Genet Med 2010;12(7):440–5.

51. Kiechl S, Kohlendorfer U, Thaler C, et al. Different clinical aspects of debrancher deficiency myopathy. J Neurol Neurosurg Psychiatry 1999;67(3):364–8.
52. Sentner CP, Caliskan K, Vletter WB, et al. Heart Failure due to severe hypertrophic cardiomyopathy reversed by low calorie, high protein dietary adjustments in a glycogen storage disease type IIIa patient. JIMD Rep 2012;5:13–6.
53. Dagli AI, Zori RT, McCune H, et al. Reversal of glycogen storage disease type IIIa-related cardiomyopathy with modification of diet. J Inherit Metab Dis 2009;32(Suppl 1):S103–6.
54. Thon VJ, Khalil M, Cannon JF. Isolation of human glycogen branching enzyme cDNAs by screening complementation in yeast. J Biol Chem 1993;268(10):7509–13.
55. Bruno C, Cassandrini D, Assereto S, et al. Neuromuscular forms of glycogen branching enzyme deficiency. Acta Myol 2007;26(1):75–8.
56. Magoulas PL, El-Hattab AW. Glycogen storage disease type IV. In: Roberta AP, editor. Gene reviews™. Seattle (WA): University of Washington; 2013 [Internet].
57. Bao Y, Kishnani P, Wu JY, et al. Hepatic and neuromuscular forms of glycogen storage disease type IV caused by mutations in the same glycogen-branching enzyme gene. J Clin Invest 1996;97(4):941–8.
58. Mochel F, Schiffmann R, Steenweg ME, et al. Adult polyglucosan body disease: natural history and key magnetic resonance imaging findings. Ann Neurol 2012; 72(3):433–41.
59. Nezu J, Tamai I, Oku A, et al. Primary systemic carnitine deficiency is caused by mutations in a gene encoding sodium ion-dependent carnitine transporter. Nat Genet 1999;21(1):91–4.
60. Magoulas PL, El-Hattab AW. Systemic primary carnitine deficiency: an overview of clinical manifestations, diagnosis, and management. Orphanet J Rare Dis 2012;7:68.
61. Lefevre C, Jobard F, Caux F, et al. Mutations in CGI-58, the gene encoding a new protein of the esterase/lipase/thioesterase subfamily, in Chanarin-Dorfman syndrome. Am J Hum Genet 2001;69(5):1002–12.
62. Fischer J, Lefevre C, Morava E, et al. The gene encoding adipose triglyceride lipase (PNPLA2) is mutated in neutral lipid storage disease with myopathy. Nat Genet 2007;39(1):28–30.
63. Laforet P, Orngreen M, Preisler N, et al. Blocked muscle fat oxidation during exercise in neutral lipid storage disease. Arch Neurol 2012;69(4):530–3.
64. Bruno C, Bertini E, Di Rocco M, et al. Clinical and genetic characterization of Chanarin-Dorfman syndrome. Biochem Biophys Res Commun 2008;369(4): 1125–8.
65. Ash DB, Papadimitriou D, Hays AP, et al. A novel mutation in PNPLA2 leading to neutral lipid storage disease with myopathy. Arch Neurol 2012;69(9):1190–2.
66. Reilich P, Horvath R, Krause S, et al. The phenotypic spectrum of neutral lipid storage myopathy due to mutations in the PNPLA2 gene. J Neurol 2011; 258(11):1987–97.
67. Laforet P, Vianey-Saban C. Disorders of muscle lipid metabolism: diagnostic and therapeutic challenges. Neuromuscul Disord 2010;20(11):693–700.
68. Wang ZQ, Chen XJ, Murong SX, et al. Molecular analysis of 51 unrelated pedigrees with late-onset multiple acyl-CoA dehydrogenation deficiency (MADD) in southern China confirmed the most common ETFDH mutation and high carrier frequency of c.250G>A. J Mol Med 2011;89(6):569–76.
69. Izumi R, Suzuki N, Nagata M, et al. A case of late onset riboflavin-responsive multiple acyl-CoA dehydrogenase deficiency manifesting as recurrent rhabdomyolysis and acute renal failure. Intern Med 2011;50(21):2663–8.

70. Olsen RK, Olpin SE, Andresen BS, et al. ETFDH mutations as a major cause of riboflavin-responsive multiple acyl-CoA dehydrogenation deficiency. Brain 2007;130(Pt 8):2045–54.

71. Antozzi C, Garavaglia B, Mora M, et al. Late-onset riboflavin-responsive myopathy with combined multiple acyl coenzyme A dehydrogenase and respiratory chain deficiency. Neurology 1994;44(11):2153–8.

72. Gempel K, Topaloglu H, Talim B, et al. The myopathic form of coenzyme Q10 deficiency is caused by mutations in the electron-transferring-flavoprotein dehydrogenase (ETFDH) gene. Brain 2007;130(Pt 8):2037–44.

73. Horvath R. Update on clinical aspects and treatment of selected vitamin-responsive disorders II (riboflavin and CoQ 10). J Inherit Metab Dis 2012;35(4):679–87.

74. Liang WC, Nishino I. Lipid storage myopathy. Curr Neurol Neurosci Rep 2011;11(1):97–103.

75. Bonnefont JP, Djouadi F, Prip-Buus C, et al. Carnitine palmitoyltransferases 1 and 2: biochemical, molecular and medical aspects. Mol Aspects Med 2004;25(5–6):495–520.

76. Orngreen MC, Duno M, Ejstrup R, et al. Fuel utilization in subjects with carnitine palmitoyltransferase 2 gene mutations. Ann Neurol 2005;57(1):60–6.

77. Joshi PR, Young P, Deschauer M, et al. Expanding mutation spectrum in CPT II gene: identification of four novel mutations. J Neurol 2013;260(5):1412–4.

78. Bonnefont JP, Bastin J, Laforet P, et al. Long-term follow-up of bezafibrate treatment in patients with the myopathic form of carnitine palmitoyltransferase 2 deficiency. Clin Pharmacol Ther 2010;88(1):101–8.

79. Laforet P, Acquaviva-Bourdain C, Rigal O, et al. Diagnostic assessment and long-term follow-up of 13 patients with Very Long-Chain Acyl-Coenzyme A dehydrogenase (VLCAD) deficiency. Neuromuscul Disord 2009;19(5):324–9.

80. Andresen BS, Olpin S, Poorthuis BJ, et al. Clear correlation of genotype with disease phenotype in very-long-chain acyl-CoA dehydrogenase deficiency. Am J Hum Genet 1999;64(2):479–94.

81. Liang WC, Nishino I. State of the art in muscle lipid diseases. Acta Myol 2010;29(2):351–6.

82. Djouadi F, Aubey F, Schlemmer D, et al. Bezafibrate increases very-long-chain acyl-CoA dehydrogenase protein and mRNA expression in deficient fibroblasts and is a potential therapy for fatty acid oxidation disorders. Hum Mol Genet 2005;14(18):2695–703.

83. Harris TE, Finck BN. Dual function lipin proteins and glycerolipid metabolism. Trends Endocrinol Metab 2011;22(6):226–33.

84. Michot C, Hubert L, Romero NB, et al. Study of LPIN1, LPIN2 and LPIN3 in rhabdomyolysis and exercise-induced myalgia. J Inherit Metab Dis 2012;35(6):1119–28.

85. DiMauro S, Schon EA, Carelli V, et al. The clinical maze of mitochondrial neurology. Nat Rev Neurol 2013;9(8):429–44.

86. Horvath R, Kemp JP, Tuppen HA, et al. Molecular basis of infantile reversible cytochrome c oxidase deficiency myopathy. Brain 2009;132(Pt 11):3165–74.

87. Crooks DR, Natarajan TG, Jeong SY, et al. Elevated FGF21 secretion, PGC-1alpha and ketogenic enzyme expression are hallmarks of iron-sulfur cluster depletion in human skeletal muscle. Hum Mol Genet 2014;23(1):24–39.

88. Suomalainen A, Elo JM, Pietilainen KH, et al. FGF-21 as a biomarker for muscle-manifesting mitochondrial respiratory chain deficiencies: a diagnostic study. Lancet Neurol 2011;10(9):806–18.

89. Spinazzola A, Zeviani M. Disorders of nuclear-mitochondrial intergenomic communication. Biosci Rep 2007;27(1–3):39–51.
90. Lara MC, Valentino ML, Torres-Torronteras J, et al. Mitochondrial neurogastrointestinal encephalomyopathy (MNGIE): biochemical features and therapeutic approaches. Biosci Rep 2007;27(1–3):151–63.
91. Suomalainen A, Isohanni P. Mitochondrial DNA depletion syndromes–many genes, common mechanisms. Neuromuscul Disord 2010;20(7):429–37.
92. Mollet J, Delahodde A, Serre V, et al. CABC1 gene mutations cause ubiquinone deficiency with cerebellar ataxia and seizures. Am J Hum Genet 2008;82(3): 623–30.
93. Gerards M, van den Bosch BJ, Danhauser K, et al. Riboflavin-responsive oxidative phosphorylation complex I deficiency caused by defective ACAD9: new function for an old gene. Brain 2011;134(Pt 1):210–9.
94. Nouws J, Nijtmans L, Houten SM, et al. Acyl-CoA dehydrogenase 9 is required for the biogenesis of oxidative phosphorylation complex I. Cell Metab 2010; 12(3):283–94.
95. Mochel F, Knight MA, Tong WH, et al. Splice mutation in the iron-sulfur cluster scaffold protein ISCU causes myopathy with exercise intolerance. Am J Hum Genet 2008;82(3):652–60.
96. Linderholm H, Muller R, Ringqvist R, et al. Hereditary abnormal muscle metabolism with hyperkinetic circulation during exercise. Acta Med Scand 1969; 185:153–66.
97. Taivassalo T, Jensen TD, Kennaway N, et al. The spectrum of exercise tolerance in mitochondrial myopathies: a study of 40 patients. Brain 2003;126(Pt 2): 413–23.
98. Christian BE, Spremulli LL. Mechanism of protein biosynthesis in mammalian mitochondria. Biochim Biophys Acta 2012;1819(9–10):1035–54.
99. Bykhovskaya Y, Casas K, Mengesha E, et al. Missense mutation in pseudouridine synthase 1 (PUS1) causes mitochondrial myopathy and sideroblastic anemia (MLASA). Am J Hum Genet 2004;74(6):1303–8.
100. Riley LG, Cooper S, Hickey P, et al. Mutation of the mitochondrial tyrosyl-tRNA synthetase gene, YARS2, causes myopathy, lactic acidosis, and sideroblastic anemia–MLASA syndrome. Am J Hum Genet 2010;87(1):52–9.
101. Uusimaa J, Jungbluth H, Fratter C, et al. Reversible infantile respiratory chain deficiency is a unique, genetically heterogenous mitochondrial disease. J Med Genet 2011;48(10):660–8.
102. Taivassalo T, Haller RG. Implications of exercise training in mtDNA defects–use it or lose it? Biochim Biophys Acta 2004;1659(2–3):221–31.
103. Murphy JL, Blakely EL, Schaefer AM, et al. Resistance training in patients with single, large-scale deletions of mitochondrial DNA. Brain 2008;131(Pt 11): 2832–40.

Muscle Channelopathies

Jeffrey Statland, MD[a], Lauren Phillips, MD[b], Jaya R. Trivedi, MD[b],*

KEYWORDS

- Channelopathies • Ion channel • Nondystrophic myotonia • Periodic paralysis
- Congenital myasthenic syndrome

KEY POINTS

- Skeletal muscle channelopathies are rare heterogeneous disorders and include nondystrophic myotonia, congenital myasthenic syndrome, and periodic paralyses.
- Clinical diagnosis is confounded by marked phenotypic heterogeneity.
- Electrodiagnostic testing can aid in diagnosis, but genetic testing is confirmatory.
- Treatment options are few and not approved by the US Food and Drug Administration.

INTRODUCTION

Skeletal muscle ion channelopathies are rare disorders characterized by episodic and fluctuating symptoms, exacerbation by environmental factors, and frequently autosomal dominant inheritance patterns. However, there is major genotypic and phenotypic heterogeneity of ion channelopathies. For instance, a sodium channel mutation of the skeletal muscle can cause paramyotonia congenita (PMC), sodium channel myotonia, hyperkalemic periodic paralysis, or hypokalemic periodic paralysis. Myotonic disorders can similarly be caused by sodium channel or chloride channel defects. Skeletal muscle channelopathies, in particular nondystrophic myotonias (NDMs), represent some of the first known examples and best studied ion channelopathies.[1] This article reviews clinical features, diagnostic testing, pathophysiology, and treatment options in NDM, congenital myasthenic syndrome, and periodic paralyses.

NDM

NDM has a prevalence of less than 1 per 100,000.[2,3] NDM is caused by mutations in the skeletal muscle sodium (SCN4A) and chloride (CLCN1) channels and includes

Funding Sources: MDA Clinical Research Training Grant (J. Statland); none (L. Phillips, J.R. Trivedi).
Conflict of Interest: Consultant for Cytokinetics (J. Statland); no conflict (L. Phillips, J.R. Trivedi).
[a] Department of Neurology, University of Rochester, 601 Elmwood Drive, Rochester, NY 14607, USA; [b] Department of Neurology and Neurotherapeutics, UT Southwestern Medical Center, 5323 Harry Hines Boulevard, Dallas, TX 75390, USA
* Corresponding author.
E-mail address: jaya.trivedi@utsouthwestern.edu

myotonia congenita (MC), PMC, hyperkalemic periodic paralysis with myotonia, and a diverse group of sodium channel myotonias.[2-9]

Clinical Features

The most characteristic symptom in NDM is muscle stiffness generated by voluntary movement. A brief voluntary contraction elicits a sustained burst of action potentials originating from the muscle fiber, which persists for several seconds after motor neuron activity has ceased. This sustained activity results in myotonia, or an involuntary delay in the relaxation of muscle contraction; patients describe this as stiffness.[4] Other commonly reported symptoms include transient or prolonged weakness, pain associated with myotonia, and fatigue. Environmental factors that may increase myotonia include pregnancy, dietary potassium, cold temperature, hunger, fatigue, and emotional stress; some of these have traditionally been thought to help distinguish some of the NDM subtypes.[10-13] Clinical manifestations may range in severity from severe neonatal myotonia with respiratory compromise[14] to milder late-onset myotonic muscle stiffness. Myotonic dystrophy type 2 can present with a pure myotonic phenotype that may be clinically indistinguishable from MC.[5]

MC

MC is the most common skeletal muscle channelopathy and is caused by a mutation in the CLCN1 gene encoding for the main skeletal muscle chloride channel ClC-1. MC may be inherited as an autosomal dominant (Thomsen disease) or recessive (Becker disease) trait, with a more severe phenotype in the latter.[5,15,16] Clinical heterogeneity within a family is common. These patients typically have hypertrophic muscles, action myotonia, and percussion myotonia.[17] Patients experience muscle stiffness that is most evident during rapid voluntary movements following a period of rest; stiffness improves with several repetitions of the same movement, a finding referred to as a warm-up phenomenon.[18] The most common site of stiffness is the legs, whereas the face is less commonly affected.[19] Patients with Becker disease classically have transient weakness that improves with exercise. This transient weakness is unique to MC and is not seen with PMC.[20]

PMC

PMC is autosomal dominant and is caused by mutations of the sodium channel SCN4A gene on chromosome 17. Cold-induced, prolonged, painful myotonia and episodic weakness are the hallmarks of PMC.[4,21-23] Paradoxic myotonia, or myotonia appearing during muscle activity and increasing with continued exercise, is associated with PMC. Facial stiffness and eye closure myotonia are more common, and paradoxic eye closure myotonia is typically exclusive to PMC.[19] Although myotonia typically lasts seconds or minutes, muscle weakness following prolonged exercise can last from several hours to 2 days in PMC[24]; this is in contrast with the transient weakness that can be seen in the recessive form of MC. Interattack weakness is common and some patients go on to require assistive devices such as a wheelchair or wheeled walker.[23] Paramyotonia is triggered by rest after exercise, fasting, and cold; these characteristics are also seen in hyperkalemic periodic paralysis, which is allelic with PMC.[25,26]

Sodium channel myotonias

The sodium channel myotonias (SCMs) include acetazolamide-responsive myotonia, myotonia fluctuans, and myotonia permanens. Common features include autosomal dominant inheritance pattern, absence of episodic weakness or cold sensitivity, and potassium aggravation; they are also known as potassium-aggravated myotonias.

Other pure myotonic syndromes with cold sensitivity have also been linked to the SCN4A gene.[13,21,27–29] Presence of warm-up phenomenon and variable cold sensitivity can make these patients difficult to distinguish from patients with MC.

Diagnosis

Creatine kinase can be normal to mildly increased. Thyroid function should be checked because hypothyroidism can cause clinical and electrical myotonia.[30] Electromyography reveals myotonia in proximal and distal limb muscles, and is useful in confirming a myotonic disorder.[19] The short exercise and long exercise test have been used in further characterization of NDM. For the short exercise test, the patient is asked to perform maximum voluntary contraction for 5 to 10 seconds and compound muscle action potential amplitude (CMAP) is recorded immediately after exercise (eg, stimulating the ulnar nerve at the wrist, recording over the abductor digiti minimi). CMAPs are subsequently recorded every 10 seconds up to 1 minute after exercise. This test is repeated 3 times with 60 seconds in between trials and may help distinguish CLCN1 and SCN4A mutations. CMAP reduction of greater than 10% is considered abnormal.[31,32] On the short exercise test, 3 patterns have been recognized:

- Pattern I: seen in PMC in which there may be a reduction in CMAP, facilitated by repetition or cold.
- Pattern II: patients with recessive MC can have a transient reduction in CMAP that rapidly returns to baseline.
- Pattern III: patients with dominant MC and SCM may have no change in CMAP.

For the long exercise test, patients are instructed to contract the abductor digiti minimi (usually alternating 15-second contractions with 3–4 seconds of rest) for up to 5 minutes against fixed resistance and then CMAPs are recorded every 1 to 2 minutes for up to 50 minutes. Characteristic reductions in CMAP amplitude (>20%) are considered abnormal. After prolonged exercise, patients with MC have none to a slight decrease in CMAP, whereas patients with PMC have a persistent CMAP decrement that starts immediately after exercise.[31] However, electrophysiologic testing has limitations: (1) some CLCN1 mutations are associated with both dominant and recessive inheritance of MC; (2) certain SCN4A mutations can manifest either as SCM or PMC; (3) there is significant overlap with the short exercise test, suggesting that these patterns might not be sensitive or specific enough to make a definitive diagnosis.

CLCN1 and SCN4 are both large genes with 23 and 24 exons, respectively. More than 100 CLCN1 mutations and more than 20 SCN4 mutations have been identified.[21,33] Genetic testing is the gold standard in making a definitive diagnosis of NDM. However, cost is a limitation and an argument could be made that, from a clinical standpoint, available treatment strategies are similar for all NDM subtypes. However, knowledge of the specific mutation is important in distinguishing NDM from myotonic dystrophy; mutation-specific characteristics might help improve understanding of the disease pathophysiology, and lead to accurate genetic counseling to affected individuals.

Pathophysiology

Bryant and colleagues[34] showed a greatly diminished sarcolemmal chloride conductance in affected muscle fibers from myotonic goats and this has been established as the basis for the enhanced muscle excitability in MC. In the absence of the chloride conductance, the repolarizing influence of the chloride current is lost and the length constant of the sarcolemma is significantly increased, allowing summation of electrical potentials.[34] Therefore, increases of the potassium concentration in the T-tubular lumen during electrical activity cause a greater depolarized shift in the resting potential of the sarcolemmal membrane, which leads to muscle hyperexcitability and myotonic discharges.[35]

Distinct allelic mutations in CLCN1 have been identified in a large number of autosomal dominant and autosomal recessive myotonia cases.[36,37] Several CLCN1 mutations have been reported to cause both autosomal dominant and autosomal recessive forms in different families.[9,38–41] The exact mechanism by which mutations in the same gene cause both dominant and recessive diseases remains unclear. The chloride channel CLC-1 exists as a homodimer with each individual subunit forming a gated pore. The channel has 2 main gating modes, referred to as the fast gate, which can operate the 2 pores independently, and the slow gate, which regulates the open probability of both pores simultaneously.[42] The dominant forms of MC occur because of effects of the mutated subunit when dimerized with the wild type (WT) subunit (dominant negative effect), whereas recessive MC occurs because of loss of function of the mutated subunit.[43] Recessive mutations are more common than dominant mutations.

In the 1980s, electrophysiologic studies on human muscle revealed that chloride conductance was normal in patients with PMC and with hyperkalemic periodic paralysis.[44,45] These patients had an anomalous persistent inward current that was blocked by tetrodotoxin, suggesting a voltage-gated sodium channel defect. Missense mutations in the muscle sodium channel gene SCN4A are responsible for PMC, potassium-aggravated myotonia, and hyperkalemic periodic paralysis.[46,47]

Therapeutic Options in NDM

Table 1 presents various treatment options in NDM. There is no treatment approved by the US Food and Drug Administration (FDA) at this time. Patients with NDM experience constant, lifelong symptoms and their impact on quality of life is comparable with that of some muscular dystrophies.[55,56] A quarter of subjects in a natural history study of NDM were disabled or unemployed because of NDM.[19]

Physicians rely on off-label use of antiepileptic, anesthetic, and antiarrhythmic drugs to treat myotonia (see **Table 1**). Anecdotal data support the use of quinine,[57] procainamide,[57,58] and phenytoin[58] in patients with myotonia. There is also evidence for class 1B antiarrhythmics, tocainide (withdrawn from the market) and mexiletine, which may be more effective than quinine, procainamide, or phenytoin for autosomal recessive myotonia and PMC.[17,59] In a prospective multinational NDM study, about 40% patients were not on any antimyotonic treatment.[19] A randomized double-blind placebo-controlled study was subsequently performed to study effects of mexiletine in NDM. Mexiletine 200 mg 3 times a day significantly reduced stiffness, in addition to improving severity of graded myotonia on electromyography and quality-of-life measures.[48] However, 15% of subjects experienced gastrointestinal side effects and a third of the subjects had suboptimal or no response. Use of mexiletine is further limited by a black box warning about increased mortality in asymptomatic non–life-threatening ventricular arrhythmias in patients who had a myocardial infarction more than 6 days but less than 2 years previously. All patients using mexiletine should have QTc interval monitoring because of its proarrhythmogenic potential.

Other possible treatment avenues in NDM require better understanding of the biophysical behavior of different disease-causing mutations, and this can be done through functional expression studies. Targeting the biophysical abnormalities could lead to mutation-specific treatments that may better control myotonia and transient muscle weakness.

Table 1
Antimyotonic drugs used to treat symptoms of NDM

Antimyotonic Drugs	Dosage	Side Effects	Monitoring
Mexiletine[48]	Start 150 mg BID with slow titration to 200–300 mg TID	GI distress, tremor, ataxia	LFTs, ECG
Quinine[49]	200–1200 mg/d	Cardiac arrhythmias, hypersensitivity reactions, bone marrow suppression, liver damage, GI distress, visual disturbance	CBC with platelet count, LFTs, blood glucose, ECG, ophthalmologic evaluation
Procainamide[49,50]	125–1000 mg/d	Rash, GI distress, positive ANA	ECG, creatinine, CBC, ANA
Phenytoin[49,50]	300–400 mg/d	Gingival hypertrophy, agranulocytosis, pancytopenia, rash, cognitive impairment, liver damage	CBC, LFTs
Tocainide[50]	Withdrawn from the market	Potentially fatal agranulocytosis[51]	NA
Flecainide[52]	Start 100 mg/d, titrate to 100 mg BID	Cardiac arrhythmias, dizziness, rash	ECG, periodic drug serum concentrations
Carbamazepine[53]	20 mg/kg divided TID	Rash, agranulocytosis, pancytopenia, liver damage	LFTs, CBC, TSH
Acetazolamide[49,54]	125 mg BID with slow titration to goal dose 250 mg TID	GI distress, electrolyte abnormalities (hypokalemia, hyponatremia), paresthesias, nephrolithiasis, rash, agranulocytosis	Serum electrolytes, LFTs, CBC

Abbreviations: ANA, antinuclear antibodies; BID, twice a day; CBC, complete blood count; GI, gastrointestinal; LFTs, liver function tests; NA, not applicable; TID, 3 times a day; TSH, thyroid-stimulating hormone.

CONGENITAL MYASTHENIC SYNDROMES

The congenital myasthenic syndromes (CMSs) are rare and can be caused by presynaptic, synaptic, or postsynaptic genetic defects of the neuromuscular junction; postsynaptic defects account for 75% of cases.[60] Most postsynaptic CMSs are associated with mutations in nicotinic acetylcholine receptor (nAChR) subunit genes, leading to a deficiency of functional channels or abnormal channel gating kinetics.[4] Antibodies to nAChR, P/Q-type calcium channels, or muscle-specific kinase are not detected in CMS. CMS associated with nAChR subunit gene mutations can be further characterized by slow-channel and fast-channel variants.[4] Symptoms may be evident at birth or develop in adulthood. Physical examination typically reveals fatigable weakness of ocular and extraocular muscles and, in severe cases, limb muscles; clinical myotonia is not seen.[4]

Slow-channel CMS

This autosomal dominant disorder is characterized by weakness and fatigability affecting primarily the neck, scapular, and distal upper extremity muscles. Nerve conduction studies reveal oscillatory CMAP afterdepolarizations following a single stimulus as well as a decremental response to repetitive nerve stimulation at 2 Hz.[4] Treatment options include quinidine sulfate (starting dose, 200 mg 3 times a day titrating up to serum level of 1–2.5 μg/mL),[61,62] fluoxetine (80–100 mg/d),[61] and salbutamol (6 mg/d).[63] There is typically no long-term response to acetylcholinesterase inhibitors.

Fast-channel CMS

Ocular and neck muscle weakness is more common in this autosomal recessive disorder. Repetitive nerve stimulation at 2 Hz reveals a decremental response after exercise.[4] Symptoms in this disorder caused by fast-channel closure respond to acetylcholinesterase inhibitors.

PERIODIC PARALYSES

The primary periodic paralyses include the disorders hyperkalemic periodic paralysis, hypokalemic periodic paralysis, and Andersen-Tawil syndrome (ATS).[64] The following features are common to the hereditary periodic paralyses:

- Episodic attacks of flaccid weakness
- Symptoms that typically start in the first 2 decades of life
- Autosomal dominant inheritance
- Attacks brought on by triggers that include diet or rest after exercise
- Often associated with changes in extracellular potassium (high or low)
- Initially normal strength between attacks, but often a fixed proximal weakness later in the disease course
- Reduction of attack frequency or severity with carbonic anhydrase inhibitors

In addition, thyrotoxic periodic paralysis has been associated with mutations in a thyroid hormone-regulated potassium channel gene but, unlike the other heritable periodic paralyses, is caused by a combination of environmental and genetic factors.[65]

Clinical Features

Hyperkalemic periodic paralysis

Hyperkalemic periodic paralysis (HyperPP) is a rare autosomal dominant disorder with prevalence less than 1 in 200,000 and is caused by mutations in the SCN4A gene on chromosome 17. HyperPP lies on one end of a spectrum of allelic SCN4A disorders that include PMC (discussed earlier). HyperPP typically presents in the first decade of life with transient episodic muscle paralysis precipitated by fasting, by rest after exercise, or by ingestion of potassium-rich foods.[22,66] Attacks most commonly last minutes to hours and can occur as frequently as 16 times per month. Attack frequency usually peaks in the young adult years then gradually decreases with age. Respiratory and cardiac muscles are typically spared; however, rarely during severe attacks respiratory muscles may become involved. Approximately three-quarters of patients show myotonia electrographically or grip and/or percussion myotonia on clinical examination. Strength is typically normal between attacks but up to half of patients develop fixed proximal weakness later in life.

- HyperPP should be considered in any patient presenting with attacks of flaccid weakness and myotonia on electrodiagnostic testing or clinical examination

Hypokalemic periodic paralysis

Hypokalemic periodic paralysis (HypoPP) is a rare autosomal dominant muscle disorder caused by mutations involving mostly the muscle calcium (CACNA1S, chromosome 1), less frequently the sodium (SCN4A, chromosome 17), channel genes and rarely the KCNE3. HypoPP is characterized by episodic attacks of weakness associated with low serum potassium beginning in the first or second decade of life and without clinical or electrical myotonia. The prevalence of genetically confirmed HypoPP is approximately 0.13 per 100,000.[67] Patients experience attacks of variable severity, from mild weakness to profound paralysis, occurring at a frequency of around 7 to 9 episodes per month, each lasting from hours to days.[22] Carbohydrate-rich foods, stress, alcohol, and rest after exercise can trigger attacks, and potassium levels during attacks can decrease to less than 3.0 mmol/L. Ocular, bulbar, and respiratory muscles can, rarely, be involved in severe attacks. Attack frequency usually peaks in the early adult years and decrease in frequency after age 40 years. Although many attacks are mild, patients still experience significant lifetime morbidity because of the unpredictable and disabling nature of attacks, and variable degrees of fixed weakness that occur over time.[68,69]

ATS

ATS is a rare autosomal dominant disorder with a prevalence of approximately 1 per 1,000,000 characterized by the clinical triad[70]:

- Episodic flaccid muscle weakness, in the setting of high, low, or normal potassium
- Ventricular arrhythmias and prolonged QT interval
- Dysmorphic features

Approximately 60% of patients with ATS have a mutation in a potassium inward rectifier KCNJ2 on chromosome 17. Attacks of weakness usually start in the first or second decade of life, and duration and frequency are variable, with potassium levels low, high, or normal during attacks.[66] Patients are short statured with any combination of low-set ears, wide-set eyes, broad nasal bridge, small mandible, abnormally bent or curved fifth finger, and toes joined at the base. Cardiac arrhythmias consist of premature ventricular contractions, prominent U wave, and polymorphic or multifocal ventricular tachyarrhythmia. Most cardiac arrhythmias remain asymptomatic; however, some patients experience palpitations or syncope, or, very rarely, sudden cardiac death.[71]

Diagnosis

Diagnosis in the primary periodic paralyses is based on:

- Clinical history of attacks of flaccid paralysis
- Positive family history
- Characteristic ictal changes in serum potassium (high or low)
- Characteristic reduction in CMAP amplitude after long periods of exercise on electrodiagnostic testing
- Genetic testing

One of the most useful diagnostic procedures is the neurologic examination during an acute attack. Patients should have a flaccid paralysis and typically lose muscle stretch reflexes in affected limbs.

In all cases of periodic paralysis the first step is verifying that the disorder is primary and not secondary to metabolic disorders resulting in low or high potassium and secondary paralysis (**Box 1**). At the minimum, basic electrolyte studies and thyroid studies are indicated in all patients. Alterations in serum potassium during attacks can be useful in characterizing the periodic paralyses but are not required for diagnosis: in HypoPP serum potassium is often less than 3.0 mmol/L; in HyperPP increases in potassium greater than 5 mmol/L or increases greater than 1.5 mmol/L are often seen; and in ATS potassium can be low, high, or normal during attacks. Nonspecific increases in serum creatine kinase are often seen during attacks. An electrocardiogram (ECG) can show abnormalities: prominent U waves, long QT interval, or ventricular arrhythmias in ATS; sinus tachycardias in thyrotoxic periodic paralysis. Muscle biopsies are not typically required for diagnosis but show nonspecific myopathic changes, including variability in fiber size, rounding of fibers, internal nuclei, and vacuoles. Tubular aggregates can occasionally be seen in HypoPP and ATS.

In the recovery phase and interictally closer to an attack, electrodiagnostic long exercise testing is a sensitive test routinely performed diagnostically before genetic testing and is based on the principle of provoked attacks of focal paralysis with exercise. During testing, patients are instructed to contract the muscles of their hands (usually alternating 15-second contractions with 3–4 seconds of rest) for up to 5 minutes against fixed resistance and then CMAPs are recorded every 1 to 2 minutes for up to 1 hour. Characteristic reductions in CMAP amplitude (>20%) are considered diagnostic.[31]

ATS is suggested by clinical history, positive long exercise test, and the clinical triad that includes cardiac conduction abnormalities and dysmorphic features in addition to attacks of paralysis. However, family history can sometimes be difficult to determine

---

Box 1
Conditions associated with secondary periodic paralysis

Low potassium

Thyrotoxic

Primary hyperaldosteronism

Renal tubular acidosis

Juxtaglomerular apparatus hyperplasia

Gastrointestinal potassium wastage

Laxative abuse

Licorice

Corticosteroids

Potassium-depleting diuretics

High potassium

Addison disease

Hypoaldosteronism

Potassium-sparing diuretics

Excessive potassium supplementation

because affected family members may not show all of the classic clinical triad. HyperPP is suggested by changes on long exercise testing and myotonia on electromyography. The diagnosis for all the primary periodic paralyses is ultimately confirmed by commercial genetic testing, which identifies a mutation in approximately 60% to 70% of patients with a clinical history and electrodiagnostic testing suggesting this diagnosis.

Pathophysiology

HyperPP is one of several allelic disorders caused by missense mutations in the alpha pore forming unit of the SCN4A gene. Overall, mutations lead to depolarized sarcolemma but clinically form a spectrum from no weakness with increased excitability (myotonia) to inexcitable membrane (paralysis). HyperPP shows both ends of the spectrum, myotonia and paralysis, in the same patient. Modeling studies have suggested that whether patients experience myotonia or paralysis depends on the extent of persistent inward sodium currents.[4] Most mutations alter the rate of sodium channel inactivation, but mutations associated with HyperPP also result in incomplete inactivation and thus larger persistent inward depolarizing currents. When inward currents are large enough to shift the resting membrane to depolarized potentials SCN4A channels switch to an inactive configuration, resulting in paralysis.

In contrast, HypoPP caused by SCN4A mutations show no abnormal current through the conducting pore. Almost all mutations associated with HypoPP in both calcium and sodium channels occur at arginine residues in the fourth transmembrane (S4) segment of the voltage sensor domains.[72] Recent studies have shown that, in response to changes in membrane potential, the S4 segment translocates through a crevasse, or gating pore, in the channel protein. In patients with HypoPP, mutations in the S4 region cause this gating pore to conduct ions at rest. This gating pore current is typically small, but in low potassium conditions the size of the depolarizing gating pore current becomes large compared with the repolarizing potassium current, which causes the membrane to depolarize and sodium channels to switch to an inactive configuration, making the sarcolemma inexcitable. This anomalous gating pore current has been shown in mouse models for both sodium and calcium channel HypoPP.[73,74]

The exact pathophysiologic mechanism of ATS is not known. The potassium inward rectifier (Kir 2.1) helps set the resting membrane potential. Mutations are thought to result in a loss of function: decreased potassium conductance depolarizes the membrane, which shifts sodium channels to an inactive configuration.[70]

Therapeutic Options

Treatment strategies for the primary periodic paralyses are usually divided into treatments to abort ongoing attacks of paralysis and chronic therapies intended to reduce overall attack frequency or severity (**Table 2**). For all the periodic paralyses, mild exercise at the attack onset can help prevent a full-blown attack of paralysis. Acute treatment strategies depend on whether attacks are associated with low or high serum potassium. For HypoPP or ATS (with low potassium during attacks) potassium supplementation is the main abortive therapy. The preferred method for potassium supplementation is oral. If attacks are severe and patients cannot take medication orally, potassium should be given in 5% mannitol rather than saline or glucose because these solutions can worsen paralysis. Patients should be monitored in an inpatient setting on telemetry if repeated doses of potassium are required. For HyperPP, mild exercise or oral carbohydrate snacks are usually enough to abort attacks, but, if attacks persist or are severe, inhaled beta agonist or intravenous calcium gluconate can be used. As in

Table 2
Treatment strategies for primary periodic paralyses

Treatment	HypoPP	HyperPP	ATS
Acute Therapy			
Behavioral	Mild exercise at attack onset	Mild exercise at attack onset	Mild exercise at attack onset
Oral potassium	0.2–0.4 mEq/kg every 30 min not to succeed 200–250 mEq per day	Not indicated	If potassium low during attacks: 0.2–0.4 mEq/kg every 30 min not to succeed 200–250 mEq per day
Oral carbohydrate	Not indicated	Oral carbohydrate up to 2.0 g/kg	Not typically indicated
Intravenous potassium	Only if cannot take orally: 40 mEq/L in 5% mannitol solution to run at maximum of 20 mEq/h; not to exceed 200–250 mEq per day	Not indicated	If potassium low during attack and cannot take orally: 40 mEq/L in 5% mannitol solution to run at maximum of 20 mEq/h and not to exceed 200–250 mEq per day
Beta agonist	Not indicated	1–2 puffs inhalation 0.1 mg albuterol	Not typically indicated
Intravenous calcium gluconate	Not indicated	If attack severe and associated with high potassium: 0.5–2.0 g	Not typically indicated
Chronic Therapy			
Diet	Low salt, low carbohydrate; avoid alcohol	Avoid potassium-rich foods	Low salt, low carbohydrate; avoid alcohol
Oral potassium	10–20 mEq up to TID	Not indicated	If potassium low during attacks: 10–20 mEq up to TID
Carbonic anhydrase inhibitor	Acetazolamide 125–1000 mg/d; or dichlorphenamide[a] 50–200 mg/d	Acetazolamide 125–1000 mg/d; or dichlorphenamide[a] 50–200 mg/d	Acetazolamide 125–1000 mg/d; or dichlorphenamide[a] 50–200 mg/d
Potassium-sparing diuretic	Triamterene 50–150 mg/d; spironolactone 25–100 mg/d	Not indicated	If potassium low during attack: triamterene 50–150 mg/d; spironolactone 25–100 mg/d
Oral hydrochlorothiazide	Not indicated	25 mg; monitor potassium	Not typically indicated

[a] Not available in the United States.

HypoPP, severe attacks requiring repeat interventions should be monitored on telemetry.

Chronic therapy to reduce the frequency or severity of attacks usually consists of a combination of diet modification and daily medications. Diet modifications can help reduce attack frequency or severity in both HypoPP and HyperPP. In HypoPP, patients should be encouraged to maintain a low-salt, low-carbohydrate diet, and avoid alcohol. For HyperPP, patients should be encouraged to avoid potassium-rich foods and fasting; eating multiple carbohydrate snacks during the day can help reduce the frequency of attacks. Carbonic anhydrase inhibitors can be used daily to reduce the attack frequency or severity in HypoPP, HyperPP, and ATS (acetazolamide or dichlorphenamide; for dosing, see **Table 2**).[75,76] For patients who cannot tolerate or do not respond to carbonic anhydrase inhibitors, potassium-sparing diuretics may prove useful for HypoPP. For HyperPP, hydrochlorothiazide may be effective.

ATS requires a multidisciplinary approach to patient care, with yearly follow-up with cardiology. Patients may require yearly Holter monitor evaluation, and, if symptomatic arrhythmias develop, they may require implantable cardioverter-defibrillators.

SUMMARY

Despite advances in understanding molecular pathology of skeletal muscle channelopathies, the diverse genetic and phenotypic manifestations remain a challenge in diagnosis, therapeutics, genetic counseling, and research planning. These limitations are compounded by the rarity of these disorders. Electrodiagnostic testing is useful in directing the diagnosis, but has several limitations: it involves patient discomfort, is time consuming, is not reimbursed by insurance carriers, and there is a significant overlap of findings in muscle channelopathies. Genetic testing is the gold standard in making a definitive diagnosis, but cost is an issue. There are no FDA-approved therapies for NDM, periodic paralyses, and CMS; apart from mexiletine,[48] available options are few and unvalidated. However, research networks now facilitate the study of mutation-specific treatment responses in randomized clinical trials.[77]

REFERENCES

1. Fahlke C. Molecular mechanisms of ion conduction in ClC-type chloride channels: lessons from disease-causing mutations. Kidney Int 2000;57(3):780–6.
2. Emery AE. Population frequencies of inherited neuromuscular diseases–a world survey. Neuromuscul Disord 1991;1(1):19–29.
3. Pinessi L, Bergamini L, Cantello R, et al. Myotonia congenita and myotonic dystrophy: descriptive epidemiological investigation in Turin, Italy (1955-1979). Ital J Neurol Sci 1982;3(3):207–10.
4. Cannon SC. Pathomechanisms in channelopathies of skeletal muscle and brain. Annu Rev Neurosci 2006;29:387–415.
5. Fialho D, Schorge S, Pucovska U, et al. Chloride channel myotonia: exon 8 hotspot for dominant-negative interactions. Brain 2007;130(Pt 12):3265–74.
6. Hoffman EP, Wang J. Duchenne-Becker muscular dystrophy and the nondystrophic myotonias. Paradigms for loss of function and change of function of gene products. Arch Neurol 1993;50(11):1227–37.
7. Lehmann-Horn F, Rudel R. Channelopathies: the nondystrophic myotonias and periodic paralyses. Semin Pediatr Neurol 1996;3(2):122–39.
8. Ptacek LJ, George AL Jr, Griggs RC, et al. Identification of a mutation in the gene causing hyperkalemic periodic paralysis. Cell 1991;67(5):1021–7.

9. Sun C, Tranebjaerg L, Torbergsen T, et al. Spectrum of CLCN1 mutations in patients with myotonia congenita in Northern Scandinavia. Eur J Hum Genet 2001; 9(12):903–9.

10. Basu A, Nishanth P, Ifaturoti O. Pregnancy in women with myotonia congenita. Int J Gynaecol Obstet 2009;106(1):62–3.

11. Fialho D, Kullmann DM, Hanna MG, et al. Non-genomic effects of sex hormones on CLC-1 may contribute to gender differences in myotonia congenita. Neuromuscul Disord 2008;18(11):869–72.

12. Lacomis D, Gonzales JT, Giuliani MJ. Fluctuating clinical myotonia and weakness from Thomsen's disease occurring only during pregnancies. Clin Neurol Neurosurg 1999;101(2):133–6.

13. Orrell RW, Jurkat-Rott K, Lehmann-Horn F, et al. Familial cramp due to potassium-aggravated myotonia. J Neurol Neurosurg Psychiatry 1998;65(4): 569–72.

14. Lion-Francois L, Mignot C, Vicart S, et al. Severe neonatal episodic laryngospasm due to de novo SCN4A mutations: a new treatable disorder. Neurology 2010;75(7):641–5.

15. Colding-Jorgensen E. Phenotypic variability in myotonia congenita. Muscle Nerve 2005;32(1):19–34.

16. Raja Rayan DL, Hanna MG. Skeletal muscle channelopathies: nondystrophic myotonias and periodic paralysis. Curr Opin Neurol 2010;23(5):466–76.

17. Streib EW. AAEE minimonograph #27: differential diagnosis of myotonic syndromes. Muscle Nerve 1987;10(7):603–15.

18. Becker PE, Knussmann R, Kuhn E. Topics in human genetics. Stuttgart (Germany): Georg Thieme Publishers; 1977.

19. Trivedi JR, Bundy B, Statland J, et al. Non-dystrophic myotonia: prospective study of objective and patient reported outcomes. Brain 2013;136(Pt 7): 2189–200.

20. Trip J, Drost G, Ginjaar HB, et al. Redefining the clinical phenotypes of non-dystrophic myotonic syndromes. J Neurol Neurosurg Psychiatry 2009;80(6): 647–52.

21. Matthews E, Fialho D, Tan SV, et al. The non-dystrophic myotonias: molecular pathogenesis, diagnosis and treatment. Brain 2010;133(Pt 1):9–22.

22. Miller TM, Dias da Silva MR, Miller HA, et al. Correlating phenotype and genotype in the periodic paralyses. Neurology 2004;63(9):1647–55.

23. Ptacek LJ, Johnson KJ, Griggs RC. Genetics and physiology of the myotonic muscle disorders. N Engl J Med 1993;328(7):482–9.

24. Fontaine B. Periodic paralysis, myotonia congenita and sarcolemmal ion channels: a success of the candidate gene approach. Neuromuscul Disord 1993; 3(2):101–7.

25. Ptacek LJ, Trimmer JS, Agnew WS, et al. Paramyotonia congenita and hyperkalemic periodic paralysis map to the same sodium-channel gene locus. Am J Hum Genet 1991;49(4):851–4.

26. Ptacek LJ, Tyler F, Trimmer JS, et al. Analysis in a large hyperkalemic periodic paralysis pedigree supports tight linkage to a sodium channel locus. Am J Hum Genet 1991;49(2):378–82.

27. Ptacek LJ, George AL Jr, Barchi RL, et al. Mutations in an S4 segment of the adult skeletal muscle sodium channel cause paramyotonia congenita. Neuron 1992;8(5):891–7.

28. Ricker K, Moxley RT 3rd, Heine R, et al. Myotonia fluctuans. A third type of muscle sodium channel disease. Arch Neurol 1994;51(11):1095–102.

29. Trudell RG, Kaiser KK, Griggs RC. Acetazolamide-responsive myotonia congenita. Neurology 1987;37(3):488–91.
30. Venables GS, Bates D, Shaw DA. Hypothyroidism with true myotonia. J Neurol Neurosurg Psychiatry 1978;41(11):1013–5.
31. Fournier E, Arzel M, Sternberg D, et al. Electromyography guides toward subgroups of mutations in muscle channelopathies. Ann Neurol 2004;56(5):650–61.
32. Fournier E, Viala K, Gervais H, et al. Cold extends electromyography distinction between ion channel mutations causing myotonia. Ann Neurol 2006;60(3): 356–65.
33. Wu FF, Ryan A, Devaney J, et al. Novel CLCN1 mutations with unique clinical and electrophysiological consequences. Brain 2002;125(Pt 11):2392–407.
34. Bryant SH, Morales-Aguilera A. Chloride conductance in normal and myotonic muscle fibres and the action of monocarboxylic aromatic acids. J Physiol 1971;219(2):367–83.
35. Adrian RH, Bryant SH. On the repetitive discharge in myotonic muscle fibres. J Physiol 1974;240(2):505–15.
36. George AL Jr, Crackower MA, Abdalla JA, et al. Molecular basis of Thomsen's disease (autosomal dominant myotonia congenita). Nat Genet 1993;3(4): 305–10.
37. Koch MC, Steinmeyer K, Lorenz C, et al. The skeletal muscle chloride channel in dominant and recessive human myotonia. Science 1992;257(5071):797–800.
38. George AL Jr, Sloan-Brown K, Fenichel GM, et al. Nonsense and missense mutations of the muscle chloride channel gene in patients with myotonia congenita. Hum Mol Genet 1994;3(11):2071–2.
39. Meyer-Kleine C, Steinmeyer K, Ricker K, et al. Spectrum of mutations in the major human skeletal muscle chloride channel gene (CLCN1) leading to myotonia. Am J Hum Genet 1995;57(6):1325–34.
40. Papponen H, Toppinen T, Baumann P, et al. Founder mutations and the high prevalence of myotonia congenita in northern Finland. Neurology 1999;53(2): 297–302.
41. Zhang J, George AL Jr, Griggs RC, et al. Mutations in the human skeletal muscle chloride channel gene (CLCN1) associated with dominant and recessive myotonia congenita. Neurology 1996;47(4):993–8.
42. Saviane C, Conti F, Pusch M. The muscle chloride channel ClC-1 has a double-barreled appearance that is differentially affected in dominant and recessive myotonia. J Gen Physiol 1999;113(3):457–68.
43. Pusch M, Steinmeyer K, Koch MC, et al. Mutations in dominant human myotonia congenita drastically alter the voltage dependence of the ClC-1 chloride channel. Neuron 1995;15(6):1455–63.
44. Lehmann-Horn F, Rudel R, Dengler R, et al. Membrane defects in paramyotonia congenita with and without myotonia in a warm environment. Muscle Nerve 1981;4(5):396–406.
45. Lehmann-Horn F, Rudel R, Ricker K, et al. Two cases of adynamia episodica hereditaria: in vitro investigation of muscle cell membrane and contraction parameters. Muscle Nerve 1983;6(2):113–21.
46. Ebers GC, George AL, Barchi RL, et al. Paramyotonia congenita and hyperkalemic periodic paralysis are linked to the adult muscle sodium channel gene. Ann Neurol 1991;30(6):810–6.
47. Fontaine B, Khurana TS, Hoffman EP, et al. Hyperkalemic periodic paralysis and the adult muscle sodium channel alpha-subunit gene. Science 1990;250(4983): 1000–2.

48. Statland JM, Bundy BN, Wang Y, et al. Mexiletine for symptoms and signs of myotonia in nondystrophic myotonia: a randomized controlled trial. JAMA 2012;308(13):1357–65.
49. Dunø M, Colding-Jørgensen E. Myotonia congenita. In: Pagon RA, Adam MP, Bird TD, et al, editors. GeneReviews [Internet]. Seattle (WA): University of Washington; 2005 [updated 2011 Apr 12].
50. Aichele R, Paik H, Heller AH. Efficacy of phenytoin, procainamide, and tocainide in murine genetic myotonia. Exp Neurol 1985;87(2):377–81.
51. Volosin K, Greenberg RM, Greenspon AJ. Tocainide associated agranulocytosis. Am Heart J 1985;109(6):1392–3.
52. Desaphy JF, Modoni A, Lomonaco M, et al. Dramatic improvement of myotonia permanens with flecainide: a two-case report of a possible bench-to-bedside pharmacogenetics strategy. Eur J Clin Pharmacol 2013;69(4):1037–9.
53. Berardinelli A, Gorni K, Orcesi S. Response to carbamazepine of recessive-type myotonia congenita. Muscle Nerve 2000;23(1):138–9.
54. Shapiro B, Ruff R. Disorders of skeletal muscle membrane excitability: myotonia congenita, paramyotonia congenita, periodic paralysis, and related disorders. In: Katirji B, Kaminski H, Preston D, et al, editors. Neuromuscular disorders in clinical practice. Boston: Butterworth-Heinemann; 2002. p. 987–1020.
55. Rose MR, Sadjadi R, Weinman J, et al. Role of disease severity, illness perceptions, and mood on quality of life in muscle disease. Muscle Nerve 2012;46(3):351–9.
56. Sansone VA, Ricci C, Montanari M, et al. Measuring quality of life impairment in skeletal muscle channelopathies. Eur J Neurol 2012;19(11):1470–6.
57. Leyburn P, Walton JN. The treatment of myotonia: a controlled clinical trial. Brain 1959;82(1):81–91.
58. Griggs RC, Davis RJ, Anderson DC, et al. Cardiac conduction in myotonic dystrophy. Am J Med 1975;59(1):37–42.
59. Kwiecinski H, Ryniewicz B, Ostrzycki A. Treatment of myotonia with antiarrhythmic drugs. Acta Neurol Scand 1992;86(4):371–5.
60. Engel AG, Ohno K, Shen XM, et al. Congenital myasthenic syndromes: multiple molecular targets at the neuromuscular junction. Ann N Y Acad Sci 2003;998:138–60.
61. Engel AG. The therapy of congenital myasthenic syndromes. Neurotherapeutics 2007;4(2):252–7.
62. Harper CM, Engel AG. Quinidine sulfate therapy for the slow-channel congenital myasthenic syndrome. Ann Neurol 1998;43(4):480–4.
63. Finlayson S, Spillane J, Kullmann DM, et al. Slow channel congenital myasthenic syndrome responsive to a combination of fluoxetine and salbutamol. Muscle Nerve 2013;47(2):279–82.
64. Fontaine B. Periodic paralysis. Adv Genet 2008;63:3–23.
65. Ryan DP, da Silva MR, Soong TW, et al. Mutations in potassium channel Kir2.6 cause susceptibility to thyrotoxic hypokalemic periodic paralysis. Cell 2010;140(1):88–98.
66. Venance SL, Cannon SC, Fialho D, et al. The primary periodic paralyses: diagnosis, pathogenesis and treatment. Brain 2006;129(Pt 1):8–17.
67. Horga A, Raja Rayan DL, Matthews E, et al. Prevalence study of genetically defined skeletal muscle channelopathies in England. Neurology 2013;80(16):1472–5.
68. Dalakas MC, Engel WK. Treatment of "permanent" muscle weakness in familial Hypokalemic Periodic Paralysis. Muscle Nerve 1983;6(3):182–6.

69. Links TP, Zwarts MJ, Wilmink JT, et al. Permanent muscle weakness in familial hypokalaemic periodic paralysis. Clinical, radiological and pathological aspects. Brain 1990;113(Pt 6):1873–89.

70. Plaster NM, Tawil R, Tristani-Firouzi M, et al. Mutations in Kir2.1 cause the developmental and episodic electrical phenotypes of Andersen's syndrome. Cell 2001;105(4):511–9.

71. Tristani-Firouzi M, Jensen JL, Donaldson MR, et al. Functional and clinical characterization of KCNJ2 mutations associated with LQT7 (Andersen syndrome). J Clin Invest 2002;110(3):381–8.

72. Cannon SC. Voltage-sensor mutations in channelopathies of skeletal muscle. J Physiol 2010;588(Pt 11):1887–95.

73. Wu F, Mi W, Burns DK, et al. A sodium channel knockin mutant (NaV1.4-R669H) mouse model of hypokalemic periodic paralysis. J Clin Invest 2011;121(10):4082–94.

74. Wu F, Mi W, Hernandez-Ochoa EO, et al. A calcium channel mutant mouse model of hypokalemic periodic paralysis. J Clin Invest 2012;122(12):4580–91.

75. Sansone V, Meola G, Links TP, et al. Treatment for periodic paralysis. Cochrane Database Syst Rev 2008;(1):CD005045.

76. Tawil R, McDermott MP, Brown R Jr, et al. Randomized trials of dichlorphenamide in the periodic paralyses. Working Group on Periodic Paralysis. Ann Neurol 2000;47(1):46–53.

77. Hoffman EP, Kaminski HJ. Mexiletine for treatment of myotonia: a trial triumph for rare disease networks. JAMA 2012;308(13):1377–8.

Distal Myopathies

Mazen M. Dimachkie, MD[a],*, Richard J. Barohn, MD[b]

KEYWORDS

- Distal myopathy • Welander myopathy • Myoshi myopathy • Nonaka myopathy
- Laing myopathy • Markesbery-Griggs myopathy • Udd distal myopathy
- Myofibrillar myopathy

KEY POINTS

- Except for hand extension weakness in Welander myopathy, the classic distal myopathies manifest as distal leg weakness beginning in early or late adult life.
- Myoshi myopathy, manifesting as calf muscle weakness and atrophy after a hypertrophic phase, is allelic to LGMD2B, because both diseases are caused by mutation in the gene encoding for dysferlin.
- Patients with myofibrillary myopathy present in the third to fifth decade with distal myopathy, frequent cardiomyopathy, and pathologic evidence of myofibrillary degradation.
- Mutation in genes encoding for αBC, desmin, myotilin, ZASP, filamin C, BAG3, and SEPN1 are responsible for myofibrillary myopathies.
- Myotonic dystrophy is the most common adult muscular dystrophy; early in the disease, wrist and finger extensors and ankle dorsiflexors are weaker than proximal muscles.

APPROACH

In approaching patients with distal weakness, we have to consider disorders affecting motor neurons, peripheral nerves, neuromuscular junction, or muscle[1] and the reader is referred for a full discussion to the article an the approach to muscle disease elsewhere in this issue by Barohn and colleagues. Some myopathies with pattern 2 have predominantly distal presentations, including distal muscular dystrophies, myofibrillar myopathies, myotonic dystrophy type 1, and some forms of hereditary inclusion body myopathies (hIBM). Pattern 3 or scapuloperoneal pattern has proximal arm and distal leg involvement. In the presence of facial weakness, fascioscapulohumeral (FSH)

This publication was supported by an Institutional Clinical and Translational Science Award, NIH/National Center for Advancing Translational Sciences Grant Number UL1TR000001. Its contents are solely the responsibility of the authors and do not necessarily represent the official views of the NIH.

[a] Neuromuscular Section, Neurophysiology Division, Department of Neurology, University of Kansas Medical Center, 3901 Rainbow Boulevard, Mail Stop 2012, Kansas City, KS 66160, USA; [b] Department of Neurology, University of Kansas Medical Center, 3901 Rainbow Boulevard, Mail Stop 2012, Kansas City, KS 66160, USA
* Corresponding author.
E-mail address: mdimachkie@kumc.edu

muscular dystrophy is considered likely. Emery-Dreifuss muscular dystrophy is usually associated with contractures and cardiac involvement. Late onset acid maltase deficiency can rarely have a scapuloperoneal presentation as well. Pattern 4 consists of distal arm involvement and proximal leg weakness, as is typical for the sporadic inclusion body myositis (IBM), in which there is prominent finger flexor, wrist flexor, and knee extensor weakness. Pattern 5 is associated with ptosis and ophthalmoplegia and includes patients with oculopharyngeal dystrophy and mitochondrial myopathy.

The presence of rimmed vacuoles (**Box 1**) significantly helps to further narrow down these diagnostic possibilities. Welander myopathy is nearly always in cases from Scandinavia and presents with distal hand involvement. The Markesbery-Griggs and Udd types are autosomal dominant (AD) late onset distal leg myopathies caused by mutations in the genes encoding Z-band alternatively spliced PDZ-motif-

---

Box 1
Muscle disorders with rimmed vacuoles on biopsy

IBM

h-IBM

- h-IBM2 or Nonaka type distal myopathy (GNE)
- IBMPFD[a] (VCP)
- h-IBM3 (myosin heavy chain IIa)[a]

Distal muscular dystrophies

- Welander type[a]
- Markesbery-Griggs type (ZASPopathy)[a]
- Udd type (titinopathy)[a]

MFM

- Myotilinopathy (LGMD1A)[a]
- ZASPopathy[a]
- Desminopathy[a]
- Filaminopathy[a]
- Bag3-opathy[a]
- αB-crystallin[a]
- SEPN1

Other muscular dystrophies/myopathies

- Reducing body myopathy (FHL1-opathy)
- Emery-Dreifuss (emerinopathy, laminopathy[a])
- LGMD2G (telethoninopathy)
- Oculopharyngeal muscular dystrophy (PABP2-GCG triplet)[a]
- Oculopharyngodistal muscular dystrophy
- Pompe disease (acid maltase deficiency)
- Danon disease (LAMP-2)
- X-linked myopathy with excessive autophagy (VMA21)

   [a] Autosomal dominant.

containing protein (ZASP) and titin, respectively.[2–4] Limb girdle muscular dystrophy 1A caused by autosomal-dominant mutations in the myotilin gene is associated with adult onset of proximal or distal weakness and rimmed vacuoles and occasional nemaline rodlike inclusions.[5] Histopathologically, myotilinopathy and ZASPopathy can be placed into the category of myofibrillar myopathy (MFM) (**Table 1**).[2–5,10] Another group of disorders with rimmed vacuoles on biopsy are the hIBM.[2] Nonaka myopathy (NM) or hIBM2 is autosomal recessive (AR) with anterior leg involvement (see **Box 1, Table 2**). Hereditary IBM3 caused by heavy chain 2 myosin mutations is associated with congenital arthrogryposis and later onset ophthalmoplegia. One AD late onset multi-system form of hIBM is variably associated with Paget disease and frontotemporal dementia (IBMPFD) and is caused by valosin-containing protein (VCP) mutations (**Table 3**). Immunostaining using VCP antibodies shows the presence of VCP-positive cytoplasmic aggregates in scattered muscle fibers, including those with no clear vacuoles or other morphologic changes.[13] Patients with IBMPFD can present with proximal, distal, scapuloperoneal, or axial weakness[14] and can have dilated cardiomyopathy with inclusion bodies.[15]

CLASSIC DISTAL MYOPATHIES
Welander Distal Myopathy: Late Adult Onset, Type 1

Welander[16] described many patients with AD distal myopathy in 72 Swedish families with symptoms onset in the mid-fifth decade (range <30–77 years). Although Welander distal myopathy (WDM) is mainly seen in Sweden, 12 Finnish families with onset in the long extensor muscles of the hands and fingers were reported to cosegregate to chromosome 2p13 haplotype.[17,18] Proximal limb involvement rarely occurs in WDM, even with advanced disease, except in severe homozygous cases. Ankle dorsiflexion weakness occurs in 25% of cases and may be the initial presenting symptom in 10%. Flexor muscles of wrists and fingers are affected later on in 40% of cases but to a lesser extent than extensors. Tendon reflexes remain present except for loss of ankle and brachioradialis reflexes late in the disease. Although sensation is normal, deficits on quantitative temperature and vibration testing are detectable.[19]

Serum creatine kinase (CK) level has been shown to be normal or slightly increased.[20,21] Motor and sensory nerve conduction studies (NCS) are typically normal, and needle electromyography (EMG) shows occasional spontaneous activity comprised of fibrillation potentials, and myopathic motor units potentials (MUP), although some investigators have reported a mixed myopathic and neuropathic recruitment pattern.[20–23] T1 and T2 magnetic resonance imaging (MRI) of muscle in 11 patients showed signal abnormalities in the distal anterior and posterior compartments of the legs, including the gastrocnemius, soleus, tibialis anterior (TA), and extensor digitorum longus (EDL), as well hamstrings and posterior compartment muscles of the legs.[24]

Muscle biopsy shows slight to severe myopathic features, including variability in fiber size, increased connective tissue and fat deposition, central nuclei, and split fibers.[16] Vacuoles, a common feature in several of the distal dystrophies, have been noted by some[16,21,25] but not all investigators,[23,26,27] and they are not generally a conspicuous histologic feature. A disorganization and loss of myofibrils with accumulation of Z-disk material are noted at the ultrastructural level.[25] Since then, rimmed vacuoles and 15-nm to 18-nm cytoplasmic and nuclear filaments have been noted by electron microscopy (EM)[20,21] indicating that these are not specific to IBM. The main pathologic feature that distinguishes IBM from WDM is inflammatory cell infiltration in the former,[21] besides the clinical phenotype. Groups of small angular fibers can occur,

Table 1
Classification of myofibrillar myopathies

Type	Inheritance	Gene Localization	Initial Weakness	CK	Biopsy
Desmin adult onset (hIBM1& LGMD1D/E)[a] MFM1	AD or AR (6%)	2q35	Hands or legs	Moderately increased, <5× normal	Myopathy, occasional rimmed vacuoles; subsarcolemmal granules, desmin bodies
αB-crystallin early–mid-adult MFM2	AD or AR	11q22	Proximal and leg distal	Mild increase	Myopathy, desmin increase
Myotilin adult (LGMD1A)[b] MFM3	AD or sporadic	5q31.2	Proximal or distal nasal, dysarthria	Normal to 15× increased	MFM, rimmed vacuoles, hyaline/rod inclusions, desmin
ZASP late adult MFM4	AD	10q23.2	Proximal or in 9% distal	Normal or mild increase	MFM, small vacuoles, desmin aggregates
Myofibrillar with cardiomyopathy adult	AD	10q22.3 Similar to ZASP	Distal	Normal or mild increase	MFM
Filamin C Mid-adult to late adult MFM5 (see **Table 3**)	AD	7q32.1	Proximal and respiratory	2–8× increase	Myopathy, hyaline mass, vacuoles, rods, and desmin aggregates
BAG3 childhood MFM6	AD	10q25.2-q26.2	Proximal > distal, cardiac	3–15× increase	Myopathy, congophilia, desmin accumulation, small vacuoles
Scapuloperoneal also known as hyaline body myopathy adult	AD	Xq26 FHL1	Distal legs, scapular winging	1.5–10× increase	Myopathy, hyaline bodies with focal desmin inclusions
SEPN1 child also known as congenital muscular dystrophy with desmin inclusions	AR	1p36-p35	Proximal, rigid spine and cardiac	Normal or mild increase	Myopathy, vacuoles, desmin inclusions

Abbreviations: BAG3, BCL2-associated athanogene 3; CK, creatine kinase; FHL1, four-and-a-half-LIM protein 1; LGMD, limb girdle muscular dystrophy; SEPN1, selenoprotein N, 1; ZASP, Z-band alternatively spliced PDZ-motif-containing protein also known as LDB3 (Lim domain-binding 3).

[a] AD hereditary IBM1, with early quadriceps muscle involvement and later ankle dorsiflexion weakness, has been linked to a mutation in the desmin gene.[11] AD LGMD1D/E, with cardiac conduction defect and dilated cardiomyopathy, is also linked to the desmin gene.[151] A dominant neurogenic Kaeser-type scapuloperoneal phenotype also been described to harbor a desmin gene mutation.[12]

[b] AD LGMD1A has been linked to a mutation in myotilin, the causative gene of MFM3.

Table 2
Classification of classic distal myopathies

Type	Inheritance	Gene Localization	Initial Weakness	CK	Biopsy
Welander late adult type 1	AD	2p13	Hands, fingers, wrist extensors	Normal or mild increase	Myopathic; rimmed vacuoles in some
Udd late adult type 2a	AD	2q31 titin	Legs, anterior compartment	Normal or mild increase	Myopathic; rimmed vacuoles in some cases
Markesbery-Griggs late adult type 2b	AD	10q22.3-q23.2 ZASP	Legs, anterior compartment	Normal or mild increase	Vacuolar myopathy; myofibrillar features
Nonaka early adult onset or sporadic type 1 (hIBM2)[a]	AR	9p13.3 GNE	Legs, anterior compartment	Mild to moderate increase, <5× NL	Vacuolar myopathy
Miyoshi early adult onset type 2 (LGMD 2B)[b]	AR or sporadic	2p13 dysferlin	Legs, posterior compartment	10–150× NL	Myopathic, usually no vacuoles; end-stage gastrocnemius
Laing early adult onset type 3 (MPD1)	AD	14q11.2 MYH7	Legs, anterior compartment, neck flexors	Mild increase, <3× NL	Moderate myopathic changes; no vacuoles in most

Abbreviations: CK; creatine kinase; LGMD, limb girdle muscular dystrophy; NL, normal.
    [a] AR familial hereditary IBM2, also known as quadriceps sparing myopathy, has been genetically linked with the Nonaka distal myopathy.[6–8]
    [b] LGMD type 2B has been genetically linked with Miyoshi distal myopathy.[9]

suggestive of a neurogenic component.[25] Sural nerve biopsy can show a moderate reduction in myelinated nerve fibers without any axonal degeneration or demyelination and remyelination.[25]

The clinical progression of WDM is so slow in most cases that most affected patients continue to work without a reduction in life expectancy; those with atypical relative rapid progression may be homozygous for the genetic defect.[16,18]

Tibial Muscular Dystrophy: Late Onset Distal Myopathy Type 2

In the 1970s, non-Scandinavian AD late onset distal myopathy was described in English families by Sumner and colleagues[28] and in French-English and Finnish families by Markesbery and colleagues.[29] Other large pedigrees and several sporadic cases were reported and renamed tibial distal muscular dystrophy (TMD), to emphasize the dystrophic features.[30,31] Despite phenotypic overlap, recent identification of 2 distinct gene mutations led to the definition of 2 subtypes: type 2a related to titin gene defect and type 2b caused by ZASP point mutation.

Table 3
Classification of less common distal myopathies

Type	Inheritance	Gene Localization	Initial Weakness	CK	Biopsy
Myopathy with anterior leg sparing child to young adult (see **Table 1**)	AD	7q32 Filamin C	Calf and hands	Normal or mild increase	Fiber size, variability
Myopathy with Paget and dementia young adult	AD	9p13 VCP	Proximal and distal leg	Normal to 8× increase	Myopathy with vacuoles
Distal myopathy with vocal cord and pharyngeal weakness, MPD2 late adult onset	AD	5q31 Matrin 3	Legs, hands, or vocal cords	Normal to 8 x increase	Myopathy with vacuoles
Miyoshi-like myopathy 3 early adult onset	AR	11p14.3 Anoctamin 5 (ANO 5)	Posterior legs	3–100× increased	Myopathy with sarcolemmal lesion
Distal nebulin myopathy child or adult[a]	AR	2q21.2-q22 Nebulin	Toe and finger extensor	Normal	Myopathy with small rods
LGMD2G puberty onset	AR	17q12 Telethonin	Leg: proximal and anterior distal	3–17× increase	Myopathy, rimmed vacuoles
Distal myopathy type 3 (MPD3) early adult onset	AD	8p22-q11 and 12q13-q22	Asymmetric distal leg and hand	Normal or mild increase	Myopathy with vacuoles

Abbreviations: CK, creatine kinase; LGMD, limb girdle muscular dystrophy.
  [a] Allelic with rod body myopathy.

Udd Late Onset Distal Myopathy Type 2a

The prevalence of AD TMD is 5 to 15 per 100,000 in Finland. Weakness begins in ankle dorsiflexor muscles typically after age 40 years. In non-Scandinavian cases, weakness may over time involve finger and wrist extensor muscles; later, proximal involvement can supervene. Whereas most Finnish patients progressed more slowly and rarely involved the upper extremity or proximal muscles,[32] some western Finnish cases showed severe limb girdle syndrome.[30,31,33]

Serum CK level is normal or slightly increased, and EMG shows an irritative myopathy. Muscle biopsy shows dystrophic tissue with myofibers having single and multiple vacuoles. MRI in 22 affected patients showed fatty replacement of the TA muscle and EDL in 8 and in the hamstring and posterior compartment of the legs in 14 others.[24]

Tibial muscular dystrophy 2a is a titinopathy caused by mutations in TTN, the gene encoding the giant skeletal muscle protein titin,[34] with a locus at 2q31, composed of 363 exons. Mutation in Mex6 titin leads to abnormal titin-calpain3 interaction.[35] The Finnish mutation is caused by a deletion/insertion of 11 consecutive base pairs changing 4 amino acid residues without interrupting the reading frame. One French cohort had a point mutation in Mex6 that introduced a potentially harmful praline in the β sheet structure. Mutations of the Mex6 exon correspond to M-line titin in some cases, affecting the calpain3 binding site at the N2-A line in I-band titin. There is secondary calpain3 protein reduction in the homozygous state and apoptotic myonuclei.

Markesbery-Griggs Late Onset Distal Myopathy Type 2b

TMD2b has been reported in English, French, and Finnish families. Men are marginally more severely affected compared with women. Like TMD2a, weakness in TMD2b begins in the anterior leg compartment after age 40 years. Hand weakness affects distal finger and wrist extensors and late in the course, the proximal arms and legs. Progression is faster than in TMD2a, leading to disability.

CK level is normal or mildly increased and muscle biopsy shows vacuolar myopathy with myofibrillar features. One patient described by Markesbery and colleagues[29] had a cardiomyopathy with heart block and heart failure, requiring pacemaker insertion. At postmortem examination, vacuoles were present in cardiac and skeletal muscle. Muscle imaging shows considerable involvement of posterior and anterior compartments of the lower leg at a younger age.[3] Later in the course of the disease, proximal muscles are affected, with mild to moderate fatty degeneration and atrophy of gluteus maximus, hamstring, vastus medialis, and lateralis muscles, besides severe end-stage replacement in lateral gastrocnemius, soleus, lateral peroneal, and anterior compartment muscles. Deep long toe flexor and tibialis posterior muscles are relatively preserved.

No conclusive mutation in titin or other genes was noted in the original English-Finnish cases.[29] Because the pathology was compatible with MFM, both myotilin and ZASP were sequenced. A previously identified mutation in ZASP (A165V mutation) was detected in originally affected family members,[3] with full penetrance by the age of 60 years. Immunohistochemical studies showed strong accumulation of myotilin, αB-crystallin (αBC), and desmin in affected muscle fibers, but as with myotilinopathy, abnormal myotilin aggregation was more prominent than abnormal expression of desmin, αBC, or ZASP. Although occasional punctate aberrant cytoplasmic labeling is observed, dystrophin C-terminus does not consistently localize to the accumulated aggregates. Cardiomyopathy is not a regular feature, because different isoforms are predominantly expressed in cardiac and skeletal muscle. Whereas mutations in exons 4, 6, 10, and 15, which are expressed in cardiac muscle isoforms, were associated with dilated cardiomyopathy, the A165V substitution in skeletal muscle–specific exon 6 caused a myopathy dominated by skeletal muscle involvement.

Nonaka Distal Myopathy: Early Adult Onset, Type 1, Distal Myopathy with Rimmed Vacuoles

Early adult onset AR distal muscular dystrophy was reported in Japanese families from 1963 to 1975[36,37]; however, they were not widely appreciated until later reports by Nonaka and colleagues.[38–40] Similar patients were later described in the United States,[41–43] South America,[44] and Europe.[45,46] Until identification of the responsible gene defect, weakness onset was believed to be in the second to third decade. Distal myopathy with rimmed vacuoles (DMRV) or NM is characterized by its unique distribution of muscular weakness and wasting, manifesting as foot drop and steppage gait.

The hamstring and TA muscles are most severely affected initially. Although it was initially believed even at late stages to spare knee extensors, discovery of the gene defect led to the realization that the quadriceps muscle can be involved in rare cases. Finger and hand muscles can also be involved but less than the legs. The degree of progression tends to be more aggressive in non-Japanese cases. With rare exceptions,[47] weakness remained confined to distal in the Japanese cases, whereas non-Japanese cases develop significant proximal weakness in the legs, arms, and neck muscles, with loss of ambulation.[41] Complete heart block producing syncope and requiring a pacemaker has been reported,[40] and disability may supervene within 10 to 20 years of onset.

Serum CK level is slightly or moderately increased, but not more than 5 times the upper normal limit. Needle EMG examination shows fibrillation potentials and myopathic MUP. Muscle biopsy in Japanese and non-Japanese cases shows dystrophic myopathy and rimmed vacuoles caused by the deposition therein of granular material with the characteristic of basophilia after hematoxylin-eosin (H&E), purple-red coloration with the modified Gomori trichrome, and acid phosphatase reactivity (**Fig. 1**). The autophagic vacuoles have nuclear and cytoplasmic 15-nm to 18-nm filamentous inclusions on EM,[47–49] which are not unique to IBM, because they are also seen in WDM and DMRV or NM.[50] In rare cases, there may be in addition inflammatory muscle disease with rimmed vacuoles as in sporadic IBM.[51,52]

Almost all cases of DMRV are caused by mutations in the UDP-*N*-acetylglucosamine 2-epimerase/*N*-acetylmannosamine kinase gene (GNE) located within the 1.5-Mb region between markers D9S2178 and D9S1791 on chromosome 9.[53] It is allelic to AR hIBM2, wherein several mutations have been detected, including one at M712T, which is the most common mutation in early-onset Jewish hereditary IBM type 2.[54] hIBM2, the most common form of hereditary IBM, was originally described in Persian-Jewish families with distal leg onset in the second to third decade. Weakness and atrophy progressed proximal with relative sparing of the quadriceps.[55,56] A homozygous T to C substitution at nucleotide position 2186 in the GNE gene, converting methionine to threonine at codon 712, has been found in all Middle Eastern families of both Jewish and non-Jewish descent, whereas affected individuals of other ethnicities are usually compound heterozygous or homozygous for different mutations.[57] A year later, GNE mutations were also identified in patients with DMRV, also known as NM.[58] In the Japanese patients, NM is most commonly associated with V572L homozygous or compound heterozygous mutation. However, the identification of the causative gene defect has allowed recognition of phenotypic variants of this disorder in the age of onset, degree of progression of symptoms, and distribution of muscle

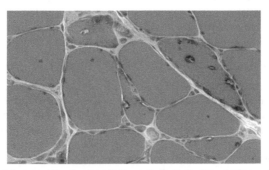

Fig. 1. Nonaka distal myopathy (early adult onset type 1). Muscle fiber size variability and rimmed vacuoles on hematoxylin-eosin.

weakness. For example, a few patients lack distal weakness or have distinctive quadriceps involvement, as well as patients with unusual facial weakness.[59] The age at onset of symptoms is sometimes delayed even to late adulthood and patients may remain asymptomatic in their sixth to seventh decade of life.[58,59]

Two individuals with DMRV and undetectable GNE mutation were postulated to be caused by mutations in the noncoding and intron sites, or abnormal transcription or translation of the GNE gene, or in other genes with a role similar to GNE.[54] Conversely, a GNE mutation detected in a non-DMRV patient showed predominant involvement of proximal leg muscles sparing the TA and gastrocnemius muscles. AD inheritance, late onset, severe cardiac involvement, and proximal leg muscle involvement distinguish DMRV from other myopathies with prominent rimmed vacuoles. Genetic analysis was instrumental in confirming the diagnosis of DMRV in 2 GNE compound heterozygote Japanese patients with the unusual feature of inflammation in muscle biopsy and otherwise typical DMRV.[51] Endomysial and perivascular inflammation is distinctly uncommon in NM but occasionally noted in hIBM.

To safely correct GNE gene function, a patient with severe hIBM2 was treated on a compassionate basis with intravenous infusion of 7 doses of liposomal wild-type GNE gene.[60] Quadriceps muscle expression of the delivered GNE, plasmid, and RNA was observed and sialic acid–related proteins were increased with stabilization in the decline of muscle strength. Further assessment of GNE gene lipoplex through a phase 1 trial in less advanced hIBM cases is in the planning stages. Because the GNE gene encodes a protein with 2 enzymatic activities in the sialic acid biosynthetic pathway, reduced sialylation of muscle glycoproteins may play a pivotal role in the h-IBM2/DMRV muscle phenotype. Oral supplementation with sialic acid metabolites in GNE knockout mice results in an increase of sialic acid in muscle to a nearly normal level and prevents development of the muscle phenotype.[61] Mice treated with sialic acid metabolites have increased strength, muscle mass, mean muscle fiber cross-sectional area, body weight, and overall survival compared with untreated control litter mates. After a phase 1 sequential dose escalation study of oral sialic acid in patients with hereditary IBM, which showed the drug to be safe and well tolerated, there is an ongoing phase 2 study to evaluate the sialic acid–extended release tablets in patients with GNE myopathy (http://clinicaltrials.gov/ct2/show/NCT01517880).

Miyoshi Distal Myopathy: Early Adult Onset, Type 2

The early reports by Miyoshi and colleagues[62,63] of this disorder went largely unnoticed for 2 decades until their cases were published in Western literature.[64] Similar patients were later reported[65–69] from the United States and Europe. Weakness in the gastrocnemii muscles begins between ages 15 and 25 years, with an AR inheritance pattern. Affected patients notice difficulty in walking on toes or climbing stairs, and calf myalgia.[70] Gastrocnemius muscle hypertrophy is followed by wasting and loss of the ankle muscle stretch reflexes at a later point (**Fig. 2**). The muscles of the leg anterior compartment and those of the arms and hands remain relatively spared early in the disease. With disease progression, there is some proximal arm and leg weakness, with the hamstring muscle group being weaker than the quadriceps.[69] Progression is variable, with some patients remaining fairly stable with distal weakness, and others experiencing a more aggressive relentless course, involving proximal and distal muscles. A consistent finding is preservation of the deltoid muscle, despite biceps atrophy.[6]

The serum CK level, which is markedly increased 10-fold to 150-fold the upper normal limit, may be a prelude to the disease in asymptomatic patients.[66] Needle EMG shows myopathic MUP and recruitment pattern. Examination of the

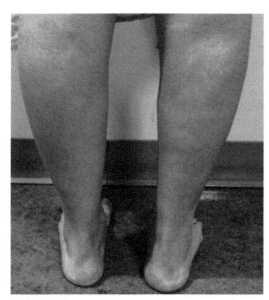

Fig. 2. Miyoshi distal myopathy. Asymmetric atrophy of posterior compartment gastrocnemii.

gastrocnemius muscle typically shows high-amplitude long-duration polyphasic MUP, with a reduced recruitment pattern, reflecting chronicity and severity. Muscle MRI confirms selective involvement of the posterior compartment muscles of the leg compared with those of the anterior compartment.[68] The diamond on quadriceps sign was present in 21 of 31 (68%) patients with dysferlinopathy, who included 62% with LGMD2B and 71% with Miyoshi myopathy (MM). The quadriceps femoris muscle had a uniform texture and smooth surface at rest, but when contracted, a portion of the muscle bulged out both clinically and radiographically toward the anterolateral aspect at midthigh.[71]

Biopsy of a severely weak and wasted gastrocnemius muscle typically shows end-stage findings, including extensive fibrosis and fatty replacement, with few if any myofibers. Biopsy of an uninvolved quadriceps muscle shows minimal myopathic changes, including variability of myofiber size and internal nuclei but absent indirect immunofluorescence for dysferlin staining of the muscle membrane.[72] If possible, the biceps femoris muscle should be biopsied, with an expectation of showing diagnostic histopathologic findings. Although perimysial and perivascular inflammation is not uncommon, vacuoles are an unexpected finding in MM.[7]

The gene for MM and LGMD2B both mapped to chromosome 2p12-14, and the protein product of this gene was found to be dysferlin.[8] It is a very large gene with 55 exons and greater than 150 kb, yielding a protein with 2080 amino acids. Although patients with both MM and LGMD2B begin in late childhood or early adulthood, with marked increase in serum CK levels, and in general, both progress slowly, the latter differs in onset in proximal not distal muscles.[73] LGMD2B accounts for 5% to 25% of all LGMD; for further discussion of MM, the reader is referred to the article on limb girdle muscular dystrophies by Wicklund and Kissel in this issue. Muscle biopsy is an excellent way to confirm MM or LGMD2B in clinically suspected cases, because they have absence of dysferlin staining, indicating a primary dysferlinopathy, whereas reduced levels of dysferlin may be secondary to a secondary disorder such as limb girdle muscular dystrophy.[74] Blood monocyte testing for dysferlin with Western blot is helpful in distinguishing truly abnormal dysferlin immunostaining in muscle from false-positive results.[75] Although the function of dysferlin is not known, it is highly expressed in skeletal muscle, where it is important for sarcolemmal maintenance. The predicted cytoplasmic component contains calcium-binding motifs homologous to C2 domains, which are believed to trigger calcium-signaled membrane fusion and trafficking,[76] suggesting a role for dysferlin in muscle membrane fusion events and repair. Consistent with this observation is that dysferlin is membrane associated[77] and it has been shown to form a protein complex with integrins at the monocyte cell membrane, and its depletion impairs cell adhesion.[78]

Laing Distal Myopathy: Early Onset, Type 3

In 1995, Laing and colleagues[79] reported affected members of a 3-generation English/Welsh family with AD distal myopathy. Age at onset was 4 to 25 years, with selective weakness of the toe and ankle extensor and neck flexor. This symptom was followed after several years by progressive weakness of the finger extensor muscles. Finger flexor and intrinsic hand muscles were relatively spared, although hip abductors and external rotator and shoulder abductor muscles were mildly affected. Tendon reflexes were preserved, and plantar responses were flexor. Disease progression was gradual, with a moderate degree of incapacity; the oldest affected member reexamined after 25 years was still ambulatory, but had difficulty maintaining an erect posture when standing. Dilated or hypertrophic cardiomyopathy (HCM) has been reported.

Serum CK levels were normal or minimally increased. Electrodiagnostic studies showed normal NCS, with occasional fibrillation potentials and positive sharp wave discharges at rest, markedly myopathic MUP in affected distal limb muscles, and early recruitment. Muscle biopsy of the quadriceps shows nonspecific myopathy, with occasional necrotic and regenerating fibers, excessive variation in fiber size, myofibers with central nuclei, without vacuoles in most cases, or fiber-type grouping. On modified Gomori trichrome, hyaline inclusions stain light green. Ultrastructural examination shows 15-nm to 20-nm intranuclear tubulofilamentous inclusions. TA muscle pathology shows end-stage myopathy with normal dystrophin and desmin immunohistochemistry. Muscle MRI studies[80] showed markedly increased signal intensity and severe atrophy of both TA and extensor hallucis longus muscles, as well as the EDL. There was selective moderately increased signal intensity and atrophy of the medial head of gastrocnemius muscles, with similar involvement of the sartorius muscles. The only abnormality in the arms was moderate symmetric atrophy, without signal change in the extensor digitorum communis muscles.

Linkage to MYH7 and D14S64 was found on chromosome 14, and later refined to the 14q11.2-q13 locus.[79,80] Two muscle genes known to lie within the linked region were the α and β cardiac myosin genes MYH6 and MYH7. Subsequent studies identified 5 novel heterozygous mutations in the light meromyosin (LMM) regions of the MYH7 tail in 6 of 7 families[9,81–84] from Europe and Western Australia. MYH7 codes for the isoform of myosin present in slow type 1 skeletal muscle fibers in skeletal and cardiac ventricle muscle, mutations of which lead to HCM. Although HCM was not present in a study cohort,[81] atrophy, grouping, and occasionally, depletion of type 1 myofibers were seen in muscle biopsies of 4 families. The pathophysiology of the mutations in MYH7 was not well understood; however, some introduced proline, which is incompatible with coiled coils. All 5 Laing mutations, including others that resulted in single amino acid deletions, significantly decreased the probability of coiled coil formation over segments of the myosin tail.

Mutation in the MYH7 rod domain at chromosome 14q has been linked to hyaline body myopathy (HBM), a rare congenital AD disorder characterized either by early nonprogressive proximal and distal weakness with significant wasting and loss of subcutaneous fat or by early progressive scapuloperoneal weakness with loss of ambulation by late teens,[9] and subsarcolemmal inclusions known as hyaline inclusion bodies exclusively in type 1 fibers. Mutation in the rod and LMM domain of myosin heavy chain IIa also leads to HBM.[85]

MYOFIBRILLAR MYOPATHY

MFM consists of a pathologic pattern of myofibrillary dissolution and degradation on EM, leading in most cases to the accumulation of myotilin, desmin, and αBC.[10,86] Myotilin is a ZASP that cross-links actin filaments and binds to α-actinin and γ-filamin.[87,88] Desmin is an intermediate filament protein of skeletal, cardiac, and some smooth muscles cells that links Z-bands with the plasmalemma and the nucleus. αBC is a member of the small heat shock protein family and is a molecular chaperone. Similar pathologic alterations are seen in spheroid body myopathy, cytoplasmic body myopathy, Mallory body myopathy, and myopathy with granulofilamentous inclusions.[89] After the first description of the inclusions and material around them reactive for desmin,[90] the term MFM was coined.[89] The first to missense mutations in desmin was described in 1998.[11] In that same year, missense mutation in αBC was first reported in a French family.[91] In 2003, Selcen and Engel[92] described the second and third mutation in αBC in 2 patients with progressive myopathy.

Clinical Manifestations

The myopathic manifestations of the disorder caused by either desmin or αBC mutations are identical, albeit with some heterogeneity. Some manifest as a relentlessly progressive adult onset myopathy with or without signs of cardiac involvement,[93,94] but in others, cardiac signs may be the leading[11] or exclusive[95] manifestation, with cardiomyopathy, congestive heart failure, heart block, and arrhythmias, often requiring pacemaker insertion. Most desmin myopathy cases show AD inheritance, but rare AR cases and sporadic cases have been reported.[86] In an adult onset multigeneration kindred of scapuloperoneal syndrome type Kaeser, desmin gene mutation was described later,[12] and the same R350P desmin mutation was identified in 4 unrelated German families. Of 13 examined cases, proximal and distal leg weakness occurred in 11 and was associated with proximal and distal arm weakness in 4, proximal arm weakness in another 4, and normal arm strength in 5. Two of 11 cases had only proximal leg weakness, and the other 2 cases, which were not examined, were also believed to have proximal leg weakness. Genotype-phenotype correlations in a total of 15 patients carrying the same mutation showed large clinical variability, even within the same family, ranging from scapuloperoneal (n = 2), limb girdle (n = 10), and distal phenotypes (n = 3). Cardiac (41%) or respiratory (41%) involvement was common, as was facial weakness, dysphagi, and gynecomastia.[12] Overall, affected men carried a higher risk of sudden cardiac death compared with affected women. Moreover, muscle biopsy histology and immunohistochemistry in 8 cases showed a wide spectrum of findings, ranging from neurogeniclike atrophy with rimmed vacuoles (n = 1) to degenerative myopathy with (n = 5) or without (n = 2) rimmed vacuoles. Accumulation of desmin was noted in 3 of 4 cases, including 1 case of degenerative myopathy without rimmed vacuoles and 2 with rimmed vacuoles. All 3 distal myopathy cases showed a degenerative rimmed vacuolar myopathy with (n = 2) or without (n = 1) neurogenic changes. One of 2 tested cases had desmin-positive inclusions on immunostaining.

Clinical Manifestations with Mutations

More recently, mutations in ZASP (allelic with Markesbery-Griggs TMD2b), myotilin (allelic with LGMD 1A), filamin C, BCL2-associated athanogene 3 (BAG3), selenoprotein N (SEPN1) and four-and-a-half-LIM protein 1 (FHL1) have been described to cause MFM (see **Table 1**). In the initial Mayo Clinic series, 2 of the 63 patients carried truncation mutations in the αBC gene, and 4 had a missense mutations in the head or tail region of desmin.[10] In a subsequent report from the Mayo Clinic, mutations in αBC, desmin, myotilin, ZASP, or filamin C were overall detected in 32 of 85 patients in the MFM cohort, with the addition of 3 BAG3 cases.[96]

Most patients develop weakness in the third to fifth decade, although there are reports of onset in infancy and later in life. The Scandinavian patients described by Edström and colleagues[90] had onset of weakness beginning at about age 40 years in the distal upper arms. The cohort of 63 cases studied at the Mayo Clinic from 1977 to 2003[10] had a mean age at onset of 54 years, but only 1 patient presented before the age of 10 years, and 3 before the age of 20 years. One-quarter of cases showed an AD mode of transmission. Of 56 patients in whom the distribution of weakness was determined, an equal number (16 patients) had similar degrees of proximal and distal myopathy or distal greater than proximal involvement. Two patients had distal myopathy alone. Ten patients had cardiomyopathy at the time of diagnosis, with congestive heart failure, arrhythmia, or dilated cardiomyopathy. Serum CK level was normal in 23 patients, and 30 patients had increased values up to 7-fold. Electrodiagnostic studies showed myogenic and high-amplitude and long-duration MUP, with occasional fibrillation potentials, positive sharp wave, complex repetitive, and rare myotonic discharges. In 2 patients, abnormal electrical irritability was the only EMG abnormality. Thirteen patients had abnormal NCS[10] consistent with polyneuropathy, including 4 with long-standing diabetes mellitus. Muscle biopsy tissue shows variability in fiber size, increased internalized nuclei, and on occasion, predominance of type 1 fiber or a few rimmed vacuoles.

Pathologic Alterations

In addition, MFM is suspected when one of the characteristic pathologic alterations is detected, best observed on H&E and modified Gomori trichrome stains. Hyaline lesions are blue to purple spherical, lobulated, or serpentine on trichrome and eosinophilic on H&E with subsarcolemmal cytoplasmic granular inclusions and amorphous granules resembling on EM cytoplasmic, spheroid, or Mallory bodies. Besides hyaline structures, trichrome also shows myofibers filled with nonhyaline lesions as dark green smudges of amorphous material and myofibers with small rimmed vacuoles and vacuoles filled with membranous material. There are also myofibers containing desmin and congophilic amyloidogenic deposits. Excessive desmin accumulation was noted in cardiac muscle of patients with associated cardiomyopathy.[97] Desmin accumulation noted in MFM is not specific, because it may also be seen in other disorders such as X-linked myotubular myopathy, spinal muscular atrophy, nemaline body myopathy, IBM, and regenerating muscle fibers.[98] Besides desmin, there is overexpression of dystrophin, αBC, gelsolin, ubiquitin, and N terminus of β-amyloid precursor protein in both lesion types in addition to cell division cycle 2 kinase and cyclin-dependent kinases 2, 4, and 7.[10,99] Neural cell adhesion molecule is overexpressed in nonhyaline lesions with depletion of actin, α-actinin, myosin, and at times, titin and nebulin. On the other hand, hyaline structures react to actin, α-actinin, filamin C, myosin, and variably to desmin, because they are composed of remnants of thick and thin filaments. Immunostains positive to αBC (MFM1, MFM2, MFM4, MFM6, and SEPN1), myotilin (MFM2, MFM4, MFM5, and MFM6), filamin C (MFM5 and SEPN1), BAG3 with gelsolin (MFM6) are noted in specific subtypes of MFM.

EM shows foci of myofibrillar destruction and hyaline structures, which appear as spheroidal bodies.[89] The foci of myofibrillary destruction consist of disrupted myofilaments, Z-disk–derived bodies, dappled dense structures of Z-disk origin, and streaming of the Z-disk. The spheroidal bodies are composed of compacted and degraded remnants of thick and thin filaments.[89] Although some[100] have shown the accumulation of 8-nm to 10-nm filaments, others[89] have not confirmed these intermediate-sized filaments, despite extensive searching. In 19 patients with different genetically proven MFMs (9 desmin, 5 αBC, 3 ZASP, 2 myotilin), an ultrastructural study showed a variety of findings that might guide efforts toward identifying the causal mutated gene.[101] On EM, 15 to 18 nm diameter tubulofilamentous inclusions (with filamentous bundles) accumulated in the sarcoplasm and nuclei of myotilinopathies. The ultrastructural findings in desminopathies and αB-crystallinopathies were similar and consisted of electron-dense granulofilamentous accumulations of predominantly reticular material and sandwich formations. This finding refers to the granulofilamentous material, which is deposited parallel to and facing the Z-lines, with mitochondria at both sides alongside these deposits, forming sandwichlike structures. Desminopathies and αB-crystallinopathies differed, in that early apoptotic nuclear changes were noted in the latter. ZASPopathies were characterized by myotilin antibody-labeled filamentous bundles and floccular accumulations of thin filamentous material.

Weakness Onset Variability

The variability in age of weakness onset in MFM is exemplified by recessively inherited SEPN1, which begins in infancy or childhood (see **Table 1**). Mutations in the SEPN1 gene have a pleomorphic presentation as congenital muscular dystrophy with spinal rigidity[102,103] multiminicore disease,[104] congenital fiber-type disproportion myopathy,[105] and desmin-related myopathy with Mallory body–like inclusions.[106] In desmin-related myopathy with Mallory body–like inclusions, muscle inclusions are immunoreactive to desmin, dystrophin, and ubiquitin,[107] and rimmed vacuoles are present.[108] Onset is in childhood for a recently identified rare severe AD, MFM6, also known as BAG3 myopathy.[96] The severe childhood onset phenotype is associated with rigid spine in 2 of 3, severe respiratory insufficiency in the teens, and hypertrophic or restrictive cardiomyopathy in all 3 cases. An adult onset isolated dilated cardiomyopathy phenotype has been described in other BAG3 gene mutations. BAG3 is a member of the antiapoptotic BAG protein family, is a ZASP, and binds heat shock protein 70, serving as a cochaperone factor controlling the chaperone activity of Hsp70.[109] Otherwise, currently described MFM are dominantly transmitted with an adult age of onset. The pattern of weakness and different levels of CK alteration are described in **Table 1**. In addition to myofibrillar changes, vacuoles are present in MFM1 to MFM6 and selenoproteinopathy (see **Box 1**).

DISTAL MYOPATHIES NOT YET CLASSIFIED
AD Inheritance Late Onset Distal Myopathy

In a multigenerational Finnish cohort with AD inheritance, a late onset distal myopathy phenotype termed MPD3 has an onset earlier in men than women, ranging from 32 to 50 years.[110,111] Early symptoms are clumsiness of the hands and steppage gait. Weakness affects the thenar and hypothenar muscles, progressing to claw hand contractures, glutei, and distally, both of the anterior and posterior leg compartments. Forearm muscles, triceps, and infraspinatus, and proximal leg muscles are involved later in the course, with frequent asymmetry. Cardiac and respiratory functions were not affected. Serum CK level was normal or slightly increased, muscle MRI showed fatty degeneration of the affected muscles, and muscle biopsy showed frequent rimmed vacuoles and dystrophic changes. The gene responsible for this phenotype remains unknown. There was no evidence of linkage to WDM or TMD. Linkage was established at 2 separate chromosomal regions, 8p22-q11 and 12q13-q22, with 2 reasonable candidate genes, including myosin light chain 1 slow-twitch muscle A (MLC1SA) on 12q13 and the muscle-specific isoform of ankyrin 1 (ANK1) on 8p11. However, sequencing excluded pathogenic mutations in the coding regions of these 2 genes.

AD Weakness of Extremities

Feit and colleagues[112] reported a southeastern Tennessee family in whom 12 of 37 members in 4 generations had AD weakness of the feet and ankles, or the hands, with an age of onset from 35 to 57 years. There was symmetric or asymmetrical peroneal weakness, with inversion of the ankles and unsteady gait, sparing the gastrocnemius muscles. There was characteristic extensor hand weakness, frequently involving the abductor pollicus brevis. Two individuals had voice change as the initial manifestation, and 10 others had later vocal cord dysfunction and pharyngeal involvement. Shoulder weakness was the only involved proximal muscle and often asymmetric. Ptosis was noted in 1 individual. Serum CK level was normal in a third of cases, and increased from 2-fold to 8-fold in the others. Electrodiagnostic studies of the vocal and pharyngeal muscles showed myopathic potentials. Muscle biopsy in one-half of the cases disclosed chronic noninflammatory myopathy with characteristic subsarcolemmal rimmed vacuoles. The syndrome of vocal cord and pharyngeal weakness with AD distal myopathy (VCPDM) was mapped to chromosome 5q, and in keeping with earlier precedent, designated MPD2. AD distal atrophy with vocal cord paralysis was previously recognized in association with spinal muscular atrophy and in neuronal forms of Charcot-Marie-Tooth disease. Two disorders that map in a similar location include LGMD2F, at 5q33-34, and LGMD1A within the linkage interval of VCPDM. In the originally reported North American family and in an unrelated Bulgarian family, Senderek and colleagues[113] identified a heterozygous C to G transversion at nucleotide 254 in exon 2 of the matrin 3 gene, which resulted in a change from serine to cysteine at codon 85. Matrin 3, an internal nuclear matrix protein, belongs to the family of nuclear matrins, a group of proteins present in the nuclear matrix of a variety of mammalian tissues and cells (see **Table 3**).

AD Adult Onset Vacuolar Distal Myopathy

Two large Italian families with AD adult onset vacuolar distal myopathy have been described[114,115] with linkage to the 19p13.3 locus. The age at diagnosis was 27 to 73 years, with a variety of severity. Asymptomatic individuals had mild scapular weakness, with normal CK levels; those mildly affected had in addition mild distal leg weakness. Severely affected individuals presented with marked ankle dorsiflexor, neck flexor, shoulder, and finger muscle weakness and wasting, with 2-fold increases in the serum CK level. Needle EMG in severely affected individuals showed myopathic MUP of proximal and distal leg more than arm muscles. Muscle biopsy showed myopathic changes and rimmed vacuoles clustered along myofiber surfaces, with basophilic granular material that stained positive for acid phosphatase, sarcolemmal protein, laminin α_2 chain, and negative for thioflavin-S, Congo red, β amyloid, tau protein. Ubiquitin was abnormally present at the surface of myofibers and in the lumen of vacuoles. Positivity was also noted for the 19S and 20S subunits of the proteasome complex on most vacuole surfaces. These findings suggested an endolysosomal origin of the vacuoles caused by abnormality in the lysosomal degradation pathway. Linkage analysis in the family reported by Di Blasi and colleagues[115] yielded positive LOD (logarithm [base 10] of odds) scores at several markers on 19p13.3.

AD distal myopathy was reported in association with mutation in the caveolin-3 gene.[116] Mutations in this gene have also been identified as a cause of LGMD1C, sporadic hyperCKemia, and rippling muscle disease.[117,118]

AD Adult Onset Slow Progression

Felice and colleagues[119] reported a family with AD adult onset slowly progressive distal myopathy without linkage to known loci. Weakness commenced in the distal anterior leg compartment, resulting in foot drop and mild proximal leg involvement. Serum CK level was 2-fold to 6-fold normal. Muscle biopsy showed nonspecific myopathic findings, including increased variation in fiber size and increased internalized nuclei.

AD Late Onset

A very late onset (around age 60 years) AD distal myopathy was described in a French kindred.[120] Serum CK level was normal or slightly increased, and muscle biopsy showed numerous rimmed and nonrimmed vacuoles accompanied by aggregates of desmin and dystrophin labeling in the cytoplasm of defective fibers.

Chinnery and colleagues[121] studied a British family with AD distal anterior compartment weakness of the legs and early respiratory muscle involvement. Age at onset varied from 32 to 75 years. Nighttime hypoventilation resulted from diaphragmatic muscle involvement. Progression of disease was variable, with loss of ambulation in some within 7 to 20 years after onset. Serum CK values were normal or slightly increased, but muscle biopsy showed myopathic dystrophic features and occasional rimmed vacuoles with some congophilic, eosinophilic, desmin, β-amyloid, and phosphorylated tau immunoreactivity. Linkage was excluded for all known distal myopathy loci.

An Australian kindred had slowly progressive symmetric, distal weakness and wasting of the anterior upper and posterior lower limbs, with sparing of TA.[122] All patients remained ambulatory and without any cardiac or respiratory muscle involvement. Serum CK levels were either normal or mildly increased, and EMG showed myopathic changes. Imaging studies showed widespread involvement of the posterior and lateral leg compartments, but proximal muscles were abnormal only in advanced disease. Muscle histopathology showed either end-stage muscle or nonspecific myopathic findings, without inflammation or vacuoles. All known distal myopathy phenotype genes and linkage regions were formally excluded.

Mitsuhashi and colleagues[123] described distal myopathy in a 52-year-old man with distal predominant slowly progressive muscle weakness since age 36 years. On muscle computed tomography, the soleus, TA, and paraspinal muscles, where type 1 fibers predominate, were almost totally replaced by fat tissue, whereas the quadriceps femoris, gastrocnemius, and upper extremity muscles were relatively spared. Quadriceps muscle biopsy showed multiminicores in addition to occasional larger cores, in about 70% of the type 1 fibers. A novel heterozygous nucleotide change c.5869T > A (p.S1957T) was identified in RYR1. Although pathogenicity was not confirmed, this nucleotide change was absent in 100 control DNA samples.

OTHER MYOPATHIES WITH DISTAL WEAKNESS

These myopathies that cause distal weakness are summarized in **Box 2**.

Box 2
Other myopathies that can have distal weakness

Myotonic dystrophy (distal myopathy)

FSH dystrophy[a]

Scapuloperoneal syndromes[a]

Oculopharyngeal dystrophy

Oculopharyngodistal myopathy (recessive)

Emery-Dreifuss humeroperonal dystrophy[a]

Inflammatory myopathy

  IBM

  Polymyositis

Metabolic myopathy

  Debrancher deficiency

  Acid maltase deficiency

  Phosphorylase b kinase

Mitochondrial myopathy

Congenital myopathy

  Nemaline myopathy[a]

  Central core myopathy[a]

  Centronuclear myopathy type 2 (dynamin 2; 19p13)

Nephropathic cystinosis

Myasthenia gravis

Cytoplasmic body myopathy (myofibrillary inclusions in type I muscle fibers; dominant)

Hyperthyroid myopathy

hIBM3 (myosin heavy chain IIa; chromosome 17p13; dominant)

hIBM and respiratory failure (6q27; dominant)

Distal weakness (distal myopathy or motor neuropathy; KLHL9; chromosome 9p22; dominant)

Distal weakness, hoarseness, and hearing loss (MYH14; chromosome 19q13.33; dominant)

  [a] Scapuloperoneal distribution of weakness can occur.

Childhood Onset Distal Myopathy

There have been reports of infants with foot drop, finger, and hand weakness before age 2 years, with predominant ankle dorsiflexor, wrist, and finger extensor muscle weakness, AD transmission, and very slow progression.[124–126] Muscle biopsy and needle EMG showed a myopathic process without vacuolization. All patients remained ambulatory.

In a large Dutch family with AD juvenile onset distal myopathy, weakness was slowly progressive, affecting flexor and extensor distal muscle groups, and without any functional limitations in adult life.[127] Myopathic and neuropathic features were found on muscle biopsy and postmortem examination. Although the reports of childhood onset distal myopathy preceded desmin immunostaining of skeletal muscle tissue, there were no clues on light microscopy to suggest excessive desmin.

Other Muscular Dystrophies

Weakness of distal muscle groups may be prominent in some forms of muscular dystrophy. In myotonic dystrophy, wrist and finger extensors and ankle dorsiflexors are typically weaker than proximal limb muscles, especially early in the disease.[128] Because the prevalence of myotonic dystrophy is 5 per 100,000, it is probably the most commonly seen myopathic condition with prominent distal weakness, especially in the young and middle-aged groups. Rare patients with the phenotypic appearance of myotonic dystrophy and distal weakness but without clinical or electrical myotonia have been described.[129]

Patients with FSH dystrophy can develop weakness of ankle dorsiflexion and wrist and finger extension, along with typical facial and scapular muscle involvement. Rarely, they can present with ankle weakness, which is part of the diagnostic criteria for FSH dystrophy.[130] FSH dystrophy type 1 has been mapped to chromosome 4q35[131] and is caused by D4Z4 contraction. For a discussion of FSHD1 and FSHD2, the reader is referred to the article elsewhere in this issue on fascioscapulomuneral muscular dystrophy by Statland and Tawil. Patients with the so-called myopathic form of the scapuloperoneal syndrome have significant ankle weakness.[132]

Patients with the X-linked Emery-Dreifuss disease, also known as humeroperoneal muscular dystrophy, present with ankle dorsiflexion, triceps, and biceps weakness, along with contractures at the elbow (**Fig. 3**) and ankle.[133] Marked contractures are also seen in an AD variant of Emery-Dreifuss muscular dystrophy caused by lamin A/C gene mutation. Some pedigrees of oculopharyngeal muscular dystrophy also have significant distal extremity weakness.[134–136]

Inflammatory Myopathies

Patients with polymyositis can manifest initial weakness in the hands and ankles,[137,138] with concurrent evidence of inflammatory myopathy on proximal muscle biopsy, and response to corticosteroid therapy. However, sporadic IBM is the more frequent cause of adult onset distal limb weakness,[139] typically after age 50 years, with early weakness and atrophy of wrist and finger flexor muscles, as well as in the quadriceps, TA, and extensor digitorum hallucis muscles, the so-called pseudo-Babinski sign. Both knee extensor and forearm and finger flexor weakness are part of the original diagnostic criteria for IBM.[140] Muscle biopsy shows endomysial

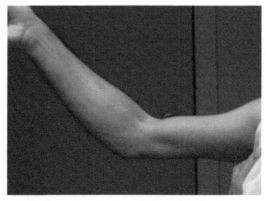

Fig. 3. X-linked Emery-Dreifuss muscular dystrophy. Atrophy of humeral compartment and elbow contracture.

inflammation with invasion of nonnecrotic muscle fibers, eosinophilic cytoplasmic in-clusions, and rimmed vacuoles within the muscle fibers, which contain amyloid de-posits. EM shows accumulation of cytoplasmic and intranuclear 15-nm to 21-nm filaments. **Box 1** lists other disorders characterized by rimmed vacuoles on biopsy. Amyloidogenic green-birefringent deposits with Congo red stain may be detected in IBM biopsies.[141] Alzheimer-characteristic proteins in vacuolated muscle fibers including β-amyloid and paired helical filament-tau are noted in IBM muscle tissue.[140] The lack of response to immunosuppressive treatment distinguishes IBM from poly-myositis and dermatomyositis.[142] For a full discussion of IBM, the reader is referred to the article elsewhere in this issue on sporadic inclusion body myositis by Dimachkie and Barohn.

Larue and colleagues[143] reported 4 patients older than 50 years with chronic myop-athy suggestive of sporadic IBM. Patients had progressive and selective weakness of the quadriceps femoris muscles and asymmetric atrophy of the forearm muscles, especially the flexor compartment. Biopsy showed granulomatous myositis, with in 1 case, evidence for systemic sarcoidosis. Corticosteroid treatment was associated with a partial but significant improvement in 2 patients.

Metabolic and Congenital Myopathies

Debrancher enzyme deficiency[144] and adult onset acid maltase deficiency can pre-sent with a scapuloperoneal pattern of weakness.[145] Patients with the AR lysosomal storage disorder, nephropathic cystinosis, develop a distal myopathy as a late compli-cation of the disease. Nonprogressive congenital muscle diseases such as nemaline rod[146,147] central core,[148] and centronuclear myopathy[149] can have significant involvement of distal limb muscles.

Myasthenia Gravis

Although most patients with myasthenia gravis present with ocular, bulbar, and prox-imal limb muscle weakness, the weakness can at times be prominent in distal limbs.[150] Of 234 myasthenic patients, 7 (3%) had primarily distal muscle weakness mainly in finger extensor and interossei muscles and another had involvement of ankle dorsi-flexor muscles, 6 of whom improved with immunosuppressive therapy.

REFERENCES

1. Barohn RJ, Watts GD, Amato AA. A case of late-onset proximal and distal mus-cle weakness. Neurology 2009;73(19):1592–7.
2. Udd B. 165th ENMC International workshop: distal myopathies 6–8 February 2009 in Naarden, the Netherlands. Neuromuscul Disord 2009;19:429–38.
3. Griggs R, Vihola A, Hackman P, et al. ZASPopathy in a large classic late-onset distal myopathy family. Brain 2007;130(Pt 6):1477–84.
4. Selcen D, Engel AG. Mutations in ZASP define a novel form of muscular dystro-phy in humans. Ann Neurol 2005;5:269–76.
5. Selcen D, Engel AG. Mutations in myotilin cause myofibrillar myopathy. Neurology 2004;62:1363–71.
6. Rosales XQ, Gastier-Foster JM, Lewis S, et al. Novel diagnostic features of dys-ferlinopathies. Muscle Nerve 2010;42(1):14–21.
7. Shaibani A, Harati Y, Amato A, et al. Miyoshi myopathy with vacuoles. Neurology 1997;47(Suppl):A195.
8. Liu J, Aoki M, Illa I, et al. Dysferlin, a novel skeletal muscle gene, is mutated in Miyoshi myopathy and limb girdle muscular dystrophy. Nat Genet 1998;20:31–6.

9. Scoppetta C, Casali C, La Cesa I, et al. Infantile autosomal dominant distal myopathy. Acta Neurol Scand 1995;92:122–6.

10. Selcen D, Ohno K, Engel AG. Myofibrillar myopathy: clinical, morphological and genetic studies in 63 patients. Brain 2004;127:439–51.

11. Goldfarb LG, Park KY, Cervenaâkova L, et al. Missense mutations in desmin associated with familial cardiac and skeletal myopathy. Nat Genet 1998;19:402–3.

12. Walter MC, Reilich P, Huebner A, et al. Scapuloperoneal syndrome type Kaeser and a wide phenotypic spectrum of adult-onset, dominant myopathies are associated with the desmin mutation R350P. Brain 2007;130(Pt 6):1485–96.

13. Watts GD, Wymer J, Kovach MJ, et al. Inclusion body myopathy associated with Paget disease of bone and frontotemporal dementia is caused by mutant valosin-containing protein. Nat Genet 2004;36:377–81.

14. Stojkovic T, Hammoud EH, Pascale Richard P, et al. Clinical outcome in 19 French and Spanish patients with valosin-containing protein myopathy associated with Paget's disease of bone and frontotemporal dementia. Neuromuscul Disord 2009;19:316–23.

15. Hübbers CU, Clemen CS, Kesper K, et al. Pathological consequences of VCP mutations on human striated muscle. Brain 2007;130(Pt 2):381–93.

16. Welander L. Myopathia distalis tarda hereditaria. Acta Med Scand Suppl 1951; 141(Suppl 265):1–124.

17. Ahlberg G, Von Tell D, Borg K, et al. Genetic linkage of Welander distal myopathy to chromosome 2p13. Ann Neurol 1999;46:399–404.

18. Von Tell D, Somer H, Udd B, et al. Welander distal myopathy outside the Swedish population: phenotype and genotype. Neuromuscul Disord 2002;12:544–7.

19. Borg K, Borg J, Lindblom U. Sensory involvement in distal myopathy (Welander). J Neurol Sci 1987;80:323–32.

20. Borg K, Tome F, Edström L. Intranuclear and cytoplasmic filamentous inclusions in distal myopathy (Welander). Acta Neuropathol 1991;82:102–6.

21. Lindberg C, Borg K, Edström L, et al. Inclusion body myositis and Welander distal myopathy: a clinical, neurophysiological and morphological comparison. J Neurol Sci 1991;103:76–81.

22. Borg K, Åhlberg G, Borg J, et al. Welander's distal myopathy: clinical, neurophysiological and muscle biopsy observations in young and middle aged adults with early symptoms. J Neurol Neurosurg Psychiatry 1991;54:494–8.

23. Edström L. Histochemical and histopathological changes in skeletal muscle in late-onset hereditary distal myopathy (Welander). J Neurol Sci 1975;26:147–57.

24. Mahjneh I, Lamminen AE, Udd B, et al. Muscle magnetic imaging shows distinct diagnostic patterns in Welander and tibial muscular dystrophy. Acta Neurol Scand 2004;110:87–93.

25. Borg K, Solders G, Borg J, et al. Neurogenic involvement in distal myopathy (Welander). J Neurol Sci 1989;91:53–70.

26. Dahlgaard E. Myopathia distalis tarda hereditaria. Acta Psychiatr Neurol Scand 1960;35:440–7.

27. Barrows HS, Duemler LP. Late distal myopathy. Report of a case. Neurology 1962;12:547–50.

28. Sumner D, Crawfurd M, Harriman DG. Distal muscular dystrophy in an English family. Brain 1971;94:51–60.

29. Markesbery WR, Griggs RC, Leach RP, et al. Late onset hereditary distal myopathy. Neurology 1974;23:127–34.

30. Udd B, Partanen J, Halonen P, et al. Tibial muscular dystrophy: late adult-onset distal myopathy in 66 Finnish patients. Arch Neurol 1993;50:604–8.

31. Partanen J, Laulumaa V, Paljärve L, et al. Late onset foot-drop muscular dystrophy with rimmed vacuoles. J Neurol Sci 1994;125:158–67.
32. Spiller WG. Myopathy of a distal type and its relation to the neural form of muscular atrophy (Charcot-Marie-Tooth type). J Nerv Mend Dis 1907;34:14–30.
33. Udd B, Kääriänen H, Somer H. Muscular dystrophy with separate clinical phenotypes in a large family. Muscle Nerve 1991;14:1050–8.
34. Hackman P, Vihola A, Haravuori H, et al. Tibial muscular dystrophy is a titinopathy caused by mutations in TTN, the gene encoding the giant skeletal-muscle protein titin. Am J Hum Genet 2002;71:492–500.
35. Udd B, Bushby K, Nonaka I, et al. 104th European Neuromuscular Center (ENMC) International Workshop: distal myopathies, 8-10th March 2002 in Naarden, The Netherlands. Neuromuscul Disord 2002;12:897–904.
36. Murone I, Sato T, Shirakawa K, et al. Distal myopathy–a case of non-hereditary distal myopathy. Clin Neurol (Tokyo) 1963;378–86.
37. Sasaki K, Mori H, Takahashi K, et al. Distal myopathy–report of four cases. Clin Neurol (Tokyo) 1969;9:627–37.
38. Nonaka I, Sunohara N, Ishiura S, et al. Familial distal myopathy with rimmed vacuole and lamellar (myeloid) body formation. J Neurol Sci 1981;51:141–55.
39. Nonaka I, Sunohara N, Satoyoshi E, et al. Autosomal recessive distal muscular dystrophy: a comparative study with distal myopathy with rimmed vacuole formation. Ann Neurol 1985;17:51–9.
40. Sunohara N, Nonaka I, Kamei N, et al. Distal myopathy with rimmed vacuole formation: a follow-up study. Brain 1989;112:65–83.
41. Markesbery WR, Griggs RC, Herr B. Distal myopathy: electron microscopic and histochemical studies. Neurology 1977;27:727–35.
42. Miller RG, Blank NK, Layzer RB. Sporadic distal myopathy with early adult onset. Ann Neurol 1979;5:220–7.
43. Krendel D, Gilchrist J, Bossen E. Distal vacuolar myopathy with complete heart block. Arch Neurol 1988;45:698–9.
44. Isaacs H, Badenhorst M, Whistler T. Autosomal recessive distal myopathy. J Clin Pathol 1988;41:188–94.
45. Scoppetta C, Vaccario ML, Casali C, et al. Distal muscular dystrophy with autosomal recessive inheritance. Muscle Nerve 1984;7:478–81.
46. Somer H. Distal myopathies: 25th ENMC international workshop, 18-20 November 1994, Naarden, The Netherlands. Neuromuscul Disord 1995;5:249–52.
47. Mizusawa H, Kurisaki H, Takatsu M, et al. Rimmed vacuolar distal myopathy: a clinical, electrophysiological, histopathological and computed tomographic study of seven cases. J Neurol 1987;234:129–36.
48. Kumamota T, Fukuhara N, Naguishima M, et al. Distal myopathy: histochemical and ultrastructural studies. Arch Neurol 1982;51:141–55.
49. Matsubara S, Tannabe H. Hereditary distal myopathy with filamentous inclusions. Acta Neurol Scand 1982;65:363–8.
50. Jongen PJ, Laak HJ, Stadhouders AM. Rimed basophilic vacuoles and filamentous inclusions in neuromuscular disorders. Neuromuscul Disord 1995;5:31–8.
51. Yabe I, Higashi T, Kikuchi S, et al. GNE mutations causing distal myopathy with rimmed vacuoles with inflammation. Neurology 2003;61:384–6.
52. Krause S, Schlotter-Weigel B, Walter MC, et al. A novel homozygous missense mutation in the GNE gene of a patient with quadriceps-sparing hereditary inclusion body myopathy associated with muscle inflammation. Neuromuscul Disord 2003;13:830–4.

53. Asaka T, Ikeuchi K, Okino S, et al. Homozygosity and linkage disequilibrium mapping of autosomal recessive distal myopathy (Nonaka distal myopathy). J Hum Genet 2001;46:649–55.

54. Tomimitsu H, Shimizu J, Ishikawa K, et al. Distal myopathy with rimmed vacuoles (DMRV): new GNE mutations and splice variant. Neurology 2004;62:1607–10.

55. Argov Z, Yarom R. "Rimmed vacuole myopathy" sparing the quadriceps. A unique disorder in Iranian Jews. J Neurol Sci 1984;64:33–43.

56. Askanas V, Engel WK. Sporadic inclusion-body myositis and hereditary inclusion-body myopathies: current concepts of diagnosis and pathogenesis. Curr Opin Rheumatol 1998;10:530–42.

57. Eisenberg I, Avidan N, Potikha T, et al. The UDP-N-acetylglucosamine 2-epimerase/N-acetylmannosamine kinase gene is mutated in recessive hereditary inclusion body myopathy. Nat Genet 2001;29:83–7.

58. Nishino I, Noguchi S, Murayama K, et al. Distal myopathy with rimmed vacuoles is allelic to hereditary inclusion body myopathy. Neurology 2002;59:1689–93.

59. Argov Z, Eisenberg I, Grabov-Nardini G, et al. Hereditary inclusion body myopathy: the Middle Eastern genetic cluster. Neurology 2003;60:1519–23.

60. Nemunaitis G, Jay CM, Maples PB, et al. Hereditary inclusion body myopathy: single patient response to intravenous dosing of GNE gene lipoplex. Hum Gene Ther 2011;22(11):1331–41.

61. Malicdan MC, Noguchi S, Hayashi YK, et al. Prophylactic treatment with sialic acid metabolites precludes the development of the myopathic phenotype in the DMRV-hIBM mouse model. Nat Med 2009;15(6):690–5.

62. Miyoshi K, Saijo K, Kuryu Y, et al. Four cases of distal myopathy in two families. Jpn J Human Genet 1967;12:113.

63. Miyoshi K, Tada Y, Iwasa M, et al. Autosomal recessive distal myopathy observed characteristically in Japan. Jpn J Human Genet 1975;20:62–3.

64. Miyoshi K, Kawai H, Iwasa M, et al. Autosomal recessive distal muscular dystrophy. Brain 1986;109:31–54.

65. Kuhn E, Schroder M. A new type of distal myopathy in two brothers. J Neurol 1981;226:181–5.

66. Galassi G, Rowland LP, Hays A, et al. High serum levels of creatine kinase: asymptomatic prelude to distal myopathy. Muscle Nerve 1987;10:346–50.

67. Barohn RJ, Miller RG, Griggs RC. Autosomal recessive distal dystrophy. Neurology 1991;41:1365–70.

68. Meola G, Sansone V, Rotondo G, et al. Computerized tomography and magnetic resonance muscle imaging in Miyoshi's myopathy. Muscle Nerve 1996;19: 1476–80.

69. Linssen WH, Notermans NC, Van der Graaf Y, et al. Miyoshi-type distal muscular dystrophy. Clinical spectrum in 24 Dutch patients. Brain 1997;120:1989–96.

70. Fallon KE, Collins Purdam C. Miyoshi myopathy–an unusual cause of calf pain and tightness. Clin J Sport Med 2004;14:45–7.

71. Pradhan S. Clinical and magnetic resonance imaging features of 'diamond on quadriceps' sign in dysferlinopathy. Neurol India 2009;57(2):172–5.

72. Soares CN, De Freitas MR, Nascimento OJ, et al. Myopathy of distal lower limbs: the clinical variant of Miyoshi. Arq Neuropsiquiatr 2003;61:946–9.

73. Aoki M, Liu J, Richard I, et al. Genomic organization of the dysferlin gene and novel mutations in Miyoshi myopathy. Neurology 2001;57:271–8.

74. Piccolo F, Moore SA, Ford GC, et al. Intracellular accumulation and reduced sarcolemmal expression of dysferlin in limb-girdle muscular dystrophies. Ann Neurol 2000;48:902–12.

75. Gallardo E, de Luna N, Diaz-Manera J, et al. Comparison of dysferlin expression in human skeletal muscle with that in monocytes for the diagnosis of dysferlin myopathy. PLoS One 2011;6(12):e29061.

76. Rizo J, Sudhof TC. C2-domains, structure and function of a universal Ca2+ binding domain. J Biol Chem 1998;273:15879–82.

77. Matsuda C, Aoki M, Hayashi YK, et al. Dysferlin is a surface membrane-associated protein that is absent in Miyoshi myopathy. Neurology 1999;53:1119–22.

78. de Morrée A, Flix B, Bagaric I, et al. Dysferlin regulates cell adhesion in human monocytes. J Biol Chem 2013;288(20):14147–57.

79. Laing NG, Laing BA, Meredith C, et al. Autosomal dominant distal myopathy: linkage to chromosome 14. Am J Hum Genet 1995;56:422–7.

80. Mastaglia FL, Phillips BA, Cala LA, et al. Early onset chromosome 14-linked distal myopathy (Laing). Neuromuscul Disord 2002;12:350–7.

81. Meredith C, Herrmann R, Parry C, et al. Mutations in the slow skeletal muscle fiber myosin heavy chain gene (MYH7) cause Laing early-onset distal myopathy (MPD1). Am J Hum Genet 2004;75:703–8.

82. Voit T, Kutz P, Leube B, et al. Autosomal dominant distal myopathy: further evidence of a chromosome 14 locus. Neuromuscul Disord 2001;11:11–9.

83. Zimprich F, Djamshidian A, Hainfellner JA, et al. An autosomal dominant early adult-onset distal muscular dystrophy. Muscle Nerve 2000;23:1876–9.

84. Hedera P, Petty EM, Bui MR, et al. The second kindred with autosomal dominant distal myopathy linked to chromosome 14q. Genetic and clinical analysis. Arch Neurol 2003;60:1321–5.

85. Bohlega S, Abu-Amero SN, Wakil SM, et al. Mutation of the slow myosin heavy chain domain underlies hyaline body myopathy. Neurology 2004;62:1518–21.

86. Goldfard LG, Vicart P, Goebel HH, et al. Desmin myopathy. Brain 2004;127:723–34.

87. Salmikangas P, van der Ven PF, Lalowski M, et al. Myotilin, the limb girdle dystrophy 1A (LGMD1A) protein, cross-links actin filaments and control sarcomere assembly. Hum Mol Genet 2003;12:189–203.

88. van der Ven PF, Wiesner S, Salmikangas P, et al. Indications for a novel muscular dystrophy pathway: gamma-filamin, the muscle-specific filamin isoform, interacts with myotilin. J Cell Biol 2000;151:235–48.

89. Nakano S, Engel AG, Waclwik AJ, et al. Myofibrillary myopathy with abnormal foci of desmin positivity. I. Light and electron microscopy analysis of 10 cases. J Neuropathol Exp Neurol 1996;55:549–62.

90. Edström L, Thornell LE, Eriksson A. A new type of hereditary distal myopathy with characteristic sarcoplasmic bodies and intermediate (Skeletin) filaments. J Neurol Sci 1980;47:171–90.

91. Vicart P, Caron A, Guicheney P, et al. A missense mutation in the αB-crystallin chaperone gene causes a desmin-related myopathy. Nat Genet 1998;20:92–5.

92. Selcen D, Engel AG. Myofibrillar myopathy caused by novel dominant negative alpha B-crystallin mutations. Ann Neurol 2003;54(6):804–10.

93. Dalakas MC, Park KY, Semino-Mora C, et al. Desmin myopathy, a skeletal myopathy with cardiomyopathy caused by mutations in the desmin gene. N Engl J Med 2000;342:770–80.

94. Dalakas MC, Dagvadorj A, Goudeau B, et al. Progressive skeletal myopathy, a phenotypic variant of desmin myopathy associated with desmin mutations. Neuromuscul Disord 2003;13:252–8.

840   Dimachkie & Barohn

95. Li D, Tapscoft T, Gonzalez O, et al. Desmin mutation responsible for idiopathic dilated cardiomyopathy. Circulation 1999;100:461–4.
96. Selcen D, Muntoni F, Burton BK, et al. Mutation in BAG3 causes severe dominant childhood muscular dystrophy. Ann Neurol 2009;65(1):83–9.
97. Muntoni F, Catani G, Mateddu A, et al. Familial cardiomyopathy, mental retardation and myopathy associated with desmin-type intermediate filaments. Neuromuscul Disord 1994;4:233–41.
98. Goebel HH. Desmin-related neuromuscular disorders. Muscle Nerve 1995; 18(11):1306–20.
99. DeBleecker JL, Engel AG, Ertl BB. Myofibrillary myopathy with abnormal foci of desmin positivity. II. Immunocytochemical analysis reveals accumulation of multiple other proteins. J Neuropathol Exp Neurol 1996;55:563–77.
100. Porte A, Stoeckel ME, Sacrez A, et al. Unusual cardiomyopathy characterized by aberrant accumulation of desmin-type intermediate filaments. Virchows Arch 1980;386:43–58.
101. Claeys KG, Fardeau M, Schröder R, et al. Electron microscopy in myofibrillar myopathies reveals clues to the mutated gene. Neuromuscul Disord 2008; 18(8):656–66.
102. Moghadaszadeh B, Petit N, Jaillard C, et al. Mutations in SEPN1 cause congenital muscular dystrophy with spinal rigidity and restrictive respiratory syndrome. Nat Genet 2001;29:17–8.
103. Lescure A, Gautheret D, Carbon P, et al. Novel selenoproteins identified in silico and in vivo by using a conserved RNA structural motif. J Biol Chem 1999;274: 38147–54.
104. Ferreiro A, Quijano-Roy S, Pichereau C, et al. Mutations of the selenoprotein N gene, which is implicated in rigid spine muscular dystrophy, cause the classical phenotype of multiminicore disease: reassessing the nosology of early-onset myopathies. Am J Hum Genet 2002;71:739–49.
105. Clarke NF, Kidson W, Quijano-Roy S, et al. SEPN1: associated with congenital fiber-type disproportion and insulin resistance. Ann Neurol 2006;59:546–52.
106. Ferreiro A, Ceuterick-de Groote C, Marks JJ, et al. Desmin-related myopathy with Mallory body-like inclusions is caused by mutations of the selenoprotein N gene. Ann Neurol 2004;55:676–86.
107. Fidzianska A, Ryniewicz B, Barcikowska M, et al. A new familial congenital myopathy in children with desmin and dystrophin reacting plaques. J Neurol Sci 1995;131:88–95.
108. Fidzianska A, Goebel HH, Osborn M, et al. Mallory body-like inclusions in a hereditary congenital neuromuscular disease. Muscle Nerve 1983;6:195–200.
109. Takayama S, Xie Z, Reed JC. An evolutionarily conserved family of Hsp70/Hsc70 molecular chaperone regulators. J Biol Chem 1999;274:781–6.
110. Mahjneh I, Haravuori H, Paetau A, et al. A distinct phenotype of distal myopathy in a large Finnish family. Neurology 2003;61:87–92.
111. Haravuori H, Siitonen HA, Mahjneh I, et al. Linkage to two separate loci in a family with a novel distal myopathy phenotype (MPD3). Neuromuscul Disord 2004; 14:183–7.
112. Feit H, Silbergleit A, Schneider LB, et al. Vocal cord and pharyngeal weakness with autosomal dominant distal myopathy: clinical description and gene localization to 5q31. Am J Hum Genet 1998;63:1732–42.
113. Senderek J, Garvey SM, Krieger M, et al. Autosomal-dominant distal myopathy associated with a recurrent missense mutation in the gene encoding the nuclear matrix protein, matrin 3. Am J Hum Genet 2009;84:511–8.

114. Servidei S, Capon F, Spinazzola A, et al. A distinctive autosomal dominant vacuolar neuromyopathy linked to 19p13. Neurology 1999;53:830–7.
115. Di Blasi C, Moghadaszadeh B, Ciano C, et al. Abnormal lysosomal and ubiquitin-protease pathways in 19p13.3 distal myopathy. Ann Neurol 2004;56: 133–8.
116. Tateyama M, Aoki M, Nishino I, et al. Mutation in the caveolin-3 gene causes a peculiar form of distal myopathy. Neurology 2002;58:323–5.
117. Fee DB, So YT, Baraza C, et al. Phenotypic variability associated with Arg26Gln mutation in caveolin3. Muscle Nerve 2004;30:375–8.
118. Sotgia F, Woodman SE, Bonuccelli G, et al. Phenotypic behavior of caveolin-3 R26Q, a mutant associated with hyperCKemia, distal myopathy, and rippling muscle disease. Am J Physiol Cell Physiol 2003;285:C1150–60.
119. Felice K, Meredith C, Binz N, et al. Autosomal dominant distal myopathy not linked to the known distal myopathy loci. Neuromuscul Disord 1999;9:59–65.
120. Penisson-Besnier I, Dumez C, Chateau D, et al. Autosomal dominant late adult onset distal leg myopathy. Neuromuscul Disord 1998;8:459–66.
121. Chinnery P, Johnson M, Walls T, et al. A novel autosomal dominant distal myopathy with early respiratory failure: clinico-pathologic characteristics and exclusion of linkage to candidate genetic loci. Neurology 2001;49:443–52.
122. Williams DR, Reardon K, Roberts L, et al. A new dominant distal myopathy affecting posterior leg and anterior upper limb muscles. Neurology 2005; 64(7):1245–54.
123. Mitsuhashi S, Nonaka I, Wu S, et al. Distal myopathy in multi-minicore disease. Intern Med 2009;48(19):1759–62.
124. Magee KE, DeJong RN. Hereditary distal myopathy with onset in infancy. Arch Neurol 1965;13:387–90.
125. Van der Does de Willebois AE, Bethlem J, Meyer AE, et al. Distal myopathy with onset in early infancy. Neurology 1968;18:383–90.
126. Bautista J, Rafel E, Castilla J, et al. Hereditary distal myopathy with onset in early infancy. J Neurol Sci 1978;37:149–58.
127. Biemond A. Myopathia distalis juvenilis hereditaria. Acta Psychiatr Neurol Scand 1955;30:25–38.
128. Morgenlander JC, Massey JM. Myotonic dystrophy. Semin Neurol 1991;11: 236–43.
129. Schotland D, Rowland L. Muscular dystrophy: features of ocular myopathy, distal myopathy, and myotonic dystrophy. Arch Neurol 1964;10:433–45.
130. Tawil R, McDermott MP, Mendell JR, et al. Fascioscapulohumeral muscular dystrophy (FSHMD): design of natural history study and results of baseline testing. Neurology 1994;44:442–6.
131. Wijmenga C, Padberg GW, Moerer P, et al. Mapping of fascioscapulohumeral muscular dystrophy gene to chromosome 4q35-qter by multipoint linkage analysis and in situ hybridization. Genomics 1991;9:570–5.
132. Thomas PK, Schott GD, Morgan-Hughes JA. Adult onset scapuloperoneal myopathy. J Neurol Neurosurg Psychiatry 1975;38:1008–15.
133. Rowland LP, Fetell M, Olarte M, et al. Emery-Dreifuss muscular dystrophy. Ann Neurol 1979;5:111–7.
134. Satoyoshi E, Kinoshita M. Oculopharyngodistal myopathy. Arch Neurol 1977;34: 89–92.
135. Fukuhara N, Kumamoto T, Tadao T, et al. Oculopharyngeal muscular dystrophy and distal myopathy: intrafamilial difference in the onset and distribution of muscular involvement. Acta Neurol Scand 1982;65:458–67.

136. Vita G, Dattola R, Santoro M, et al. Familial oculopharyngeal muscular dystrophy with distal spread. J Neurol 1983;230:57–64.
137. Hollinrake K. Polymyositis presenting as a distal muscle weakness–a case report. J Neurol Sci 1969;8:479–84.
138. Van Kasteren BJ. Polymyositis presenting with chronic progressive distal muscular weakness. J Neurol Sci 1979;41:307–10.
139. Dimachkie MM, Barohn RJ. Idiopathic inflammatory myopathies. Front Neurol Neurosci 2009;26:126–46.
140. Griggs RC, Askanas V, DiMauro S, et al. Inclusion body myositis and myopathies. Ann Neurol 1995;38:705–13.
141. Mendell JR, Sahenk Z, Gales T. Amyloid filaments inclusion body myositis: novel findings provide insight into nature of filaments. Arch Neurol 1991;48:1229–34.
142. Dimachkie MM. Idiopathic inflammatory myopathies. J Neuroimmunol 2011; 231(1–2):32–42.
143. Larue S, Maisonobe T, Benveniste O, et al. Distal muscle involvement in granulomatous myositis can mimic inclusion body myositis. J Neurol Neurosurg Psychiatry 2011;82(6):674–7.
144. DiMauro S, Hartwig G, Hays A, et al. Debrancher deficiency: neuromuscular disorder in 5 adults. Ann Neurol 1979;5:422–36.
145. Barohn RJ, McVey AL, DiMauro S. Adult acid maltase deficiency. Muscle Nerve 1993;16:672–6.
146. Hausmanowa-Petrusewicz I, Fidzianska A, Badurska B. Unusual course of nemaline myopathy. Neuromuscul Disord 1992;2:413–8.
147. Laing NG, Majda BT, Akkari PA, et al. Assignment of a gene (NEM1) for autosomal dominant nemaline myopathy to chromosome 1. Am J Hum Genet 1992;50:576–83.
148. Kratz R, Brooke MH. Distal myopathy. In: Vinken PJ, Bruyn GW, editors. Handbook of clinical Neurology, vol. 40. Amsterdam: North-Holland; 1980. p. 471–83.
149. Moxley RT, Griggs RC, Markesbery WR, et al. Metabolic implications of distal atrophy. Carbohydrate metabolism in centronuclear myopathy. J Neurol Sci 1978;39:247–59.
150. Nations SP, Wolfe GI, Amato AA, et al. Clinical features of patients with distal myasthenia gravis. Neurology 1997;48(Suppl):A64.
151. Greenberg SA, Salajegheh M, Judge DP, et al. Etiology of limb girdle muscular dystrophy 1D/1E determined by laser capture microdissection proteomics. Ann Neurol 2012;71(1):141–5.

Index

Note: Page numbers of article titles are in **boldface** type.

Neurol Clin 32 (2014) 843–857
http://dx.doi.org/10.1016/S0733-8619(14)00045-0
0733-8619/14/$ – see front matter © 2014 Elsevier Inc. All rights reserved.

neurologic.theclinics.com

I

Printed and bound by CPI Group (UK) Ltd, Croydon, CR0 4YY

03/10/2024

01040486-0012